GOLDEN'S DIAGNOSTIC RADIOLOGY

Section 7:
CLINICAL LYMPHOGRAPHY

VOLUMES OF
GOLDEN'S DIAGNOSTIC RADIOLOGY SERIES

Section 1: **Diagnostic Neuroradiology** (Taveras & Wood)
Section 2: **Radiology of The Nose, Paranasal Sinuses, and Nasopharynx** (Dodd & Jing)
Section 3: **Radiology of the Chest** (Rabin & Baron)
Section 4: **Radiology of the Heart and Great Vessels** (Cooley & Schreiber)
Section 5: **The Digestive Tract** (Golden, et al)
Section 6: **Roentgen Diagnosis of Diseases of Bone** (Edeiken & Hodes)
Section 7: **Clinical Lymphography** (Clouse, et al)
Section 8: **Urologic Radiology** (Sussman & Newman)
Section 9: **Uterotubography** (Robins)
Section 10: **Radiologic, Ultrasonic, and Nuclear Diagnostic Methods In Obstetrics** (Campbell, et al)
Section 11: **The Roentgen Diagnosis of Fractures** (Garland)
Section 12: **Dental Roentgenology** (Zegarelli)
Section 13: **The Soft Tissues of the Air and Food Passages of the Neck** (Young & Funch)
Section 14: **The Abdomen** (Taveras & Golden)
Section 15: **Pediatric Radiology** (Davis & Shearer)
Section 16: **Soft Tissue Roentgenology** (Robbins)
Section 17: **Tomography — Physical Principles and Clinical Applications** (Littleton)
Section 18: **Selective Angiography** (Hanafee, et al)
Section 19: **Mammography and Breast Diseases** (Egan)
Section 20: **Diagnostic Nuclear Medicine** (Gottschalk & Potchen, et al)
Section 22: **Radiology of the Gallbladder and Bile Ducts** (Hatfield & Wise)

CLINICAL LYMPHOGRAPHY

Edited by

Melvin E. Clouse, M.D.

Assistant Clinical Professor of Radiology, Harvard Medical School;
Chairman, Department of Radiology,
New England Deaconess Hospital,
Boston, Massachusetts

The Williams & Wilkins Company   Baltimore

SECTION 7
GOLDEN'S DIAGNOSTIC RADIOLOGY
Laurence L. Robbins, M.D., Series Editor

Made in the United States of America

Library of Congress Cataloging in Publication Data
Main entry under title:

Clinical lymphography.

   (Golden's diagnostic radiology; section 7)
   Includes index.
    1. Lymphangiography. I. Clouse, Melvin E. [DNLM: 1.
Lymphography. WN200 G6181 sect. 7]
RC78.G6 sect. 7 [RC78.7.L9] 616.07'572'08s
           [616.4'2'07572]
                            76-50804

683-01883-3

Composed and printed at the
Waverly Press, Inc.
Mt. Royal and Guilford Aves.
Baltimore, Md. 21202, U.S.A.

DEDICATED

to

Robert D. Moreton, M.D.
Laurence L. Robbins, M.D.
Mr. Robert D. Lowry

Who have always given excellent advice and whose support over the years has made this book possible.

Foreword

It is with great enthusiasm that I welcome the formation and publication of this book. As a clinician critically interested in the status of the lymph nodes and lymphatics, I have found the lymphogram a valuable asset albeit sometimes a confusing one. Interpretations of abnormalities in the lymph node architecture vary from center to center and are quite different for different diseases. This book has an excellent description of the history of studies of the lymphatics and lymph nodes. The technique of doing conventional contrast lymphography, the problems of interpretation, as well as careful review of the lymphographic findings in carcinoma and lymphoma are presented and illustrated. These will be of value, not only to the skilled diagnostic radiologist, but to the radiation, medical, and surgical oncologists dealing with these patients. These alone would be enough to justify this book. The radiation oncologist and the surgeon find lymphography useful because not only can it be used to diagnose abnormalities but it also locates the abnormalities within the patient, making them available for surgical excision or treatment by radiation. With accurate beam localization it is quite important for us to understand the location of the lymph nodes and the pattern of lymphatic drainage. The book describes in detail the normal anatomy and embryology so that these patterns can be evaluated with their anatomic variations. The book would not be complete without a discussion of the complications of lymphography. The role of radionuclide lymphangiography and the exciting experimental technique of using immunospecific radionuclide immunoglobulins for lymphography are presented for comparison with conventional techniques.

It is a great privilege to introduce this book as it is an excellent review of the history and development of lymphographic techniques, their current status, and prospects for the future.

SAMUEL HELLMAN, M.D.
Professor and Chairman
Department of Radiation Therapy
Harvard Medical School
Boston, Massachusetts

Preface

During the past 20 years diagnostic roentgenology has undergone an incredible evolution in techniques for imaging normal and abnormal anatomy. The evolution has progressed from the conventional techniques of body imaging to the use of sophisticated contrast media and equipment.

The development of lymphography is but one of the new techniques of diagnostic radiology. Study of the lymphatic system on a routine clinical basis was made possible with the startling publication by Dr. John B. Kinmonth, a British surgeon at St. Thomas Hospital, London, in 1952. The initial studies with water-soluble contrast media were of limited clinical use. The introduction of oily contrast media made lymphography applicable to the study of a large number of diseases of the lymphatic system and has produced an enormous amount of literature on the subject.

This book has been written primarily for those performing lymphography in a busy radiology department, for practicing surgeons, residents, and the oncologist. The format lends itself to easy and rapid reference beginning with history, normal anatomy, technique, interpretation, abnormal lymphatics, benign lymph node disease, lymphoma, carcinoma, complications, radionuclide studies, and immunospecific lymphography. Each chapter is accompanied by a reference list that includes the major contributors on the subject material. Harrison has written a detailed anatomic and lymphographic chapter on anatomy of the lymphatic system. The technique of pedal lymphography described in the text has proven over the years to be the least complicated and makes the most efficient use of the lymphographer's time without the need of specialized instruments.

The technique of percutaneous lymph node aspiration biopsy is also described. The more complicated techniques of cervical, testicular, and mammary lymphography have been omitted because they are time-consuming and complicated and because the diagnostic results have limited value. The importance of general interpretation of the lymphogram merits a separate chapter.

Chapter 3 is not intended as a complete reference text on the physiology of the lymphatic system but is a brief review of the formation, function, and circulation of lymph. The chapter on "Abnormal Lymphatics" by O'Donnell, a vascular surgeon, is an especially good, concise review of the lymphedemas, both congenital and acquired, describing the current clinical and surgical techniques of management. It is an up-to-date review of the subject for surgical residents and practicing surgeons as well as the radiologist.

The place of lymphography for benign diseases of the lymph node has not been clearly established, but the importance of differentiating benign from malignant disease is stressed. Lukes has written an excellent review of the classification of lymphomas for the clinician and radiologist. The chapter on "Lymphography in Lymphoma" by Hessel, Adams, and Abrams is especially clear and concise. Wallace and Jing present their vast experience with lymphography in carcinoma from the M. D. Anderson Hospital in Chapter 9, describing in detail its usefulness in staging and management of solid tumors especially in the genitourinary tract.

A review of the complications and method of management is presented in Chapter 10. Potsaid and McKusick in Chapter 11 review the use of radionuclide lymphography dealing extensively with gallium-67.

The chapter by Order on immunospecific radionuclide lymphography must be considered investigational. It has been included because of its exciting potential. Dr. Order presents a review of tumor antigenicity and possible uses of immunospecific reagents, the method of direct immunospecific lymphography — its diagnostic and therapeutic potential.

MELVIN E. CLOUSE, M.D.

Acknowledgments

The problem of acknowledgement is always difficult because so many have helped in the final product. I would like to thank Miss Ruth M. Sullivan and Mrs. Marian K. Arnoff of the Horrax Library at the New England Deaconess Hospital for obtaining a large number of reference articles and all of the staff at the Countway Library, especially Mr. Richard Wolfe, the rare book librarian, and his assistants, Mrs. Grinne Blakeslee and Mrs. Hulda Newell, for retrieving the reference books of early anatomists used in preparing Chapter 1.

The secretaries at the New England Deaconess Hospital, especially Mrs. Margo Wyner, were most helpful throughout in typing the original manuscripts. I also want to thank Sally Ann Edwards and Katherine Arnoldi for editorial assistance and final typing. Without their help the book could never have been finished on schedule. Mr. Stanley M. Bennett, Chief of the Photography Department at the Massachusetts General Hospital, and Ms. Kathleen Grady, the Photographic Assistant, were very helpful in preparing the illustrative material.

I am especially grateful and want to thank each of the contributors for their work and diligence in preparing chapters of such high quality on schedule.

M.E.C.

CONTRIBUTORS

HERBERT L. ABRAMS, M.D., Philip H. Cook Professor and Chairman, Department of Radiology, Harvard Medical School; Radiologist-in-Chief, Peter Bent Brigham Hospital, Boston, Massachusetts

DOUGLASS F. ADAMS, M.D., Associate Professor of Radiology, Harvard Medical School; Radiologist, Peter Bent Brigham Hospital, Boston, Massachusetts

MELVIN M. CLOUSE, M.D., Assistant Clinical Professor of Radiology, Harvard Medical School; Chairman, Department of Radiology, New England Deaconess Hospital, Boston, Massachusetts

DEWEY A. HARRISON, M.D., Assistant Professor of Radiology, Section of Diagnostic Oncology, Stanford University Medical Center, Stanford, California

SAMUEL J. HESSEL, M.D., Assistant Professor of Radiology and James Picker Foundation Fellow in Academic Radiology, Harvard Medical School; Radiologist, Peter Bent Brigham Hospital, Boston, Massachusetts

BAO-SHAN JING, M.D., Professor of Radiology, University of Texas System Cancer Center, M.D. Anderson Hospital and Tumor Institute, Houston, Texas

ROBERT J. LUKES, M.D., Professor of Pathology, University of Southern California School of Medicine, Los Angeles, California

KENNETH A. MCKUSICK, M.D., Assistant Professor of Radiology, Harvard Medical School; Associate Radiologist, Massachusetts General Hospital, Boston, Massachusetts

THOMAS F. O'DONNELL, JR., M.D., Formerly: Lecturer and Senior Registrar, Surgical Professorial Unit, St. Thomas Hospital, London, England; Presently: Assistant Professor of Surgery, Tufts University School of Medicine, Boston, Massachusetts; and Consulting Vascular Surgeon, National Naval Medical Center, Bethesda, Maryland

STANLEY E. ORDER, M.D., F.A.C.R., Director Radiation Oncology and Professor of Oncology and Radiological Sciences, The Johns Hopkins Hospital, Baltimore, Maryland

MAJIC S. POTSAID, M.D., Associate Professor of Radiology, Harvard Medical School; Radiologist, Massachusetts General Hospital, Boston, Massachusetts

SIDNEY WALLACE, M.D., Professor of Radiology, University of Texas System Cancer Center; Chief, Section of Clinical Diagnostic Radiology, M.D. Anderson Hospital and Tumor Institute, Houston, Texas

Contents

CHAPTER 1. History, Melvin E. Clouse, M.D. 1

CHAPTER 2. Normal Anatomy, Dewey A. Harrison, M.D. 14

CHAPTER 3. Physiology — Lymph Formation, Function, Circulation, Melvin E. Clouse, M.D. 58

CHAPTER 4. Technique, Melvin E. Clouse, M.D. 61

CHAPTER 5. Interpretation, Sidney Wallace, M.D., Bao-Shan Jing, M.D., Melvin E. Clouse, M.D., and Dewey A. Harrison, M.D. 76

CHAPTER 6. Abnormal Lymphatics .. 89
The Lymphedemas, Thomas F. O'Donnell, Jr., M.D. 89
Obstruction and Collateral Flow, Melvin E. Clouse, M.D. 108

CHAPTER 7. Benign Lymph Node Disease, Melvin E. Clouse, M.D. 122

CHAPTER 8. Lymphoma 141
The Functional Approach to the Pathology of Malignant Lymphoma, Robert J. Lukes, M.D. 141
Lymphography in Lymphoma, Samuel J. Hessel, M.D., Douglass F. Adams, M.D., and Herbert L. Abrams, M.D. 160

CHAPTER 9. Carcinoma, Sidney Wallace, M.D., and Bao-Shan Jing, M.D. 185

CHAPTER 10. Complications, Melvin E. Clouse, M.D. 274

CHAPTER 11. Radionuclide Lymphography, Majic S. Potsaid, M.D., and Kenneth A. McKusick, M.D. 285

CHAPTER 12. Immunospecific Radionuclide Immunoglobulin Lymphography, Stanley E. Order, M.D., F.A.C.R. 316

Index 323

1

History

MELVIN E. CLOUSE, M.D.

Hippocrates' description of white blood and Aristotle's description of structures containing colorless fluid make it probable that lymph and lymph vessels were observed by the Alexandrian School in ancient times. These descriptions were lost with the decline in learning during the Middle Ages but were rediscovered in late Renaissance. According to Cruikshank (1786), a student of Hunter and the personal physician of Samuel Johnson, a Roman anatomist named Eustachius discovered the thoracic duct in a horse and described it in his treatis, *De Vena Fin Pari,* in 1563. He called the thoracic duct the vena Alba thoracica.

The glory of discovering the lymphatic vessels belongs to Gasparo Asellius, Professor of Anatomy and Surgery at Pavia, who on July 23, 1622, vivisected a well fed dog before members of the Order of Physicians to observe the recurrent nerve (Fig. 1.1). According to Drinker (1942), as an afterthought he decided to observe diaphragmatic motion. On opening the abdominal cavity and pulling the stomach aside, which he noted to be full, he was astonished by small white vessels in the mesentery along with the intestine. Asellius at first thought them to be nerves, but when real nerves were seen, he incised one and observed chyle rush out. He performed the same experiment on a dog whose stomach was empty and could not demonstrate these vessels. They were observed again when the experiment was repeated on another well fed dog. Asellius called them the vasa lactea and ascribed their function to absorbing chyle from the intestines and transporting it to the liver to be mixed into the blood stream.

Asellius' discovery was completely submerged for some time by Harvey's publication, *An Anatomical Disquisition on the Motion of the Heart and Blood in Animals,* in 1628. Even at the peak of his career, however, Harvey did not believe in the existence of Asellius' lymphatics or their function.

Asellius' book, *De Lactibus sive Lacteis Venis,* which contains his excellent diagrams of the mesenteric lymphatics and lymph nodes, was not only the first book on the lymphatic system but the first to have anatomic drawings in color.

In 1651 Pecquet described the thoracic duct and the cisterna chyli (Fig. 1.2). He found the cisterna chyli while performing an autopsy on a well fed dog and observed white fluid after removal of the heart. He first thought it pus but after careful dissection found the thoracic duct. Almost simultaneously, van Horne, Professor of Anatomy at Leiden in 1652, also described the thoracic duct.

In 1652–1653 Thomas Bartholin and Olaf Rudbeck assembled the known parts of the lymphatic system and recognized them as a system (Fig. 1.3). Bartholin was the first investigator to use the term lymphatic. The chyle vessels discovered by Asellius had been thought to convey food substances to the liver, but when Bartholin ligated the portal tracts, he observed dilated lymphatics above the ligature and collapsed lymphatics below. At the same time he observed the thoracic duct, its inflow into the large veins, and the cisterna chyli. Immediately after his work was published, it became known that Rudbeck had presented essentially the same material before the Queen of Sweden at Uppsala prior to Bartholin's publication. Because of this, a violent argument erupted with each accusing the other of plagiarism. It is probable that each investigator working independently made the same discovery.

Anatomists until the time of Anton Nuck in 1685 considered the lymphatic vessels to have only one coat—the intima (Fig. 1.4). Nuck demonstrated a second fibrous coat in the thoracic

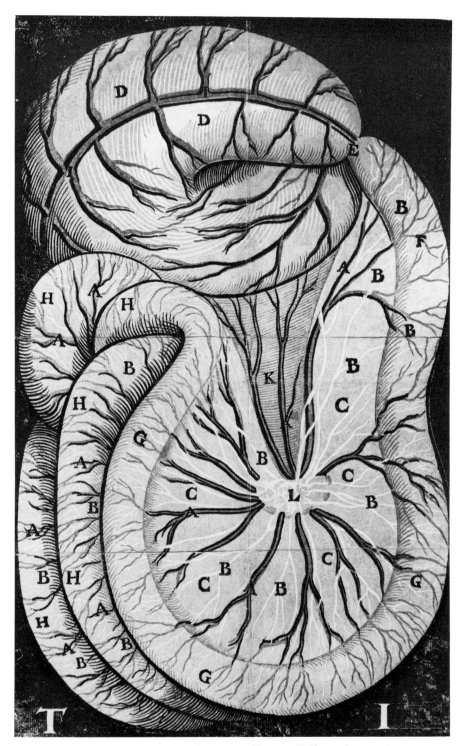

Fig. 1.1. Mesenteric Lymphatic Vessels (B Venae Lacteae)
(From Gasparo Asellius: *De Lactibus sine Lacteis Venis*. Mediolani, apud Io B. Bidellium, 1627.)

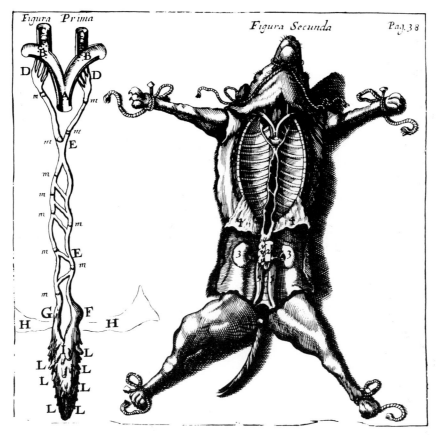

FIG. 1.2. FROM BOOK BY JEAN PECQUET, DISCOVERER OF THE THORACIC DUCT AND CISTERNA CHYLI
(From *Experimenta Nova Anatomica quibus Incognitum Chyli Receptaculum, et ab eo per Thoracem in Ramos usque Subclavis Vasa Lactea Deteguntur*. Paris, 1651, p. 38.)

duct of horses. Cruikshank in 1790 demonstrated a muscular coat as well as the intima in large lymphatics, but he could not demonstrate a muscular wall in smaller lymphatics.

According to Cruikshank the vasa vasorum in the lymphatic wall was described by William Hunter in 1762, who also noted contraction of the lymphatic vessels in response to irritation but could not demonstrate nerve innervation. Wrisberg in 1808 and Cruikshank in 1786 observed nerves in the vicinity of lymphatic vessels but could not demonstrate direct nerve innervation of the thoracic duct. It was not until 1925 that nervous innervation of the lymphatics was properly demonstrated by Lawrentjew. Dissecting cats and dogs, he described a periadventitial plexus of small ganglia surrounding the thoracic duct. Fibers from the intercostal and vagus nerves entered the thoracic duct. Branches from the lesser splanchnic nerve also supplied fibers to the lower thoracic duct and cisterna chyli.

Valves in the lymphatic vessels were almost certainly observed by Bartholin and Rudbeck,

but Frederick Ruysch (1638–1731) is considered – if not their discoveror – then the best demonstrator of the valves (Fig. 1.5).

Lymph nodes were seen by Herophilus, who noted certain veins in the mesentery that terminated in glandular bodies. These same glands were noted by Asellius, who thought them part of the pancreas because the lymph vessels were thought to pass through the pancreas on their way to the liver. For this reason they were labelled *pancreas Asellii* in *De Lacticus sive Lacteis Venis*. It was not until 1863 that His demonstrated them to be an integral part of the lymphatic system. In fact His' original description of the internal architecture and blood supply to the lymph nodes was so accurate that it has not changed.

Accurate demonstration of the course and interconnection of the lymphatic vessels was made possible by Anton Nuck in 1692. Using a time-consuming technique of injecting mercury into the lymphatics, he succeeded in visualizing practically the entire lymphatic system. It was from Nuck's technique that Mascagni in 1787

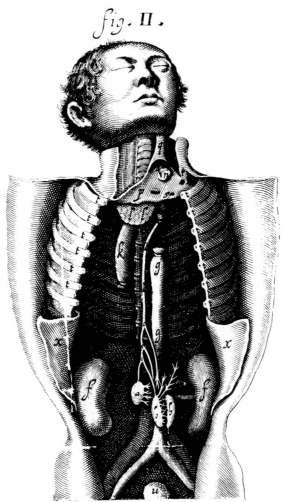

fig. II.

FIG. 1.3. HUMAN CISTERNA CHYLI AND THORACIC DUCTS
(From *The Anatomical History of Thomas Bartholinus
of the Lacteal Vein of the Thorax*. London, 1673.)

and Cruikshank in 1790 demonstrated the lymphatic topography in all parts of the body (Fig. 1.6). Gerota in 1896 introduced a new analytical technique using Prussian blue paint dissolved in turpentine and ether. On the basis of this improved technique, Jossifow in 1930 and Rouvièr in 1932 published books on the complete lymphatic system.

William Hunter was probably the first to appreciate the functional significance of the lymphatic system. He demonstrated absorption of chyle from the intestinal tract into the lymphatics. In a lecture published posthumously in 1784, he stated that lymphatic vessels all over the body (whether from the skin, lining of body cavities, or intestinal tracts) were the absorbing vessels and together with the thoracic duct transported chyle to the blood vascular system.

The mechanism of lymph formation was elu-

sive. It was generally believed until 1850 that lymph passed from the blood stream into lymphatic vessels by direct communication through thin tubules—the vasa serosa. The chief architects of the vasa serosa theory were Boerhaave (1738, 1742) and Vieussens (1705), who demonstrated canaliculi between blood vessels and the lymphatics. These were later shown to be artifacts of their primitive histologic techniques.

Virchow in 1858 contested the vasa serosa theory for lymph formation but believed there were communications through intercellular canaliculi. Von Recklinghausen in 1862 opposed the intercanalicular theory but thought the communication was direct through very small lymphatics and blood vessels. Ludwig's theory, more nearly correct, was based on simple filtration of fluid and molecular substances caused by intravascular pressure (blood pressure). Heidenhain criticized Ludwig's simple filtration theory because certain substances increased lymphatic flow. The vasa serosa theory was not abandoned, however, until after Schwann discovered the cell as the basic form of living substances within the body.

In 1894 Starling proved these theories incorrect. Starling's theory was that the blood capillary endothelium is a semipermeable membrane that is permeable to water and crystalloids but impermeable to proteins. Hydrostatic pressure in the arterial limb of the capillary induces filtration of water and crystalloids into the interstitial space. As the hydrostatic pressure in the venous limb diminishes, the plasma osmotic pressure becomes the driving force for resorption of crystalloids and water. The proteins cannot be absorbed into the blood through the semipermeable membrane (the capillary endothelium) but are absorbed by the lymphatics.

The anatomic basis for absorption of fluid and large molecules into the initial lymphatics (lymphatic capillaries) has been demonstrated by Leak and Burke (1966) and Casley-Smith (1972). Using electron microscopy these authors have demonstrated "open" junctions between the lymphatic endothelial cells for passage of fluid and large molecules. Smaller molecules may pass directly through the endothelial cell membrane into the lymphatic lumen (Figs. 1.7 and 1.8). The lymphatic endothelial cells are anchored by small fibrils to the surrounding connective tissues.

Although there have been many investigators in the field of lymphology, Cecil K. Drinker, Professor of Physiology at the Harvard School of Public Health, must be considered the father of modern lymphology because of his extensive ob-

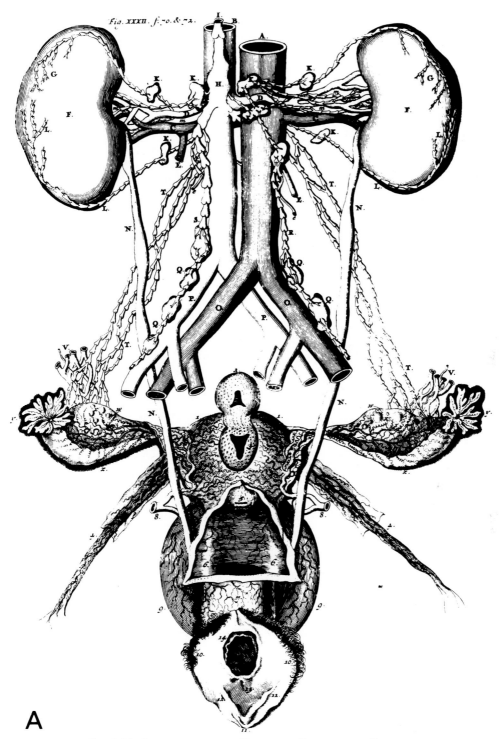

FIG. 1.4A. LYMPHATICS OF THE RENAL AND REPRODUCTIVE SYSTEMS
(From Anton Nuck: *Adenographia Curiosa et Uteri Foeminei Anatome Nova*. Lugd. B., 1692.)

servations and studies on the formation of lymph, its content, and changes in disease states (Drinker, 1942).

The concept of radiographic visualization of the lymphatics was published 35 years after Roentgen's discovery of x-rays. In 1930 and 1931 Funaoka from Japan and Carvalho of Portugal performed lymphography by injecting Thoro-

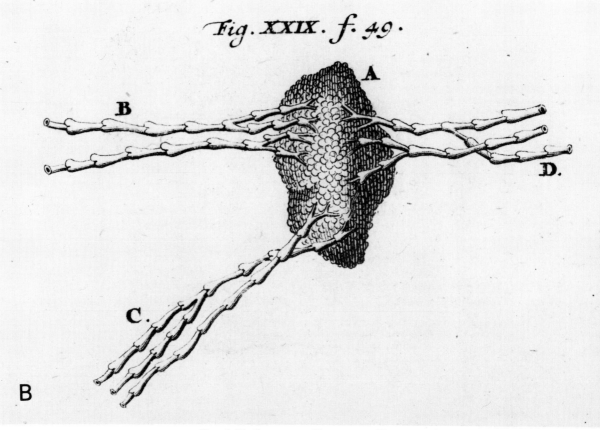

FIG. 1.4*B*. LYMPHATIC VESSELS AND NODES

An especially good drawing of valves. (From Anton Nuck: *Adenographia Curiosa et Uteri Foeminei: Anatome Nova.* Lugd. B., 1692.)

trast into the lymph nodes and subcutaneous tissues of animals and cadavers. In 1932 Pfahler showed lymphatics in a live man using the indirect method of lymphography. The indirect method of visualizing the lymphatics relies on the absorption of contrast material into the lymphatics from the connective tissue, body cavities, and organs. One week after the injection of Lipiodol into the maxillary sinuses, the lymphatics leading from the region were observed. The contrast media used for indirect lymphography were Thorotrast, oily solutions (such as Lipiodol), and water-soluble compounds (such as Urografin, Biligrafin, Joduron, and Collargol). Numerous investigators attempted to visualize the lymphatics indirectly, but this method was impractical because lymphatic vessels do not absorb the contrast material rapidly enough to adequately visualize the vessels and nodes.

The direct method of lymphography involved direct injection of contrast material into the nodes and lymph vessels. Teneff and Stoppani in 1936, and Servelle in 1945 visualized the lym-phatic channels and nodes in the pelvis by injecting Thorotrast into the inguinal nodes.

It was not until the revolutionary approach by Kinmonth in 1952 of cannulating the lymphatic vessel directly and injecting contrast material that lymphography became a useful clinical tool. The lymphatics are readily visualized for direct cannulation because of the rapid absorption of patent blue violet (11% solution) into the lymphatics from the subcutaneous tissue.

It is interesting that Hudack and McMaster in 1933 at the Rockefeller Institute outlined the cutaneous lymphatics in humans using 11% patent blue violet dye and observed the network of dermal lymphatics draining into the subcutaneous chains with channels leading into the axilla. Presumably, they did not think of directly injecting contrast material into the lymphatic vessels—hence lymphography as a useful clinical tool did not arrive until 1952!

The first studies of Kinmonth were on the pathologic changes of lymphedema using water-soluble contrast media, Biligrafin, and Uro-

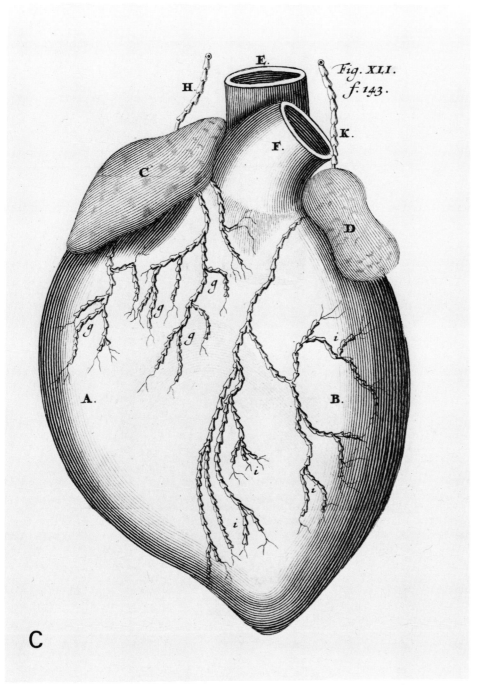

FIG. 1.4C. HEART LYMPHATICS
(From Anton Nuck: *Adenographia Curiosa et Uteri Foeminei Anatome Nova*. Lugd. B., 1692.)

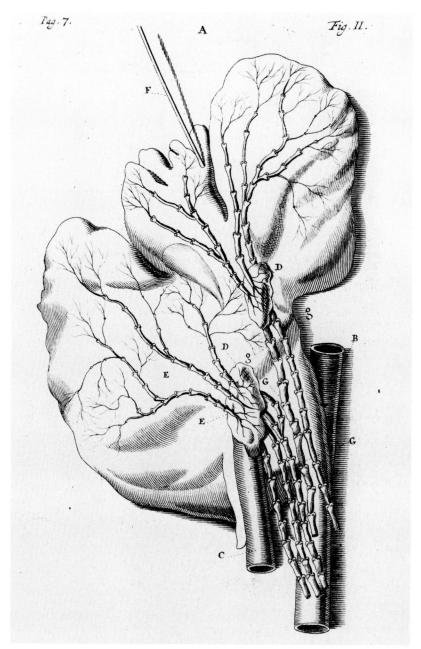

FIG. 1.5. LIVER LYMPHATIC VESSELS AND VALVES
(From Frederick Ruysch: *Dilucidatio Valvularum in Vasis Lymphaticis et Lacteis*. Hagaecomitiae, 1665, p. 7.)

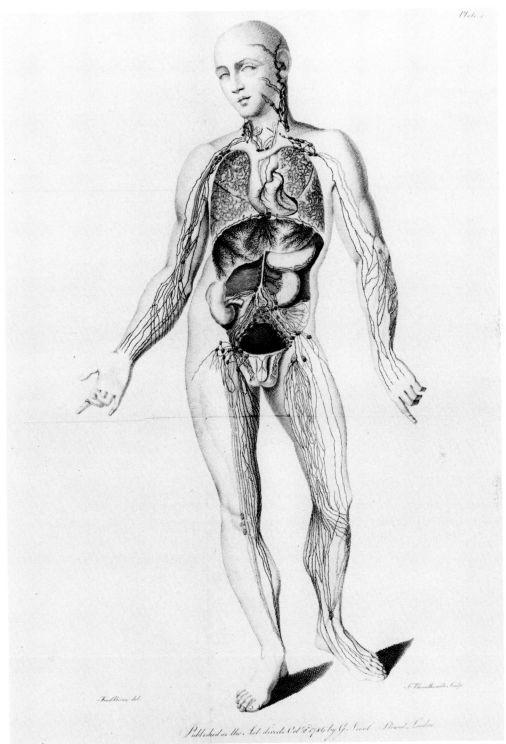

FIG. 1.6. PERIPHERAL AND VISCERAL LYMPHATIC VESSELS AND NODES
(From William Cruikshank: *The Anatomy of the Absorbing Vessels of the Human Body*. G. Nicol, London, 1786, p. 192.)

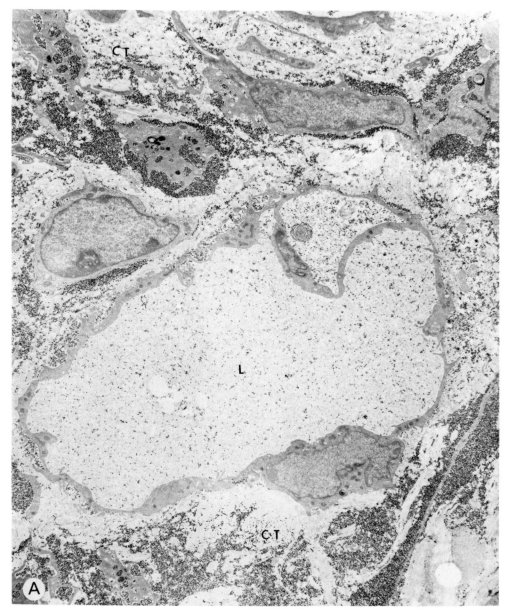

FIG. 1.7A. ELECTRON MICROGRAPH OF THE LYMPHATIC CAPILLARY AND SURROUNDING CONNECTIVE TISSUE AFTER THE
INTERSTITIAL INJECTION OF COLLOIDAL THORIUM
Note the presence of tracer throughout the connective tissue (*CT*) and within the lymphatic lumen (*L*).

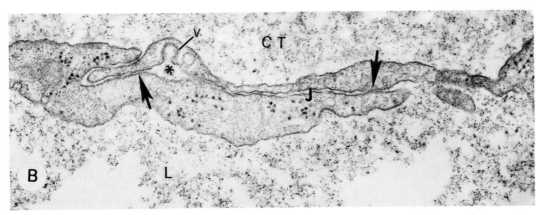

FIG. 1.7B. Although the Adjacent Endothelial Cells Are Extensively Overlapped, the Width of the Intercellular Clefts (*) Is Extremely Varied over Its Length

In addition, points of close apposition are also observed (*arrows*). Colloidal ferritin occurs in the connective tissue (*CT*) and the lumen (*L*) of the vessel. Plasmalemmal vesicles (*v*) also contain ferritin. *J*, intercellular junction.

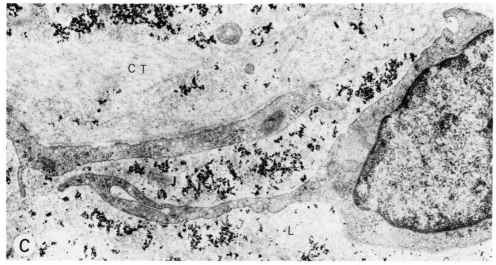

FIG. 1.7C. Electron Micrograph of a Patent Intercellular Junction (*J*) Containing Colloidal Thorium

L, lumen; *CT*, connective tissue. (Courtesy of Dr. L. V. Leak and Dr. J. F. Burke.)

grafin. Thorotrast could not be used because of its now known toxicity. Water-soluble contrast material is excellent for examination of vessels but is unsatisfactory for studying nodes, and, in addition, it is diluted by the lymph in the lumbar area.

Hreschyshyn et al. (1961), Wallace et al. (1961), and Malek (1959), all almost simultaneously (1959–61), modified the direct approach by using oil-soluble contrast material. This permits excellent visualization of the para-aortic lymph channels and nodes and the thoracic duct.

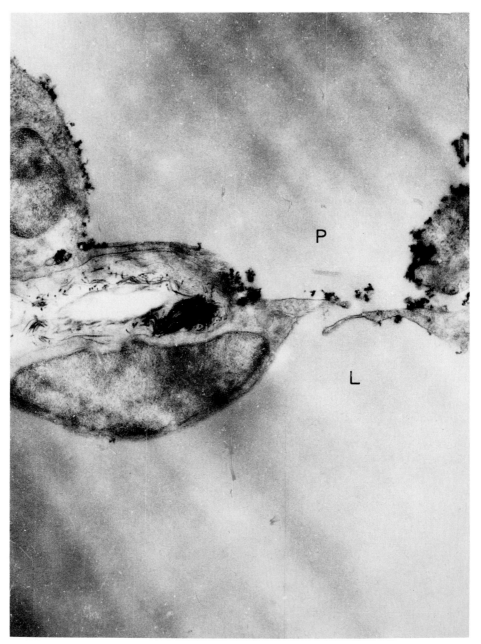

FIG. 1.8. MOUSE DIAPHRAGM

There is a gap between two lymphatic endothelial cells: *L*, lymphatic lumen; *P*, peritoneal cavity for passage of large molecules. The overlapping nature of the junction implies that it can close on diaphragmatic contraction.   ×20,000. (From Casley-Smith, J. R.: Angiologica, *9*: 106, 1972.)

REFERENCES

Asellius, G.: *De Lactibus sine Lacteis Venis.* Mediolani, apud Io B. Bidellium, 1627.

Bartels, P.: Das lymph gefasssystem. In *Handbuch d. Anatomie d. Menschen.* G. Fischer, Jena, 1909.

Bartholin, T.: *De Lacteis Thoracicis in Homine Brutisque.* M. Martzan, Hafniae, 1652.

Boerhaave, H.: Oratio de Uso Rationii Mechanicii in Medicine, habita 24 Sept 1702. In *Opusc ommnia Hagaecomitis,* 1738.

Boerhaave, H.: *Praelectiones Academiae in Proprias Institutiones Rei Medicae,* edited by A. J. Taurini, 1742.

Carvalho, R., Rodriguez, A. and Pereina, S.: Lamise en evidence por la radiographie du system lymphatique chez la vivant. Ann. Anat. Pathol. (Paris), *8:* 193, 1931.

Casley-Smith, J. R.: The role of the endothelial intercellular junctions in the functioning of the initial lymphatics. Angiologica, *9:* 106, 1972.

Cruikshank, W.: *The Anatomy of the Absorbing Vessels of the Human Body.* G. Nicol, London, 1786.

Drinker, C. K.: *The Lymphatic System: Its part in Regulating Composition and Volume of Tissue Fluid.* Stanford University Press, Stanford, 1942.

Funaoka, S., Tachikawa, R., Yamaguchi, O. and Fijita, S.: Kurz Mitteilung über die Roentgenographie dies Lymphagefässsystem souie über den Mechanismes der symphstromung. Ab Dritten Abst. Inst. Kaiserlich und Univ. Kyoto, *1:* 11, 1930.

Gerota, D.: Zur Technik der Lymph gefässinjektion. Eine nue Injektionsmasse der Lymphagefasse. Polychrome Injektion. Anat. Anz., *12:* 216 and Verh. Anat. Ges., 151-152, 1896.

Harvey, W.: *An Anatomical Disquisition on the Motion of the Heart and Blood in Animals.* In *The Works of William Harvey, M.D.,* translated by R. Willis from the Latin with a life of the author. Sydenham Society, London, 1847.

Heidenhain, R.: Versuche and Frozen zur Lehre von der Lymphbildung. Pflügers Arch., *49:* 209, 1891.

His, W.: Uber das Epithel der Lymphagefasswurzeln und uber die von Recklinghausen's schen Saftcanalchen. Z. wiss Zool., *13:* 455, 1863.

Hreschyshyn, M. M., Sheehan, F. and Holland, J. F.: Visualization of retroperitoneal lymph nodes. Lymphangiography as an aid in the measurement of tumor growth. Cancer, *14:* 205, 1961.

Hudack, S. and McMaster, P. D.: The lymphatic participation in human cutaneous phenomenon. A study of the minute lympatics of the living skin. J. Exp. Med., *57:* 751, 1933.

Jossifow, G. M.: *Das Lymphgefässsystem der menschen.* Jena, 1930.

Kinmonth, J. B.: Lymphangiography in man. Clin. Sci., *11:* 13, 1952.

Lawrentjew, A. P.: Zur Lehre von der Innervation des Lymphsystems. Über die Nerven des Ductus Thoracicus beim Hunde. Anat. Anz., *60:* 475, 1925-1926.

Leak, L. V. and Burke, J. F.: Fine structure of the lymphatic capillary and the adjoining connective tissue area. Am. J. Anat., *118:* 785, 1966.

Malek, P.: Physiologische, Pathologische und Anatomische Grundlagen der Lymphographie. IX International Congress Radiology, Munchen, 1959.

Mascagni, P.: *Vasorum Lymphaticorum Corporis Humani Historia et Ichonographia.* Siena, 1787.

Nuck, A.: *Adenographia Curiosa et Uteri Foeminei Anatome Nova.* Lugd. B., 1692.

Pecquet, J.: *Experimenta Nova Anatomica quibus Incognitum Chyli Receptaculum, et ab eo per Thoracem in Ramos usque Subclavis Vasa Lactea Deteguntur.* Paris, 1651.

Pfahler, G. G.: A demonstration of the lymphatic drainage of the maxillary sinuses. Am. J. Roentgenol., *27:* 352, 1932.

Rouvièr, H.: *Anatomie des Lymphatiques des l'homme.* Masson, Paris, 1932.

Rudbeck, O.: *Nove Exercitatio Anatomica, Exhibens Ductus Hepaticos Aquosos, et Vasa Glandularum Serosa.* Arosiae, 1653.

Ruysch, F.: *Dilucidatio Valvularum in Vasis Lymphaticis et Lacteis.* Hagaecomitiae, 1665.

Servelle, M.: A propos de la lymphographie experimentale et clinique. J. Radiol. Électro. Med. Nucl., *26:* 165, 1944-1945.

Starling, E. H.: The influence of mechanical factors on lymph production. J. Physiol. (Lond.), *16:* 224, 1894.

Teneff, S. and Stoppani, F.: Apropos de la lymphographie. J. Radiol. Électrol. Med. Nucl., *20:* 74, 1936.

van Horne, J.: *Novus Ductus Chyliferus. Nunc Primum Delineatus, Descriptus Eruditorium Examini Expositas.* Lugd. Batav., 1652.

von Recklinghausen, F. D.: *Die Lymphgefasse und ihre Beziehung zum Bindegewehe.* A. Hirschwald, Berlin, 1862.

Vieussens, R.: *Novum Vasorum Corporis Humani Systema.* Amstelod, 1705.

Virchow, R.: *Die Cellular pathologie inihrer Begründung auf physiologische gewebelehre.* Berlin, 1858.

Wallace, S., Jackson, L. and Schaffer, B.: Lymphangiograms: their diagnostic and therapeutic potential. Radiology, *76:* 179, 1961.

Wrisberg, H.: *Observations Anatomical de Nervis Vescerum Abdominis,* Part 3. Götting, 1808.

2

Normal Anatomy

DEWEY A. HARRISON, M.D.

Some familiarization with the anatomy and physiology of the lymphatic system is indispensable in assessing patients with a variety of diseases. Precise knowledge of the anatomy of the lymphatics, however, is imperative in the management of the patient with malignant disease. Clinical staging and subsequent management of malignant disease are greatly influenced by the extent of lymphatic involvement (Kaplan et al., 1973; Kirschner et al., 1974; Hays, 1975; Cutler et al., 1975; Rosenberg and Kaplan, 1975). As a clinical procedure lymphography is now most widely used and clearly defined in assessing the retroperitoneal lymphatics in patients with biopsy-confirmed neoplastic disease primary in the lymphatic system (Hodgkin's or non-Hodgkin's) (Rüttimann, 1967). Accuracy of interpretation is the overwhelming basis for such clear delineation of its use (Abrams et al., 1968; Castellino et al., 1974; Takahashi and Abrams, 1967). The normal roentgenographic anatomy of the retroperitoneal lymphatics as visualized by the dorsal pedal method, therefore, is of highest priority in discussing clinical lymphatic anatomy.

DEVELOPMENTAL AND GENERAL ANATOMIC ASPECTS OF THE LYMPHATICS

By injecting pig embryos, Florence Sabin in 1902 gave the first concepts of the developmental anatomy of the lymphatics. At approximately the sixth week of embryonic life (10-mm stage), paired jugular sacs become recognizable. The original concept postulated that lymphatic endothelium was a derivation of venous endothelium from a process of sprouting. Huntington and McClure (1906–1907) and Kampmier (1912) subsequently postulated that initial lymphatic structures originated from fusion of mesenchymal clefts and that their connection with developing contiguous veins came secondarily. Still there is disagreement on the exact mechanism of the initial derivation of the lymphatics, but otherwise the developmental anatomy of the system is clearly established (Töndury, 1967).

As differentiation continues, the lymphatics rapidly separate and grow together, anastomosing into their own system. In spite of the development into a separate system, lymphaticovenous communications have been demonstrated to persist, even in fully developed animals (Bron et al., 1963). Paired lymphatic sacs become evident in the inguinal region adjacent to the common iliac veins, and two other unpaired sacs develop along the posterior abdominal wall. One of these sacs gives rise to the cisterna chyli; the other develops into a retroperitoneal sac that extends into the lymphatic network of the mesentery, stomach, and retroperitoneal organs.

First recognition of the thoracic duct is found in embryos of approximately 23–24 mm. The embryonic thoracic duct consists of two sacs which are bilaterally symmetrical. Their starting point is in the abdominal cavity at the level of the cisterna chyli. Dorsal to the aorta, the right duct crosses at about the level of the fourth thoracic vertebra, to join the duct of the opposite side. Thus, a single trunk forms on the left side and then merges with the jugular portion of the thoracic duct. The jugular portion of the thoracic duct is a caudal outgrowth of the jugular lymph sac on the left. In the embryo the two primitive ducts are connected by numerous cross anastomoses over the course of the aorta.

The persistence and growth of a part of the embryonic duct system and the involution of other parts result in the adult anatomic structure now accepted by most authorities on the anatomy of the thoracic duct. Although the embryonic development of the thoracic duct can result in many variations, the usual adult form is that of a single duct passing into the thorax and opening into the venous system of the left side (Davis, 1915).

The lymph nodes do not appear until the vessels are well established. They are first recognized as masses of lymphoid tissue in complex networks of developing vessels. Excepting the cisterna chyli, lymphoid masses destined to be nodes develop contiguously with the primitive sacs. The lymphoid masses divide into smaller portions. Then, penetration by vessels occurs and the tissue becomes enclosed in a connective tissue capsule. The original lymphoid tissue becomes the medullary cords and cortical nodules. Enclosing lymphatic capillaries form the sinusoidal system. All of the structures of the node are present and completely arranged at birth with the exception of differentiation of germinal centers (secondary nodules) within primary nodules.

GENERAL CHARACTERISTICS OF LYMPHATIC VESSELS AND NODES

The function of the lymphatic system can be summarized as (1) production and transport of thymus-dependent small lymphocytes that function mainly in the cellular immunity mechanism; (2) production of large lymphocytes and plasma cells, which in turn produce circulating antibodies; (3) return of interstitial proteins to blood; (4) filtration of body fluids through nodal sinuses; and (5) transfer of absorbed fats from intestinal lacteals to the thoracic duct (Gowans, 1959; Kuisk, 1971; Drinker and Yoffey, 1941; Rusznyak et al., 1967).

Lymphatic Vessels

The normal lymphatic system is a closed network of vessels that commences with lymphatic capillaries in soft tissues, extends to larger vessels that pass through lymph nodes, and again collects in another network of closed vessels. Communication with the cardiovascular system predominantly is through anastomoses with neck veins by way of the thoracic duct (Davis, 1915; Brash, 1943; Clark, 1942). Lymphatic capillaries are the functional units of the system in its role of absorption and interchange of fluid substances and cells (Casley-Smith, 1967).

The capillaries are lined with endothelial cells and vary in shape throughout the body. Predominantly the capillaries form anastomotic complexes the diameters of which range from a few micra to approximately 1 mm (Fig. 2.1). Electron microscopy can demonstrate overlapping endothelial cells that interlock with fine microfibrils. This complex is cemented to interstitial tissues. The microfibrils play a crucial role in the maintenance of patency of vital endothelial interconnections, when pressure in the interstitium rises. Pappenheimer et al. (1951)

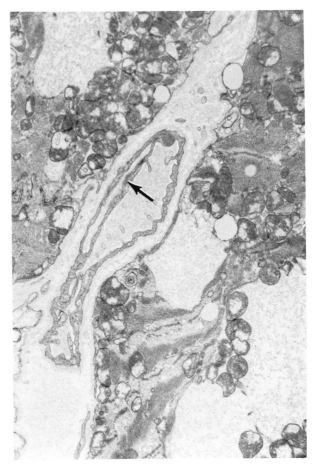

FIG. 2.1. ELECTRON MICROGRAPH OF CROSS-SECTION OF A LYMPHATIC CAPILLARY
The capillary consists of a single layer of endothelial cells blending into surrounding connective tissue. Note infolding producing valves (*arrow*). ×10,000. (Courtesy of Dr. Margaret Billingham, Department of Pathology, Stanford University Medical Center.)

elaborated on the significance of these interconnections (Pappenheimer pores) in a description of the "Pore Theory of Molecular Diffusion and Filtration." This pathway appears to be the mechanism for the movement of substances composed of large molecules. Smaller molecules pass directly through the endothelial cytoplasm.

Anatomically, larger lymphatic vessels (approximately 0.5–0.75 mm in diameter) are very similar to veins, containing three layers in their walls. The adventitia is composed of longitudinal and transverse bundles of smooth muscle and collagen fibers. Most of the medium sized vessels possess a smooth muscle media of varying muscular configurations. The intima consists of endothelium and elastic fibers, the infolding of which forms valves to prevent backflow of lymph (Ham and Leeson, 1961; Bloom and Fawcett, 1962). Differing from veins, lymphatic vessels branch into divisions of similar diameters. Vessels are classed as afferent or efferent based on their functional relationship to the nodes. The thoracic duct is the largest of the vessels (4–6 mm in diameter) (Fig. 2.2).

Alternating bands of constriction and dilatation approximately 1 cm apart are characteristic of vessel filling in lymphography. The areas of constriction are lymphatic valves that become conspicuous as the viscous oily contrast material slightly distends the surrounding portion of the vessels (Fischer and Zimmerman, 1959; Jacobsson and Johansson, 1959; Fuchs, 1969; Jackson and Kinmonth, 1974b). Although the valves influence antegrade flow, movement of fluid along the vessel is determined primarily by external forces (Drinker and Yoffey, 1941).

Lymph Nodes

The glandular structures (nodes) of the lymphatic system consist of groups of round lymphoid cells contained in a complex of reticulum

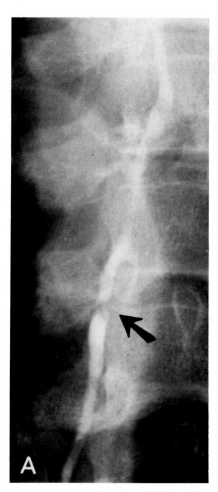 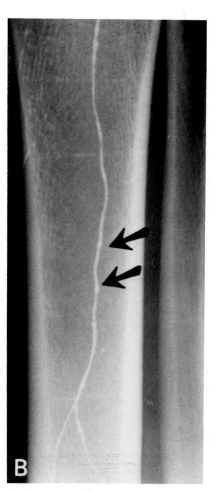

FIG. 2.2. CONTRAST FILLING OF LYMPHATIC VESSELS

A demonstrates segment of the thoracic duct. *B* shows a lower extremity vessel contrast-filled. *Arrows* indicate areas of constriction and dilatation which are characteristic of lymphatic valves during contrast infusions.

fibers (Fig. 2.3). The thymus, spleen, tonsils, other collections of lymphoid tissue (Peyer's patches), and, to some extent, bone marrow contain cells that are similar in many respects to those cells of lymph nodes. Immunity is their common bond (Drinker and Yoffey, 1941).

Nodes vary extensively in size, shape, and color and occur singly or in clusters. The specific

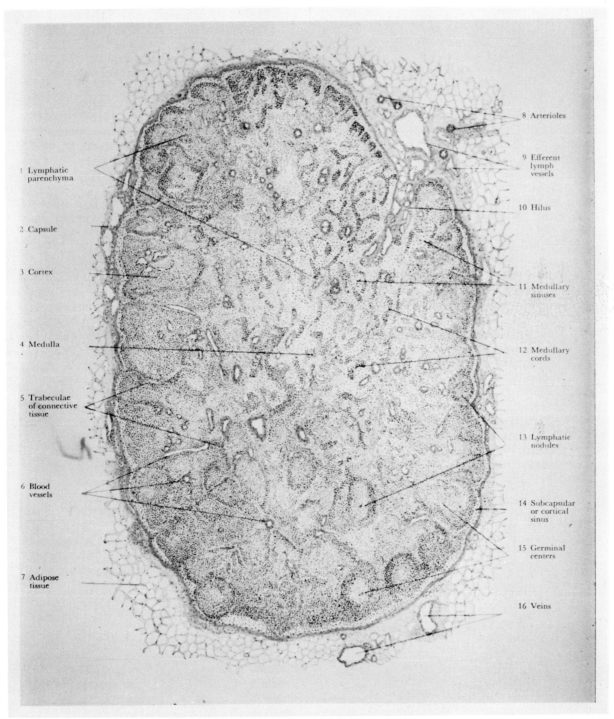

FIG. 2.3. TYPICAL LYMPH NODE ARCHITECTURE

The parenchyma is predominant and is enclosed by a fibrous capsule. The capsule is interrupted by an indentation (hilus) where the arterioles enter, and venules and efferent lymph vessels emerge. As represented, nodes often are embedded in adipose tissue.

characteristics of nodal groups depend to a large degree on the location of the node and neighboring organs (Rouviere, 1938).

Nodal parenchyma consists of a peripheral portion (cortex) and a more central core (medulla) (Fig. 2.3).

Nodal architecture has four basic features: aggregates of lymphoid tissue (nodules), lymphatic capillaries, blood vessels, and supportive tissue framework (histologic framework). Lymphoid elements predominate (Ham and Leeson, 1961; Bloom and Fawcett, 1962; Tjernberg, 1967). As noted in Figure 2.4, lymphoid nodules are encountered throughout the circumference of the periphery of the node just within the capsule and subcapsular space (marginal sinus).

The supportive tissue framework of the node is of considerable importance in lymphography (Tjernberg, 1967). Lymph nodes commonly lie in fatty tissue, but the node itself is surrounded by a capsule of dense collagenous fibers, fibroblasts, and some smooth muscle. Radiating from the capsule and hilus, extending into the substance of the node, are connective tissue strands or trabeculae. These provide nodal support and carry blood vessels. In addition to the trabeculae there is an extensive network of reticular fibers that project from the capsule and trabeculae throughout the node. These fine reticular fibers form a lacy, interdigitating communication of minute spaces (sinus system). The portion beneath the capsule is the subcapsular or marginal sinus, while those segments found in the cortical and medullary regions are named respectively (Fig. 2.4A). Physiologically these sinuses serve as areas for permeation of fluid (Ham and Leeson, 1961; Rusznyak et al., 1967). During lymphography the oily contrast material in the sinuses opacifies the nodes (Fuchs, 1969; Fischer and Zimmerman, 1959) (Fig. 2.5).

Analysis of the lymphadenogram (nodal phase) is of paramount significance during lymphography (Fig. 2.6). The roentgen appearance of the internal architecture of a node depends on the relative amounts of lymphatic tissue or other tissue of similar density, e.g., neoplasm within the node and volume of contrast material deposited in the sinuses (Tjernberg, 1967).

Lower Extremity

The roentgen description of the course and anatomic relationships of the lymphatics of the extremities was first demonstrated by Kinmonth (1952). In subsequent years, the usual or normal pathways of lymphatic drainage of the lower extremities, and their relationships to various anatomic landmarks as visualized during lymphography have been well established (Fischer et al., 1962; Jacobsson and Johansson, 1959; Fuchs, 1971b; Kinmonth et al., 1955a and 1955b; Larson and Lewis, 1967; Malek et al., 1959 and 1964; Kuisk, 1971; Browse, 1972a). It must be emphasized that a technically successful examination is imperative to obtain maximal diagnostic accuracy in assessing normal or abnormal lymphograms.

The vessels of the lower extremities consist of a superficial (subcutaneous) prefascial and deep subfascial system. Both systems accompany or are accompanied by corresponding blood vasculature. Dorsal pedal lymphatic injections (routine clinical lymphography) normally will not opacify the deep subfascial system. The superficial system is composed of anterior and posterior vessels. These vessels are usually opacified in routine clinical lymphography.

Anterior Superficial System

If a lymphatic vessel on the medial aspect of the dorsum of the foot is injected more proximally, the visualized vessels course continuously anteriorly with the greater saphenous vein. Cannulation and injection of a vessel lateral on the dorsum will opacify vessels that predominantly course anteriorly and laterally below the knee.

From approximately the midcalf to the proximal third of the lower extremity, the lateral vessels cross in a gentle curve toward the medial side. As vessel filling continues, the lateral vessels become entirely medial just proximal to the knee, and their course continues with the greater saphenous vein just as the medial chain vessels (Fig. 2.7). Therefore injection of any vessel on the dorsum results in visualization of the major portion of the superficial system, the origins (anteromedially and anterolaterally) of which ultimately accompany the greater saphenous vein and drain into the inguinal lymph nodes.

The anteromedial chain tends to originate with slightly larger vessels on the dorsum but ascends with fewer vessels below the knee as compared to the anterolateral chain. Also, the anteromedial vessels are less variable in number and character in this region. Below the knee the anterolateral vessels are serpiginous and branch frequently as they begin to course medially. Usually anterolateral vessels deviate medially; anteromedial vessels seldom become lateral. Above the knee both groups are medially placed and display frequent bifurcations. Upon

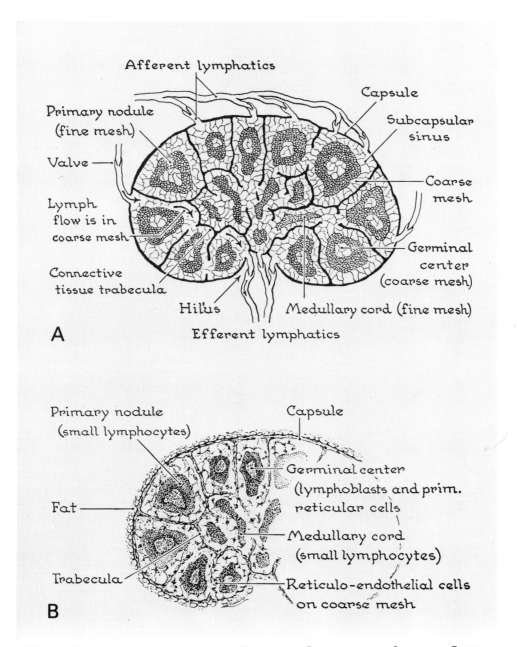

FIG. 2.4. ARCHITECTURAL RELATIONSHIP OF FUNCTIONAL CONSTITUENTS OF LYMPHATIC SYSTEM
(EXCLUDING THE CAPILLARIES)

A: Afferent vessels penetrate the surface of the node through the capsule. Note the smaller but more numerous afferent vessels. During lymphographic injections, contrast material follows a course very similar to that of lymph flow. *B*: Note the difference in appearance of the primary follicles (densely stained homogeneously) and the secondary follicle (pale stained central germinal center). Medullary cords branch and anastomose with each other and also cortical follicles. During lymphography these lymphoid elements produce the characteristic stippled radiolucencies observed in the nodes; their radiographic visualization is because of the surrounding contrast material which settles in the supportive tissue framework. (Adapted from *Histology*, 4th ed., edited by Ham and Leeson, p. 390. J. B. Lippincott Co., Philadelphia, 1961.)

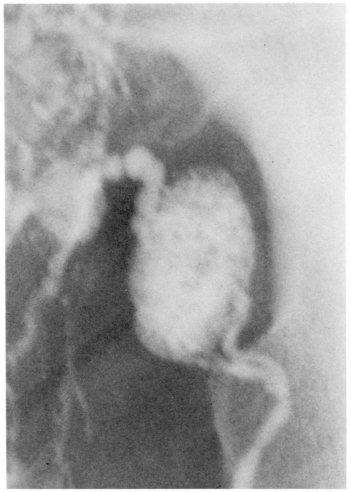

FIG. 2.5. AFFERENT VESSELS DURING CONTRAST INJECTION
Note the afferent vessels transporting the oily substance to the node. After permeating the node through the sinuses, the material exits through a large efferent vessel.

reaching their destination, the inguinal nodes, there are 10–20 vessels with similar characteristics (Fig. 2.8).

Posterior Superficial

The posterior component of the superficial prefascial lymphatics contributes far less to the system but can be visualized by cannulating and injecting a superficial vessel below the lateral malleolus. These vessels are smaller and more tortuous than the anterior component, and they contribute only one to three subcutaneous trunks. Posteriorly, these trunks accompany the lesser saphenous vein to the popliteal fossa. The afferents empty into one to three popliteal nodes. Efferent vessels then emerge, turn anteromedially, become deep subfascial vessels, and thereafter follow the deep blood vessels on the medial aspect of the thigh. Subse-

quent drainage is into deeper, more proximal inguinal nodes.

Deep Subfascial System

Valves in lymphatics of the lower extremity direct flow from the deep to the superficial system, contrasting the flow pattern in the venous system. Techniques to perform lymphangiography on the deep subfascial system of the lower extremity have been devised, hence some knowledge of its roentgen appearance has been gained (Malek et al., 1959 and 1964; Larson and Lewis, 1967).

The deep system of the lower leg and thigh collects lymph from the muscles, fascia, and joints. Some of the deep lymphatics of the thigh are demonstrated by opacification of the posterior superficial lymphatics. Once past the popliteal region, these vessels become subfascial as

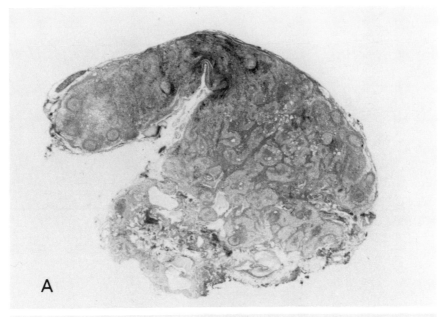

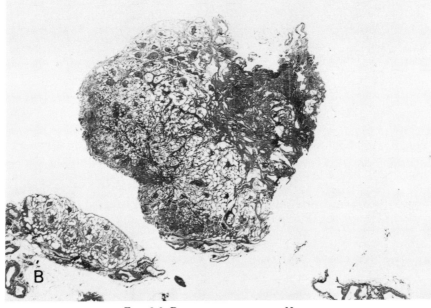

FIG. 2.6. PHOTOMICROGRAPHS OF NODES

A demonstrates mild reactive hyperplasia emphasizing the lymphoid elements of a node that has not undergone lymphography. *B* shows sections of nodes with lymphographic contrast material entrapped in the reticular network. *A*, ×8; *B*, ×9. (Courtesy of Dr. Margaret Billingham, Department of Pathology, Stanford University Medical Center.)

they continue in the thigh (see "Posterior Superficial" section). Lymphographically the ascending vessels of the superficial and deep systems do not seem to communicate extensively.

Ngu (1964) postulated an interesting concept pertaining to the lymphatic drainage of the lower leg and thigh. This postulate suggested separate pathways of drainage for each of these regions. Evidence to support this was derived from the observation that there were separate nodes of drainage for each of these areas and that in the presence of postinflammatory edema below the knee, normal thigh lymphatics were maintained. Although the observations were accurate, the postulate was not proven. No attempts were made to visualize simultaneously the deep system of the lower leg and thigh for possible communication above the knee.

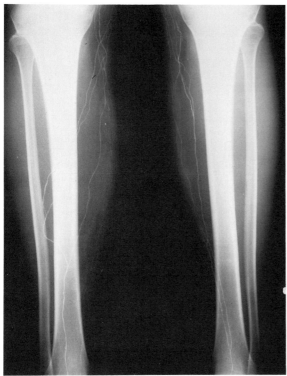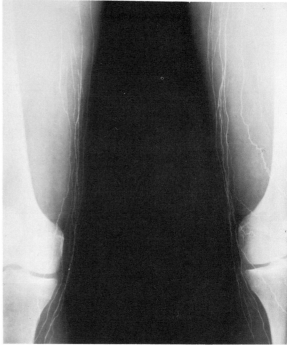

FIG. 2.7. VASCULAR PHASE OF LYMPHOGRAPHY SHOWING COURSE OF INJECTED CONTRAST MATERIAL
In *B* note that all channels have become medial.

INGUINAL REGION

Lymphographically, the lymphatics of the inguinal region are strikingly variable. Contrast filling of the inguinal lymphatics shows wide variations in number and course of the vessels with more extensive variations in the number, size, and appearance of the nodes (Fischer et al., 1962). This significant variability of nonmalignant nodes can simulate malignancy in this region (Greening and Wallace, 1963; Wallace et al., 1962; Butler, 1969; Castellino et al., 1974). Therefore it is quite tenuous to interpret the inguinal nodes as containing primary or secondary malignant disease without substantial abnormality in higher regions (Browse, 1972a; Castellino, 1974; Kuisk, 1971; Wallace et al., 1961 and 1962; Abrams et al., 1968) (Fig. 2.9).

Those nodes lymphographically considered as inguinal fall below the inguinal ligament. The nodes are divided into a superficial and deep group. Specific distinction between these groups by lymphography can be difficult. The superficial group is further subdivided into superior and inferior groups. The superior nodes are more proximal than the inferior group and thus are closer to the inguinal ligament; the inferior group is more distal and closer to the femoral canal. Lymphographically, the inferior group is visualized far more frequently than the superior group that drains the perineal structures (Fuchs, 1969 and 1971b; Kuisk, 1971).

The deep inguinal group is also located more proximal and closer to the inguinal ligament than the superficial inferior group. The most proximal nodes of the deep inguinal group are larger, more constant, and occasionally seem contiguous with the above external iliac group. In the inguinal fossa, medial to the femoral vein and immediately below the medial external iliac nodes, is a relatively large constant node (Fig. 2.10). This node has descriptively been called the node of *Rosenmüller, Pirogow,* or *Cloquet* (Kubik et al., 1967; Kuisk, 1971; Fuchs, 1971b).

The vessels from the lower nodes pass superiorly, sometimes bypassing a higher inguinal group on their way to the external iliac nodes. The efferents that emerge from the inguinals are larger and more tortuous than antecedent afferents, and lymphographically the valves become more apparent and accentuated.

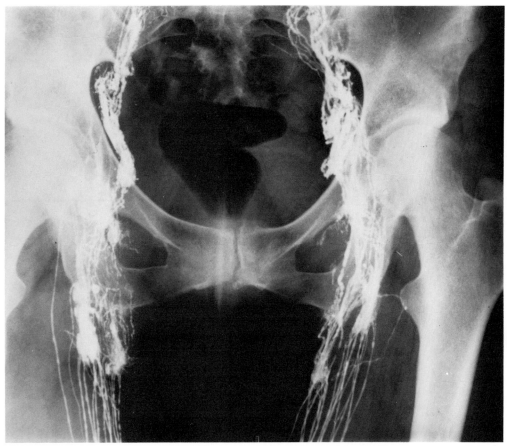

FIG. 2.8. NUMEROUS LOWER EXTREMITY VESSELS TRAVERSING INGUINAL REGION
Note the similarity in appearance, particularly in size, even after frequent divisions distally.

Pelvic Region

The next region visualized by lymphography is the pelvic (iliac) lymphatics. These nodes are located between the inguinal ligament inferiorly and the bifurcation of the common iliac blood vessels. Specific names for these lymphatics basically are those of the corresponding iliac blood vessels.

External Iliac Group

The external iliac lymphatics consist of three chains: lateral (external), intermediate (middle), and medial (internal) (Fig. 2.11). The *lateral (external) chain* is usually composed of one to three vessels that run along the lateral aspect of the external iliac artery. Lymphography usually demonstrates the most inferior node of this group. It is variously called the lateral *retrocrural node* (Herman et al., 1963) and the lateral *lacunar node* (Kubik, 1967) and is a rather constant, fairly large node. Herman et

al. (1963) describe one to three additional smaller nodes within this group.

The *intermediate (middle) chain* is less routinely demonstrated and is usually composed of fewer vessels than the lateral or medial chain (Herman et al., 1963; Kuisk, 1971). It is positioned between the artery and the vein, and anastomotic connections with the lateral and medial chains are common. The entire intermediate group is usually composed of two to four nodes. Fuchs (1969) states that the middle retrocrural node is frequently absent.

The *medial (internal) chain* contains the greatest number of vessels (Herman et al., 1963). This chain is medial to the vein, superior to the obturator nerve, and more dorsal to the vein than the other external iliac chains. Herman et al. (1963) described the dorsal location of this chain as being "prolapsed into the pelvis," and Fuchs (1969) specifically states that this group is situated close to the pelvic wall. Critical analysis of the lymphographic appearance of

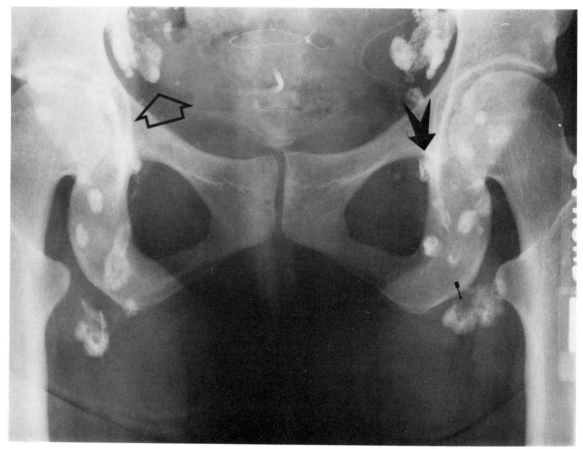

FIG. 2.9. NORMAL INGUINAL NODES
The inguinal nodes are enlarged and characteristically foamy. Striking filling defects are also typical. Left inguinal node (*small arrow*) possesses sufficient characteristics to cause a false-positive diagnosis of nodal malignancy. The more cephalad low iliac nodes (*upper arrows*) appear less ominous but still can be easily misinterpreted.

this group requires oblique and/or stereoscopic views of this region (Fig. 2.12). The most inferior node of this group is called the internal retrocrural node (Herman et al., 1963) or the medial lacunar node (Kubik, 1967; Fuchs, 1969). Although small additional nodes may be found in this chain, the middle node is the largest and most commonly opacified node of this group. This single node may represent the group in its entirety due to fusion with the node of Rosenmüller or nodes of the intermediate chain (Fuchs, 1969; Herman et al., 1963; Kuisk, 1971).

Nevertheless, whether this node is seen on the lymphogram independently or tapered toward other nodes in an apparently inseparable cluster, thorough familiarization with the regional anatomy and the internal architectural morphology of this node has high priority to the oncologic lymphologist. This node is a most important lymphatic drainage site for the majority of male and female pelvic organs and is a com-

mon site for deposition of metastatic pelvic malignancies (Rouviere, 1938; Kuisk, 1971). Optimal visualization of this node frequently requires stereoscopy and occasionally laminagraphy.

The deep femoral lymphatics communicate with the middle node through the deep inguinal chain (Kuisk, 1971).

The term *obturator node* is lost in a myriad of confusion (Fuchs, 1969; Herman et al., 1963; Kuisk, 1971), and lymphologists who use the term must specify the anatomic location of the node to which they refer. In an attempt to correlate lymphographic anatomy with surgical and pathologic anatomy, Herman et al. (1963) concluded that the lymphogram conforms more accurately with the anatomic description of Rouviere (1938), and therefore lymphographic terminology is more precise than surgical terminology. Anatomic descriptions state obturator nodes are part of the external iliac chain (Rou-

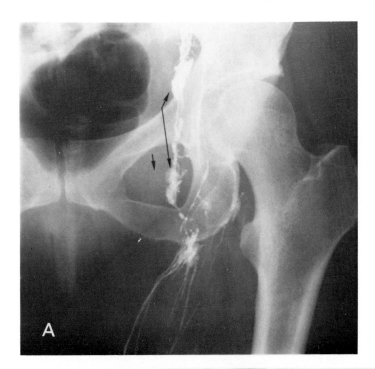

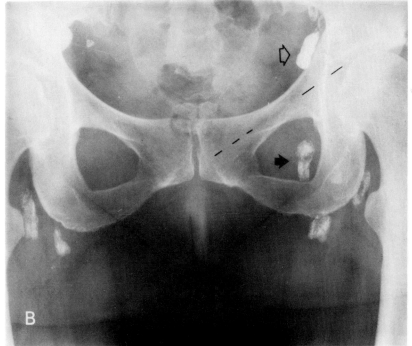

FIG. 2.10. NODE OF ROSENMÜLLER, PIROGOW, OR CLOQUET

A: The node is shown communicating with the external iliac group (*arrows*). *B*: *Open arrow* shows opacified external iliac node; *broken line* delineates area of inguinal ligament; *solid arrow* points to node of Rosenmüller. Although the presence of this node is quite constant, its appearance is quite variable.

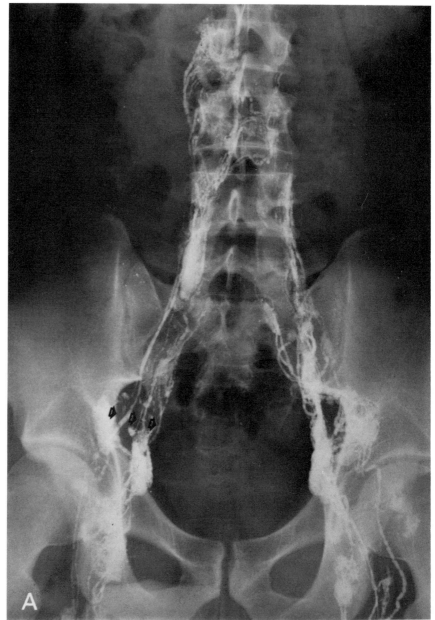

FIG. 2.11. EXTERNAL ILIAC LYMPHATICS

A: Frontal projection of vascular phase of lymphogram. Three chains are demonstrated and indicated by *arrows*: (*1*) lateral, (*2*) intermediate, and (*3*) medial. Note the normal undulating vessel appearance; observed looping and cross-over in the paralumbar region are also characteristic vessel filling patterns. *B*: Better delineation of respective chains is obtained with a posterior oblique projection. *C*: Nodal retention phase depicting external iliac chains in frontal projection. *D*: Posterior oblique projection of the nodal retention phase. Note fusion of node of Rosenmüller with internal retrocrural node (*3*).

viere, 1938; Clark, 1942). The term *obturator node* tends to designate specifically the middle node of the internal chain of the external iliac group (Herman et al., 1963) (Fig. 2.13).

Internal Iliac (Hypogastric Group)

The internal iliac (hypogastric) nodes, usually four to eight in number, are located along the distribution of the internal iliac artery and its branches (Figs. 2.14 and 2.15). This group contributes to lymphatic drainage of musculoskeletal structures of the pelvis as well as organs intrinsic to the pelvic cavity. Most of these nodes are in close proximity to their respective structures of drainage (Rouviere, 1938; Fuchs, 1969; Brash, 1943).

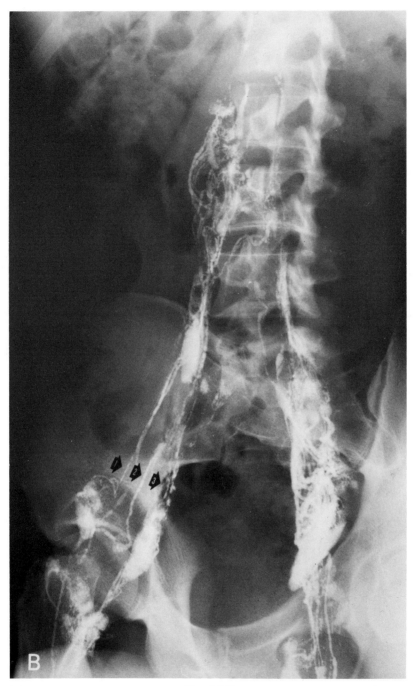

FIG. 2.11B

Topographically, two subgroups have been designated. Adjacent to internal iliac blood vasculature are the parietal nodes that service musculoskeletal portions of the pelvis; the visceral nodes are similarly related to blood vessels of the splanchnic structures of the pelvis.

The presence of specific nodes of the parietal or visceral subgroup is quite variable. When present, however, specific node clusters are named according to adjacent internal iliac blood vessel branches or tributaries.

Pedal lymphography seldom visualizes internal iliac nodes. There are data indicative of the wide anatomic variability of the nodes of the internal iliac group (Howett and Greenburg, 1966; Reiffenstuhl, 1964). Thus, nonopacification or very erratic minimal opacification of these nodes, lymphographically, is common.

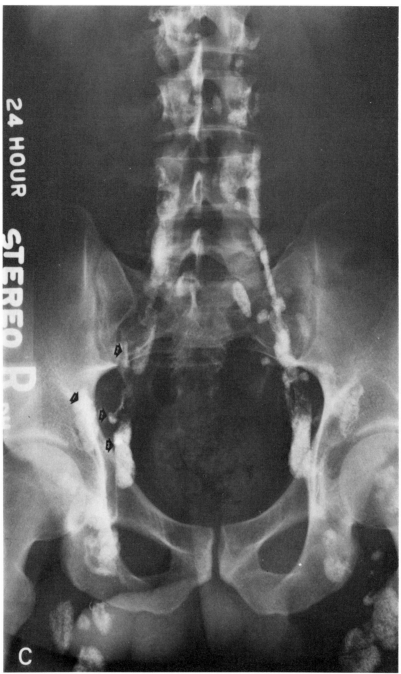

FIG. 2.11C

The most frequently opacified node of the entire internal iliac group is the lateral sacral node of the parietal subgroup and that is seen only in approximately 50% of normal lymphograms (Herman et al., 1963) (Fig. 2.15).

Common Iliac Group

The common iliac arteries begin at the aortic bifurcation, usually in the vicinity of L4. Exter-nal and internal iliac blood vessels communi-cate at approximately the level of the sacral promontory. Between these two landmarks, the adjacent lymphatic vessels and nodes are termed the *common iliacs*.

The lateral chain of the external iliacs contin-ues as the lateral chain of the common iliac group. It is lateral and slightly posterior to the artery. The intermediate chain can be found

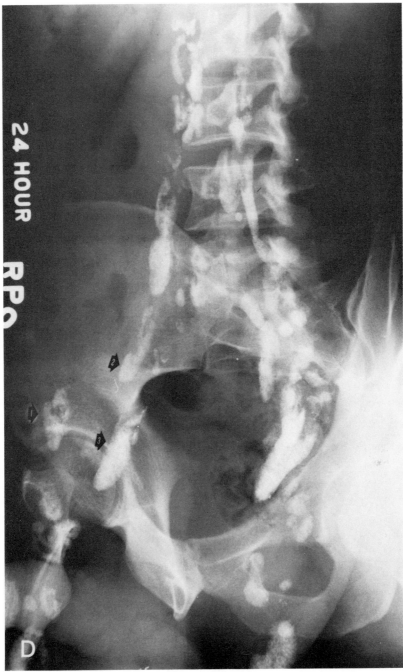

Fig. 2.11D

both anterior and posterior between the artery and the vein. The medial chain is dorsal and medial to the blood vessels. The three chains communicate extensively with each other. Cross communication between left and right common iliacs occurs with 50% frequency (Fuchs, 1969 and 1971b; Herman et al., 1963) (Fig. 2.14).

The aortic bifurcation influences the ana-tomic relationships of the common iliac vessels and nodes. The connection of the medial com-mon iliac chain is influenced far more by the aortic bifurcation than the intermediate or lat-eral chains. Influencing factors are (1) the pre-cise lumbar vertebral level and acuteness of the angle of the bifurcation and (2) the distortion of the bifurcation by arterial atherosclerotic dis-ease. The tendency, however, is for the right

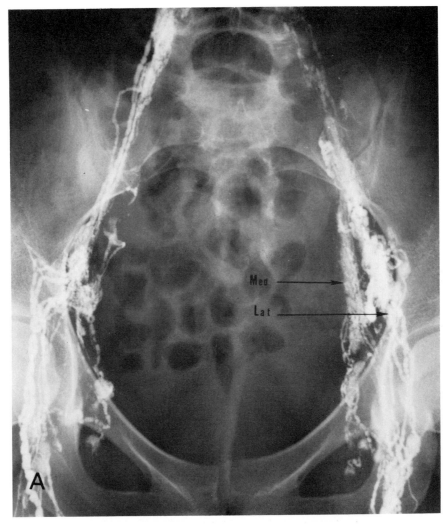

FIG. 2.12. MEDIAL AND LATERAL EXTERNAL ILIAC LYMPHATICS

A: Frontal projection of vascular filling phase. In this projection the extensive superimposition of vessels and nodes is typical. *B*: Nodal retention phase in the frontal projection. Stereoscopic or oblique projections are imperative for adequate assessment. *C*: Left posterior oblique coned view delineates the respective nodal groups. The lateral and medial chains are endowed with more numerous, larger, and better opacified nodes. Commonly the intermediate group is the least endowed. The configuration of the larger nodes is elongated and ovoid. Smaller nodes tend to be more round. The medial (internal) chain is fused extensively into a single cluster. This cluster is fused with the *middle node* of the medial chain which is the *obturator* node according to Rouviere and Herman et al.

and left medial chains to complete their course just inferior to the aortic bifurcation, forming an inverted "V" (Fig. 2.14).

The medial chain is important because it serves as one of the important pathways of communicaton between the pelvic visceral structures (e.g., ovary, fallopian tubes, uterus, bladder and prostate, and the abdominoaortic region) (Fuchs, 1969; Browse, 1972a). From the pelvic viscera, efferents connect with the medial common iliac chain that connects with the ab-

dominoaortic channels through intermediate chains that anastomose freely with each other.

Generally, a continuous series of vessels and nodes progress up to the aortic bifurcation. The number of nodes along each chain ranges from approximately three to six nodes with the medial chain of the left containing the least (Fuchs, 1969). Few gaps are found and lymphographically, coarse opacification and sharp delineation of nodes in this region should be expected (Browse, 1972a) (Fig. 2.15). These nodes

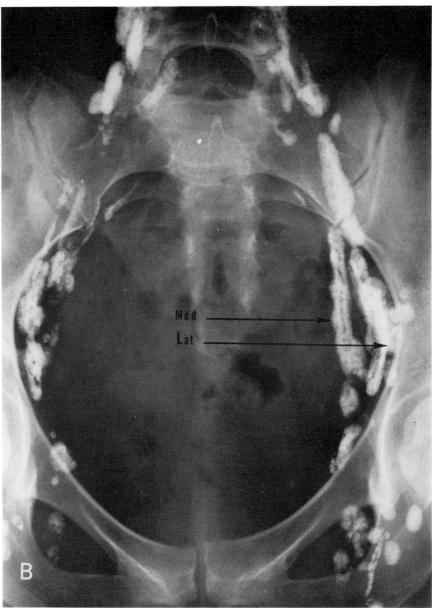

FIG. 2.12B

are much less misleading in diagnostic oncology than nodes more caudally positioned (see Chapter 9 on neoplasms). Even in this area nebulous filling defects in a single node or few nodes can genuinely frustrate lymphographic attempts to confirm or negate the presence of metastatic neoplasms (Parker et al., 1974a; Castellino et al., 1973).

Most common iliac nodes, especially the lateral and intermediate groups, are oval (Fig. 2.16). The medial chain nodes usually are slightly smaller and rounder. From the author's studies of normal lymphograms with histologic correlation, an elongated "transitional" node in the right lateral chain was observed frequently at the point of transition between the common iliacs and lumbar (abdominoaortics) (D. A. Harrison, unpublished data). The normal internal architecture of this node is compact and homogeneous (Fig. 2.17B).

In patients less than 20 years of age, the roentgen appearance of the internal architecture of common iliac nodes can differ slightly and falsely suggest lymphoma (Castellino et al., 1975). Nodes in these patients present a more reticulated or "foamy" pattern (relatively more

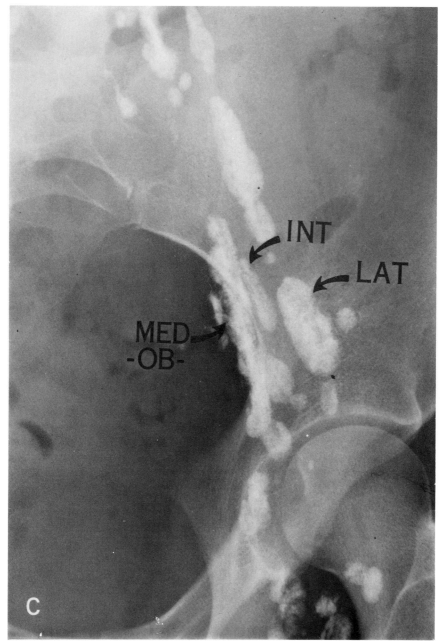

Fig. 2.12C

lucent to opaque areas) than in adults. When normal, foaminess is not striking and tends to be generalized and uniform throughout the intra-abdominal nodes (Figs. 2.17 and 2.18). Also, a significant increase in size of the nodes is not present with normal foaminess. Histologically, relatively more collections of lymphatic components to sinusoidal spaces can be found (Butler, 1969). Therefore, relatively less contrast material settles in the nodes.

Lateral chain nodes are positioned on the lat-eral aspect of the common iliac artery. Lymphography usually demonstrates three densely opacified nodes. The most superior node not uncommonly represents the entire chain (elongated "transitional" node at the aortic bifurcation).

The *intermediate chain* becomes slightly more posterior to the artery and vein than its predecessors of the external iliac group. Having become more posterior, and therefore closer to the nodes of the medial chain, clear delineation

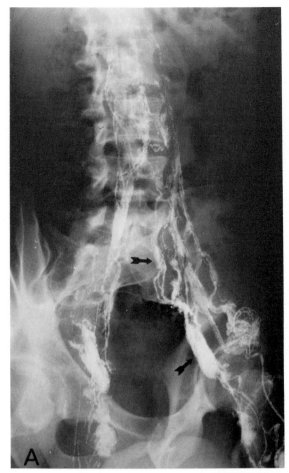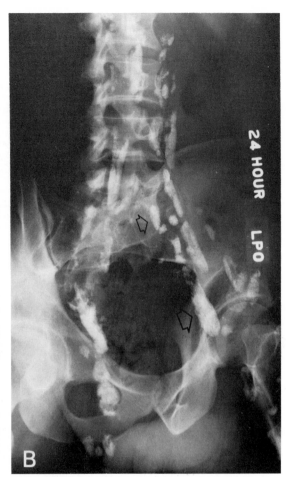

FIG. 2.13. OBTURATOR NODE

A: Posterior oblique projection of the filling phase demonstrates a dominant medial chain (*upper arrow*). Fusion of the middle node and Rosenmüller's node is demonstrated (*lower arrow*). *B*: Nodal retention phase in the posterior oblique projection shows subsequent opacification of the large fused node. Continuation of the medial chain is shown by cephalad *arrows*.

and precise localization of individual intermediate nodes can be quite difficult. Some separation of these individual nodes for "critical evaluation" and interpretation can be accomplished with proper radiographic technique (see "External Iliac Group"). The intermediate chain averages two to four more nodes than the lateral or medial chains and thus produces a continuous sequence of nodes devoid of a gap. The lymphographic appearance of a succession of nodes in an uninterrupted column may not be simple continuity of a single chain, however, but actually may be the confluence and superimposition of intermediate and medial chains (Fuchs, 1969).

The medial common iliac chain is deep in the pelvis and medial to the artery and vein. Included in this chain are the subaortic or "promontory" nodes (Rouviere, 1938; Herman et al.,

1963). Marked asymmetry between left and right medial common iliac nodes is characteristic. Predominantly this chain contains one to two chain nodes that are on the right. Other nodes superimposed over the lumbosacral area may have this appearance, and differentiation from incidentally filled nodes of the internal iliac group sometimes can be difficult. On frontal roentgenograms, medial nodes are frequently superimposed over the sacral promontory. Rouviere (1938) described these nodes as "subaortic nodes" or "nodes of the promontory" (Fig. 2.15).

Testicular Lymphatics

In males between the ages of 20–35 years, testicular malignancies rank first (Twito and Kennedy, 1975). However, current methods of therapy control effectively a significant number

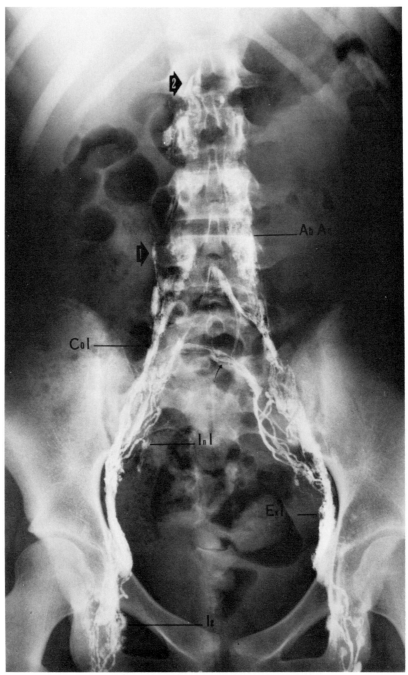

FIG. 2.14. WELL OPACIFIED LYMPHATIC VESSELS

These vessels demonstrate with clarity the commonly described characteristic vascular filling patterns. *Ig*, inguinals; *ExI*, external iliacs; *InI*, internal iliacs or hypogastrics; *CoI*, common iliacs; *small arrow*, extensive vessel communication between contralateral and ipsilateral. Also note inverted "V" appearance of connecting right and left medial chains at the aortic bifurcation (*Ab Ao*, abdominal aortic, i.e., paralumbar), the left chain being the most richly endowed of the three (*arrow 1*, right paralumbar "skip channel"; *arrow 2*, cisterna chyli).

of these neoplasms. With treatment some forms have an overall 5-year control rate of greater than 90%. In that these neoplasms are particularly prone to disseminate by the lymphatics, lymphography can be quite useful in efforts to stage the lymphatic extension of the disease (Von Keiser, 1967; Fuchs, 1971a; Safer et al., 1975).

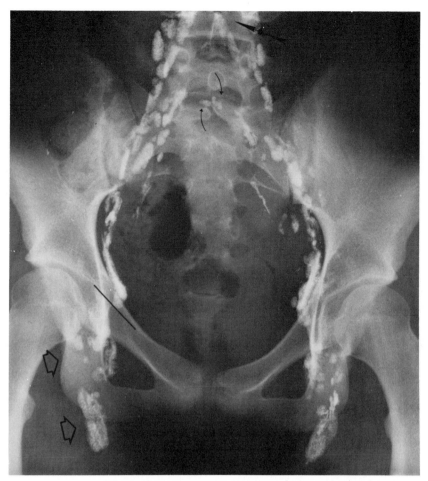

FIG. 2.15. FRONTAL PROJECTION OF PATIENT IN FIGURE 2.14

External iliac nodes are above *line* delineating inguinal ligament. The lateral sacral nodes of the right internal iliac chain are opacified, but it is difficult to distinguish between these nodes and the nodes of the medial common iliac chain in this projection. Stereoscopic views and/or oblique projections assist greatly in this distinction. Vessel filling patterns are helpful also. *Open arrow*, inguinal nodes; *small curved arrows*, "nodes of the promontory"; *top arrow*, aortic bifurcation.

Standard Anatomy

Anatomic descriptions of testicular lymphatics have emphasized the character and course of the vessels (Rouviere, 1938; Clark, 1942; Brash, 1943). Two sets of efferent vessels emanate from each testicle: a superficial system drains the tunica vaginalis; a deep system drains the epididymis and the body of the gland. The superficial and deep systems travel from each testicle as a unit of six to eight trunks that ascend in the spermatic cord, through the inguinal ring, and follow the testicular blood vessels (i.e., along the psoas major muscle). These lymph vessels empty into the corresponding lumbar lymph nodes. Vessels that drain only the glandular portion of each testicle empty into the lateral aortic nodes adjacent to the renal bed (preaortic)

nodes. Vessels that drain the ductal portion of the testicle (epididymis) preferentially terminate in the distal aortic or proximal common iliac nodes. Vessels draining the serosal covers and scrotum differ and usually terminate in the external iliac or inguinal nodes (Chavez, 1967). Embryologic development explains the range of terminal drainage sites of the testicular region (Lemeh, 1960). The glandular portion of the testicle originated as an organ high in the posterior abdominal cavity. The ductal system joined the organ in its descent into the pelvis. Hence, ductal drainage is comparable to that of organs of the pelvic region because these organs arise simultaneously and in the same position. Drainage of the more superficial enveloping tissue follows patterns of structures more in contiguity with the abdominal wall and scrotum (an

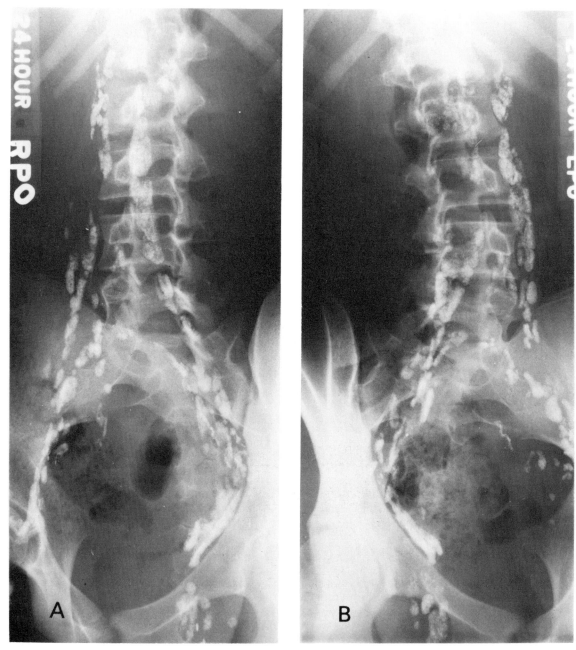

FIG. 2.16. POSTERIOR OBLIQUE PROJECTIONS OF SAME LYMPHOGRAM
Pelvic and paralumbar (abdominoaortic) nodes can be visualized far more discreetly. Right posterior oblique separates the more posterior right lateral sacral nodes from the medial chain nodes of the common iliac group.

outpouching of the abdominal wall) following the more superficial lymphatic vascular pathways (inguinals) (Fig. 2.19).

Lymphographic Anatomy

Chiappa et al. (1966) elucidated the lymphographic anatomy of the entire testicle through the sequential use of both injection techniques.

Lymphographically, six to eight lymphatic vessels course from each testicle to their respective primary drainage sites. These vessels turn medially and empty into primary drainage sites located variously between T11-12 to L4-5 (Wahlqvist et al., 1966; Chiappa et al., 1966). Cross-over is common. In some series demonstration of cross-over occurred in at least 50% of

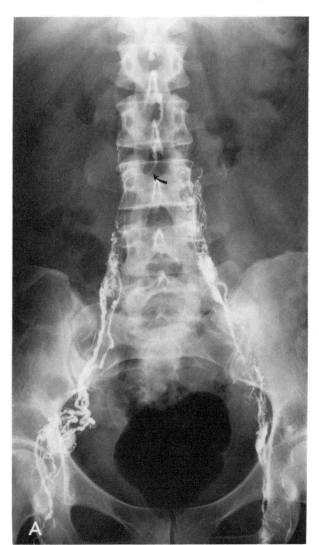
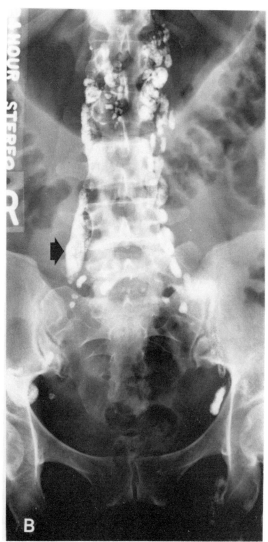

FIG. 2.17. BENIGN NODAL HYPERPLASIA

A: Vascular filling of a lymphogram that shows asymmetry of pelvic vessels. Paralumbar cross-over is demonstrated superiorly (*arrow*). *B*: Nodal retention phase of the same lymphogram. *Arrow* illustrates the large elongated, homogeneously opacified right common iliac node (transitional node). More superior abdominoaortic nodes are slightly larger than usual and have relatively more lucencies dispersed throughout their internal architecture than usual (foaminess). Oblique projections (*C* and *D*) display this appearance with distinctness. Postlaparotomy histologic examination proved these nodes to contain benign follicular hyperplasia. This entity can simulate lymphomata and is the basis of most false lymphographic interpretations.

testicular lymphograms (Wahlqvist et al., 1966). Right to left cross-over is more common. Nevertheless evidence for the reverse course has been well established. Regardless of course cross-over is observed most frequently between L2 and L5.

Nodal opacification should demonstrate a primary testicular drainage center that is adjacent to the renal pedicle of either side. On the right, this is in the region of L1-3; on the left, it is in the L2 region. Although no constant pattern is

observed, secondary testicular nodal drainage in the lumbar aortic region can be opacified by testicular injections. These are the nodes usually well opacified by dorsal pedal lymphography (Chiappa et al., 1966).

Retrograde opacification of pelvic nodes was not a finding of some authors (Busch and Sayegh, 1963), but evidence supporting retrograde flow has resulted from other studies (Wahlqvist et al., 1966). Definite statements implicating physiologic flow patterns derived from lympho-

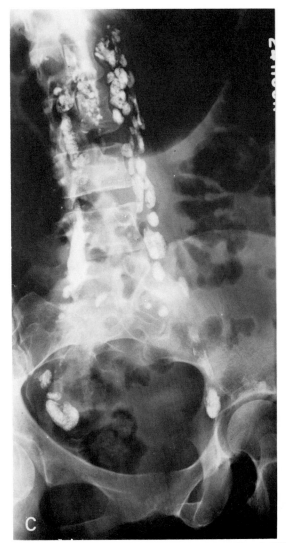

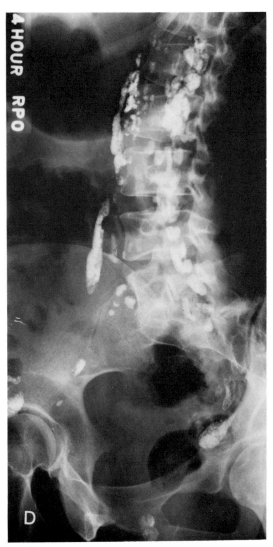

Fig. 2.17C and D

graphic data should not be considered conclusive, however, because of the unphysiologic nature of the procedure. Nevertheless, retrograde flow should be a consideration of clinical importance because there is inferential evidence of its occurrence. Opacification of mediastinal nodes is common (Busch et al., 1965; Wahlqvist et al., 1966), and thoracic duct filling with minimal aortic nodal filling also occurs (Wahlqvist et al., 1966). Opacification of supraclavicular nodes in the region of the termination of the thoracic duct is a common feature also.

Separate injections within a few days, using both techniques, outlines with precision the ex-

tent of lymphatic dissemination of testicular neoplasms. Testicular injections visualize with far more definity the primary sites of drainage of the deeper testicular tissues than dorsal pedal injections. This method can delineate early lymphatic metastases of locally noninvasive neoplasms more efficiently. Dorsal pedal lymphography, the more comprehensive technique, better delineates more progressive testicular neoplasms. Testicular neoplasms that have disseminated distally can be demonstrated with greater precision by dorsal pedal lymphography than testicular injections (Chiappa et al., 1966; Kuisk, 1971).

NORMAL ANATOMY AND COMMON VARIATIONS OF AORTIC REGION

The abdominoaortic lymphatics are those vessels and nodes immediately above the common

iliacs along the course of the lumbar vertebrae, inferior vena cava, and the abdominal aorta.

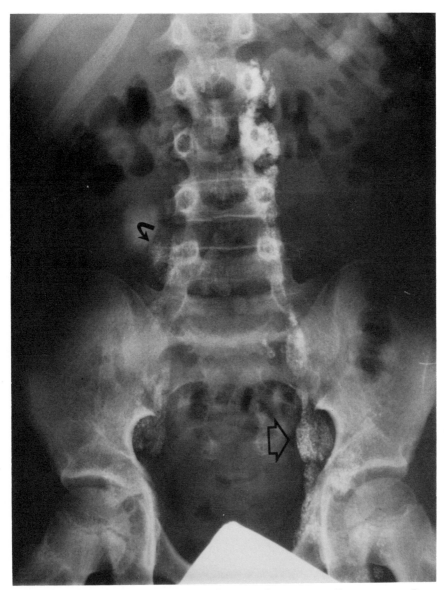

FIG. 2.18. FRONTAL PROJECTION OF NODAL RETENTION PHASE OF LYMPHOGRAM PERFORMED ON PEDIATRIC PATIENT
Arrows show nodes that were extensively foamy but were without histologic evidence of neoplasm.

These lymphatics are also commonly termed para-aortics, periaortics, lumbar, and paralumbar lymphatics. The terms right and left juxta-aortic groups also have been used (Herman et al., 1963). Although location of these vessels and nodes are related to major regional blood vessels (i.e., inferior vena cava and aorta), radiographic visualization of the vertebral bodies enables the radiologist to use the vertebral column quite conveniently as a landmark. The functional anatomy of the abdominoaortic nodes and the architecture of their interconnections enables one to anticipate which nodes should be more routinely demonstrated by clinical lym-

phography. Also knowledge of actual anatomy enables one to better appreciate the potential for many lymphographic variations. Although the lymphographic flow patterns cannot be rigidly correlated with physiologic flow patterns, analysis of sequentially visualized lymphatic vessels can be quite informative in attempts to anticipate routes of lymphatic dissemination of neoplasms (Wallace, 1968; Busch et al., 1965).

Lymph Vessel Anatomy and Significance in Lymphography

According to Rouviere's (1938) anatomic descriptions, the vessels in this region are contin-

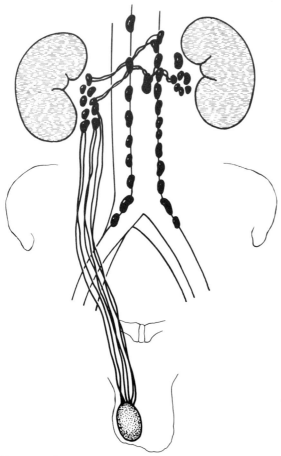

Fig. 2.19. Lymphatic Vessels and Nodes of Primary Drainage to the Glandular Tissue of Testicles

Diagram is according to descriptions by Rouviere. Vessels emanate from the gland, by-passing the nodes usually demonstrated by clinical lymphography. Note the clusters of nodes in the region of the renal pedicles bilaterally. Also illustrated is cross communication. The relationship of the gonadal center nodes to the paralumbar (paracaval/para-aortic) nodes as represented has been confirmed by simultaneous dorsal pedal and testicular lymphography (Chiappa et al., 1966).

anatomy and function more than the highly variable structural arrangement of the lymphatic vessels (Rosenberg, 1968; Kaplan et al., 1973). Takahashi and Abrams (1967) were instrumental in the development of lymphography as it is used currently in neoplastic disease and established criteria for distinguishing the normal from abnormal para-aortic lymphatic vessels and nodes. Their original criteria indicate the far greater significance of nodal characteristics in the determination of the presence of malignant disease. Vessel aberrations, including lymphaticovenous communications that indeed prove to be abnormal, rarely are the sole indicators of an abnormal lymphogram (Wallace and Jackson, 1968) (Fig. 2.20).

Lymphographic Vascular Anatomy

In general, para-aortic vessels ascend along the sides of the aorta (Herman et al., 1963). A middle chain is filled occasionally from the right common iliac vessels but rarely contains as much contrast media as either lateral chain. The usual course of either chain is within 2-3 cm of the lateral edge of the vertebral body or within the confines of the transverse processes of the vertebral body (Abrams et al., 1968; Jackson and Kinmonth, 1974b).

Approximately 30% of confirmed normal lymphograms exhibit right lower para-aortic "skip channels" (Jackson and Kinmonth, 1974b; Jackson, 1972) (see Fig. 2.14). Lymphographic-pathologic correlations have produced convincing evidence that the position of these looping channels is unrelated to deviation either by normal or abnormal lymphatics or other structures. Reasonable explanations for these phenomena have been elusive thus far. On the lateral projection, most of the vessels and nodes usually are anterior to the anterior edge of the vertebral body but within 3-4 cm (Abrams et al., 1968) (Fig. 2.21).

Contralateral opacification of the para-aortic chains occurs in approximately half of normal lymphograms. Cross-filling is most often demonstrated in the L4-5 region (Fuchs, 1971b; Jackson and Kinmonth, 1974a). The para-aortic vessels terminate at the level of L1-2. Two lumbar trunks and an intestinal trunk connect with the cisterna chyli which fills with contrast media unpredictably.

Standard Lymph Node Anatomy

Approximately 25-30 abdominoaortic (lumbar) nodes surround and are in direct contiguity with the aorta and inferior vena cava (Rouviere, 1938; Clark, 1942; Brash, 1943; Gray, 1959). An-

uations of the common iliacs that ascend the borders of the aorta. Para-aortic vessels, however, also communicate extensively and receive drainage from other intra-abdominal sources. Organs that commonly drain directly into the para-aortic lymphatics are the testes, ovaries, fallopian tubes, corpus uteri, kidneys, adrenals, and abdominal wall lymphatics (Rouviere, 1938; Reiffenstuhl, 1964).

Coursing superiorly along the wall of the aorta the para-aortic vessels empty into the cisterna chyli near the first to second lumbar vertebral bodies. More common clinical indications for lymphography presently emphasize nodal

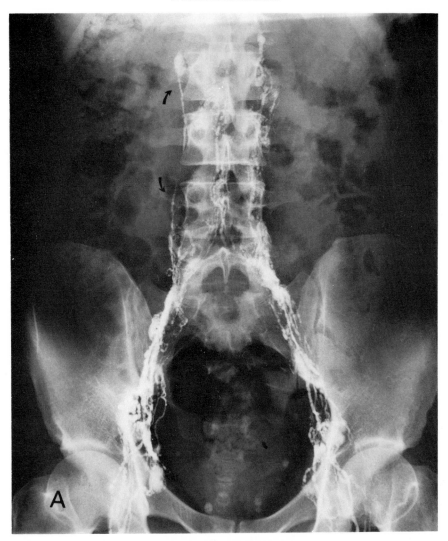

FIG. 2.20. LYMPH VESSEL ABERRATION

A: Vascular filling of a vessel that is atypical because of the looping course taken along the right paralumbar region (*arrows*). Lateral (*B*) and (*C*) frontal projections of the same lymphogram in the nodal phase. The region traversed by looping vessel is devoid of opacified nodes. Laparotomy revealed no nodal abnormalities or other apparent reasons for this phenomenon. Histologic examination of the opacified nodes was normal.

atomically, these nodes can be grouped according to their specific relationships to the adjacent major blood vessels: the right aortic, midaortic, and left aortic nodes. The right aortic nodes extensively encompass the inferior vena cava and can be subgrouped according to their specific relationships with the cava: precaval, interaorticocaval, retrocaval, and laterocaval nodes. Pre- and retroaortic nodes (midaortic) are located approximately at the midpoint of the diameter of the aorta, either anteriorly (pre-) or posteriorly (retro-). Left aortic nodes are situated more along the course of the left lateral aspect of the aorta (Fig. 2.21).

The lymphographic anatomy of the right aor-

tic chain does not conform to classical descriptions. Anatomically, right aortic (paracaval) chain nodes are more numerous than the mid- or left aortic chains (Rouviere, 1938). The right aortic nodes that are anterior to the vena cava are situated near the termination of the renal vein. Posteriorly positioned nodes are concentrated at the origin of the psoas major muscle and on the right crus of the diaphragm.

Preaortic nodes of the midaortic group lie directly on the anterior surface of the abdominal aorta at levels that correspond to the celiac artery, renal arteries, and superior and inferior mesenteric arteries. Retroaortic nodes of the midaortic group lie on the dorsal aspect of the

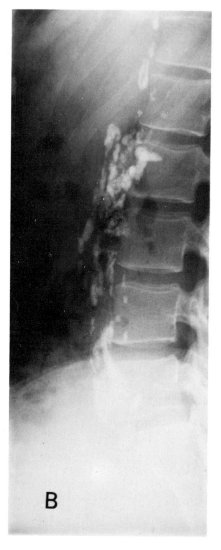

Fig. 2.20B

abdominal aorta, somewhat toward the left. Strict separation of some of the more lateral retroaortic nodes from left aortic nodes can be difficult.

Left aortic nodes form a continuous chain on the left lateral border of the aorta, anterior to the psoas major muscle and the left crus of the diaphragm. The two lateral chains receive drainage from the following areas: (1) the common iliacs; (2) the testes or ovaries, fallopian tubes, and uterine corpus; (3) the kidney and perirenal tissues; (4) adrenals; and (5) lymphatics that drain the abdominal wall. Afferents to the preaortic group of the midaortic chain emanate from the lymphatics of regions corresponding to the three major regional visceral arteries.

Some communication with the two lateral nodal groups can be demonstrated although it is seldom prominent. Retroaortic nodes of the midaortic group receive drainage from the intermediate chain of the common iliac lymphatics and the two lateral aortic groups.

A great deal of communication exists among the nodes of the lumbar group. Lumbar nodes, as functionally positioned, are the terminal abdominal lymphatic drainage areas of virtually all structures below the diaphragm. From this final common pathway, abdominal lymphatic flow enters the cisterna chyli and leaves the abdomen through the thoracic duct. These nodes are of the same significance to lymphatic drainage as is the aorta to arterial blood flow

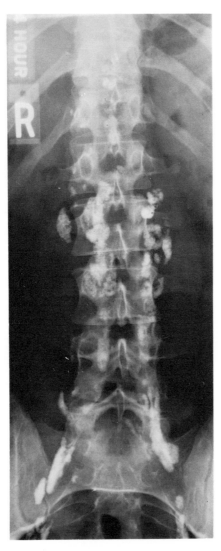

Fig. 2.20C

and the inferior vena cava is to venous return below the diaphragm.

In spite of their importance, however, paralumbar nodes do not represent the primary nodal drainage sites of all intra-abdominal groups.

Lymphographic Nodal Anatomy

The lymphographic appearance of the lumbar nodes can produce diagnostically reliable data that is most contributory in the assessment of neoplastic disease of the retroperitoneal nodes (Abrams et al., 1968; Wallace and Jackson, 1968; Baum et al., 1963; Castellino et al., 1974; Viamonte et al., 1963; Kuisk, 1971; Fuchs, 1969).

Therefore, skillful analysis of the position, size, and appearance of each para-aortic/paracaval node and correlation with the total lymphographic pattern will produce the diagnostic accuracy of which the procedure is capable. Individually and as a group, these nodes are more constant than pelvic nodes; nevertheless, some variability is most often present as normal anatomy. Thorough assessment of the nodes should include stereoscopic views, multiple projections, and, if necessary, laminagraphy.

Normal Lymphographic Nodal Characteristics

Lymphographically, paralumbar nodes are usually oval, vertically oriented, and with

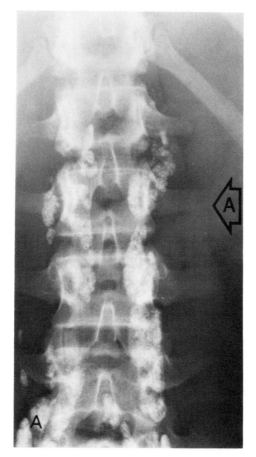
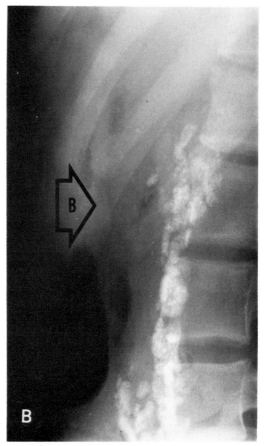

FIG. 2.21. CONED VIEWS OF ABDOMINOAORTIC NODES IN FRONTAL, LATERAL, AND BOTH OBLIQUE POSITIONS
A: More opacified nodes are observed in the left chain, and the height to which these nodes are seen exceeds that of the middle and right chains. Most of the midchain nodes are visualized poorly because of superimposition over the vertebral column; therefore, differentiating between pre- and retroaortic nodes in this projection is virtually impossible. The right chain contains few opacified nodes between L2–4. Note the nodal size and position to concur with described criteria of normal lymphographic anatomy (*arrow A*). *B*: This projection demonstrates the paralumbar nodes to be within the confines of established criteria of normal position (less than 3 cm anterior to the vertebral bodies) (*arrow B*). *C* and *D*: Oblique projections separating the nodal chains giving a more three-dimensional picture of the abdominoaortic group.

sharp margins around the vertical edges. Small nodes tend to be more round. Abrams et al. (1968) and Takahashi and Abrams (1967) established a limit for size in normal nodes. Normal para-aortic nodes proved seldom to be greater than 3 cm in their greatest diameter (Fig. 2.22). Prior to Takahashi and Abrams' study, Wiljasalo (1965) devised what was termed a "projection difference index" as a measure of normal nodal size. Currently, few lymphographers consider it of significant clinical value.

The internal lymphographic architecture of nodes is mostly determined by the amount of oily contrast material that permeates the subcapsular or marginal sinus, the intermediate sinus, and the medullary sinuses. Contrast material cannot permeate the follicular tissue; thus, minute lucencies are interspersed among contrast-filled sinuses. The node assumes a fine granular but homogeneous appearance with sharp, distinct margins. Of the patients with malignant lymphoma who undergo lymphography and in whom nodal opacification shows this characteristic internal architecture, less than 1% will have occult retroperitoneal disease (Castellino et al., 1974). presently there are some data to suggest that approximately 20–25% of patients evaluated for metastatic malignancy who have normal nodal internal architecture by lymphography can have occult nodal metastases (Parker et al., 1974b; Castellino, 1975). Various stimuli unrelated to neoplasm, however, can incite a variety of reactive responses within the node; hence, normal nodes

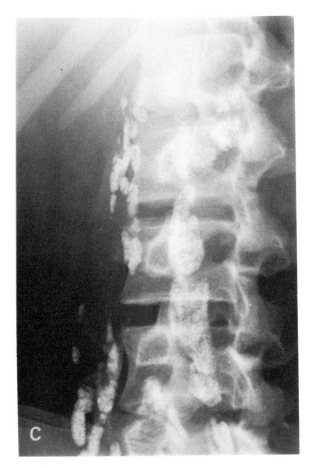 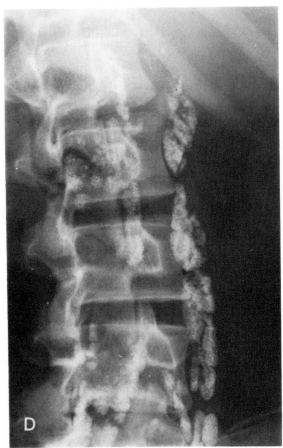

FIG. 2.21C AND D

can lymphographically appear somewhat reticular, occasionally described as "foamy" (relatively more lucencies), and not contain lymphoma. Nodes that are reactive and without intrinsic malignancy tend to be uniform, individually and as a group (see Fig. 2.17). In spite of this, however, follicular hyperplastic responses of nodes have been shown to be the greatest source of diagnostic error when one attempts to determine the presence or absence of lymphoma (Hodgkin's or non-Hodgkin's) by lymphography (Castellino, 1974).

Similarly, complete contrast filling of the sinuses seldom occurs in every lymph node on the lymphogram. Although the para-aortic nodes have proved to be the most reliable group to show features of high diagnostic accuracy, even these nodes can be misleading. Incomplete contrast filling of the sinuses can be unrelated to any disease entity. Benign processes, especially fibrolipomatous disease, frequently produce incomplete nodal filling although not to the degree found in iliac and inguinal nodes. Also,

small filling defects in the node can be produced by normal nodal hilar vessels (Wallace and Jackson, 1968; Viamonte et al., 1963).

Densely opacified, homogeneous, sharply delineated lymphadenograms should not be expected routinely above the second lumbar vertebral body, and rarely above the first vertebral body. Clusters of nodes near the first and second lumbar vertebrae most often will contain minute areas of incomplete filling.

Right Aortic Chain and Its Variations

Left and midaortic chains have been shown lymphographically to contain many more nodes than the right aortic chain because many paracaval nodes are not in the pathway of the vessels transporting the greatest volume of contrast media (Jackson and Kinmonth, 1974b; Fuchs, 1971c; D. A. Harrison, unpublished data). Contrast-bearing common iliac vessels continue superiorly along the aortic wall. The major chains generally do not extend beyond 2–

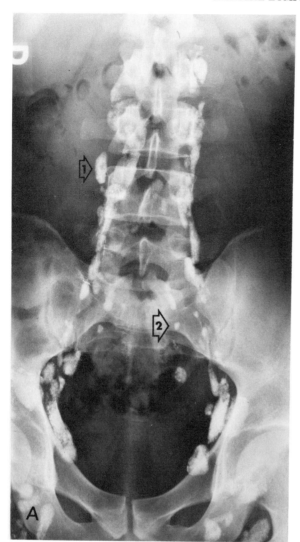 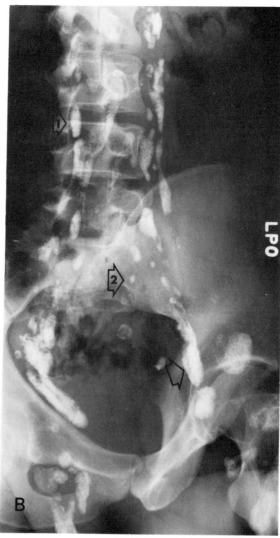

FIG. 2.22. FRONTAL, LEFT, AND RIGHT POSTERIOR PROJECTIONS OF NODAL RETENTION PHASE OF USUAL NORMAL
LYMPHOGRAPHIC ANATOMY

Note the larger, less uniform, more caudad nodes. The internal architecture is more reticular (foamy), and these nodes contain multiple filling defects. The inguinal nodes display this pattern most floridly. The more inferior external iliacs are of similar character but become somewhat more uniform than the inguinal nodes. *A* demonstrates the marked superimposition of most of the nodes either over other nodes or osseous structures, thus limiting their visualization. *B* and *C* clearly emphasize the value of the oblique views to assist visualization maximally of all regional nodes. Fusion of the middle (obturator) node and the internal retrocrural node on the right becomes obvious (*open arrow*, in *C*). The hilus of the middle node on the left becomes apparent (*open arrow* in *B*). *Arrow 2* in *A*, *B*, and *C* gives attention to a small node in the medial chain of the common iliac group. Oblique views clearly delineate this node from the larger though less opacified, more caudad node (lateral sacral node of the internal iliac group (hypogastric)). Increased uniformity of these more cephalad nodes is apparent. The strikingly typical appearance of the three chains (dominant left chain) is shown. The position, size, and internal architecture of one of the paralumbar nodes are indicated (*arrow 1* in *A*, *B*, and *C*). All of the criteria of a normal paralumbar node are well emphasized by this node in the three projections.

3 cm of the lateral border of the vertebral column and thus ascend as para-aortic vessels.

This route of lymphatic transport of contrast media leads to visualization of nodes near the aorta. Although some filling of aberrant vessels is not rare, nodes along their routes seldom are

optimally opacified. A large number of caval nodes are located more laterally and/or more anteriorly to the lymphatic vessels transporting the greatest volume of contrast media (see Fig. 2.20). This mechanism of contrast transport accounts for nonvisualization of paracaval nodes

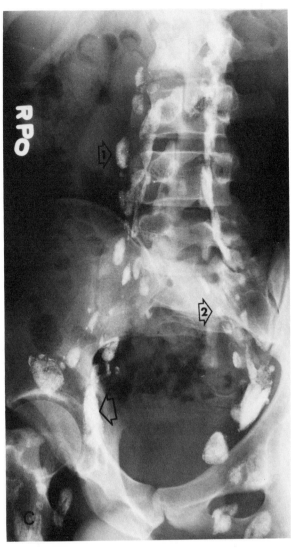

Fig. 2.22C

35–40% of lymphograms (Fuchs, 1969; Kuisk, 1971; Jackson and Kinmonth, 1974b). Lymphographic differentiation of anterior from posterior nodes can be difficult. Whether positioned anterior or posterior on the aortic surface, these lymph nodes universally project over the spine. Stereoscopic views and laminagraphy are quite useful in delineating individual nodes, but in most clinical circumstances complete separation of each node of this column is not necessary.

The quality and quantity of nodes in this chain vary widely. Jackson and Kinmonth (1974b) have reported absence of the entire chain in 40% of lymphograms but others report total absence as a rare occurrence (Fuchs, 1969; D. A. Harrison, unpublished data). The difficulty is precise localization of each individual node. Occasionally, nodes of both lateral chains are slightly more medially positioned; conversely, midchain nodes may be more laterally positioned, particularly toward the left. Since there are no criteria of lymphographic anatomy that can infallibly localize each individual node in subtle situations, a conclusion of complete absence of this chain can become quite arbitrary.

The Left Aortic Chain and Its Variations

The left aortic chain is the most constant of the three chains and regularly contains more nodes considered characteristic of the abdominoaortic group. From their origin (immediately superior to the common iliac nodes) to their termination (seldom below L2), these homogeneous, well opacified nodes form an almost uninterrupted column along the left lateral border of the vertebrae. Lateral extension can be influenced by the state of the aorta, but the column is usually within 2 cm of the lateral edge of the vertebrae (Fuchs, 1969; Abrams et al., 1968; Jackson and Kinmonth, 1974b).

The nodes superior to the renal pedicle become fewer and less homogeneously opacified than the nodes in the caudal cluster. With few exceptions, the left chain is the most constant of the three abdominoaortic (paralumbar) chain. Nodes in this chain are visualized to L2 with frequencies up to 90% (Fuchs, 1969; D. A. Harrison, unpublished data). Some nodal opacification is demonstrated at the level of L1 in 30% of lymphograms (Fuchs, 1969). Nodes at this level in either chain become less densely opacified and form clusters that are almost inseparable. These clusters often simulate large nodes with filling defects that appear ominous.

known to exist, but it does not explain the "skip channels" in the L4–5 region. Evidence exists to confirm the absence of any nodes adjacent to these vessels (Jackson and Kinmonth, 1974b). The top of the column of the right chain reaches the level of L2 in approximately 30% of lymphograms (Fuchs, 1969 and 1971b).

The Midaortic Chain and Its Variations

The midaortic chain (preaortic and retroaortic) is formed by a column of nodes that are superimposed over the vertebral column near the midline. Usually nodes are more opacified in this chain than in the right chain but less than in the left chain. The inferior nodes of this chain are found in the region of L3–4, often in clusters; the chain terminates at the L2 level in

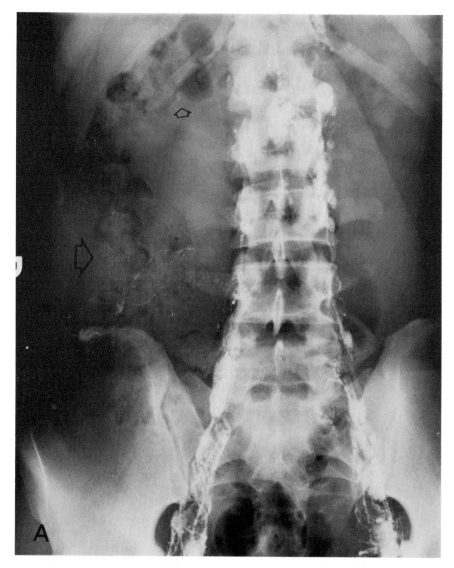

FIG. 2.23. UNCOMMON NODAL VARIATION

A is a display of aberrant vessel filling during contrast injection. The large inferior *arrow* indicates the multiple tortuous, serpiginous vessels widespread in the right hemiabdomen. Vessels are opacified above and below the right iliac crest. The smaller superior *arrow* denotes filling of subcostal lymph vessels. In *B*, the nodal retention phase shows opacification of nodes (*arrows*) that received contrast material from aberrantly filled vessels.

The Roentgen Appearance and Significance of Uncommon Nodal Variations

Those nodes that are visualized uncommonly are situated extrinsic to usual lymphographic regions. One such area is the pelvic-lower lumbar region. Opacification of these nodes occurs from vessels low in the pelvis that course superiorly and quite lateral. These nodes are found over the region of the iliac crest (Figs. 2.23 and 2.24). Occasionally nodal opacification is ob-

served beyond the terminal points of the abdominoaortic lymphatics (superior to the cisterna chyli) but still adjacent to the vertebral column (Fig. 2.25). Such nodes have been observed bilaterally and also superimposed over the vertebral column. Other nodes that occasionally fill are popliteal (Fig. 2.26), mediastinal, bilateral hilar, paratracheal, supraclavicular, and even nodes in the axilla. Although an aberration from usual nodal filling, opacification of these nodes can be a normal variant. Therefore, interpretation of these nodes utilizing abdominoaortic criteria can produce dubious diagnostic conclusions. Concrete data on the spectrum of normal lymphographic anatomy of any of these nodes are not presently available (Yee et al., 1969; Wallace and Jackson, 1968; Fuchs, 1969; Negus et al., 1970; Baltaxe and Constable, 1968; Kuisk, 1971).

THORACIC DUCT

The thoracic duct is the principal lymphatic vessel in the body (Fig. 2.27). With the exception of the convex surface of the liver, lymphatic flow from all structures below the diaphragm is transmitted to the thoracic duct. Above the diaphragm it receives lymphatic flow from all of the structures on the left when joined by the left bronchial, mediastinal, subclavian, and jugular trunks. Lymph flow enters the blood system as the thoracic duct ends its course, usually anas-

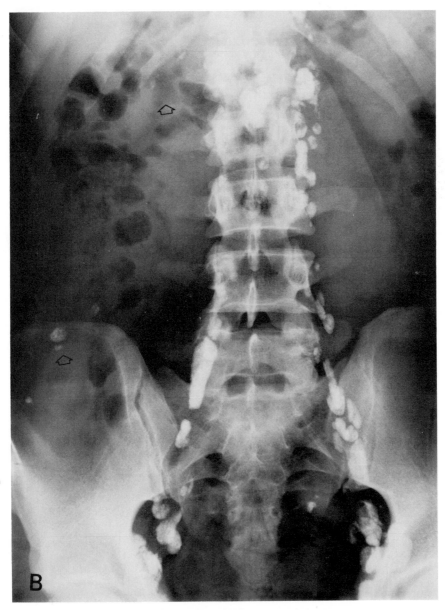

FIG. 2.23B

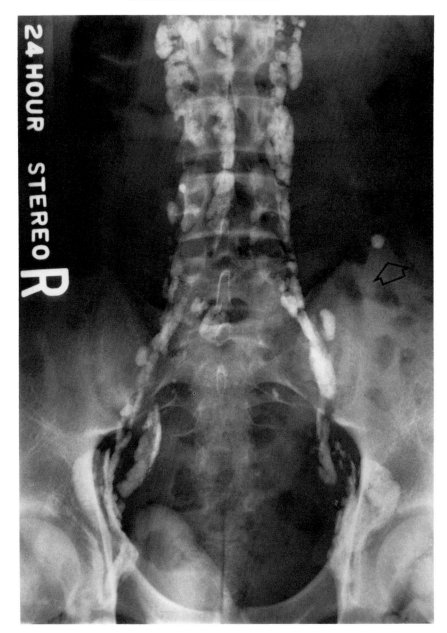

FIG. 2.24. OPACIFICATION OF NODE OVER REGION OF LEFT ILIAC CREST (*ARROW*)

tomosing into the left subclavian vein. The significance of the thoracic duct to the function of the lymphatic system in healthy and diseased states becomes readily apparent.

Although good visualization of the thoracic duct lymphographically would be of enormous value in many clinical situations, routine satisfactory delineation without excess risk as yet is not technically feasible. Various modifications of antegrade and retrograde techniques have been reported (Shieber, 1974; Nusbaum et al., 1964; Pomerantz et al., 1963; Cox and Kin-

month, 1975; Göthlin et al., 1975), but substantial evidence supporting their efficacy is not available presently. Since present methods do not routinely opacify the entire thoracic duct, the exact role of lymphography in the evaluation of the thoracic duct is unclear.

Anatomy

Anatomic studies by Davis (1915) have depicted the usual adult structure and frequency of anatomic variations. It was shown that in 14 of 22 dissections, the thoracic duct was single

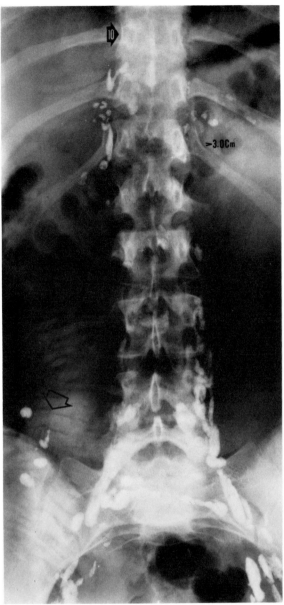

FIG. 2.25. ABERRANTLY OPACIFIED NODES
These nodes are over the right iliac crest (*open arrow*) and adjacent to the thoracic vertebral column to T10 (*arrow 10*). Left parathoracic nodes extend beyond 3 cm of the edge of the vertebral body.

1969; Wirth and Frommhold, 1970): the abdominal, thoracic, and cervical segments. Its abdominal segment begins as two lumbar trunks which combine to form the cisterna chyli. Lymphographic demonstration of this relationship occurs in 50-72% of observed lymphograms (Rosenberger and Abrams, 1971; Wirth and Frommhold, 1970; Fuchs, 1969). Visualization of the cisterna chyli by these same authors occurred in 30-87% of lymphograms. The position of the cisterna chyli occurs most often at the level of L1-2 with frequencies of 38-91% of lymphographic studies by Rosenberger and Abrams, Fuchs, and Wirth and Frommhold, respectively. The morphologic character of the cisterna chyli also varies widely. Even within the same patient the character of the cisterna chyli can vary when examined by consecutive filming techniques (Rosenberger and Abrams, 1971). Usually, however, a saccular structure less than 5 cm in length but of greater width than the adjacent thoracic duct is characteristic. The configuration also can be round, ovoid, or linear (Fuchs, 1969; Wirth and Frommhold, 1970).

Leaving the cisterna chyli the thoracic duct continues into the thoracic segment emerging through the aortic hiatus of the diaphragm. It courses then between the aorta and the azygous vein. Contrast filling of the entire thoracic segment of the duct is infrequent. The cephalad portion of the duct visualizes more frequently than the caudad section bcause there are more valves above the sixth thoracic vertebra and at the termination of the duct as it enters the venous system (Nusbaum et al., 1964). These valves delay contrast emptying into the venous system by the cephalad portion. Simultaneously, the caudad portion permits uninhibited antegrade flow of contrast media. Retrograde flow of contrast media does not occur in the presence of intact valves (Kinmonth, 1972; Nusbaum et al., 1964). The flow of contrast media (lymph) along the course of the thoracic duct does not appear to be assisted by active peristalsis (Dumont, 1967; Pomerantz et al., 1963; Nusbaum et al., 1964).

Although the aorta can greatly influence the course of the thoracic duct, the usual course observed roentgenographically correlates with classical anatomic descriptions. On the frontal projections the initial or caudad subsection is superimposed over the vertebral body, either midline or somewhat to the right of the spinous processes. This correlates with the right lateral aortic wall. On the lateral projection, it lies immediately anterior to the vertebrae.

From approximately T10-12, the thoracic

and traveled cephalad into and through the thorax on the right lateral aspect of the aorta. At the level of the fifth thoracic vertebra it crossed to the left side and opened into and through the venous system of the left side. Lymphographic studies have corroborated these postmortem studies (Wirth and Frommhold, 1970; Pomerantz et al., 1963; Kinmonth, 1972).

Three subdivisions of the thoracic duct are based on embryologic development (Fuchs,

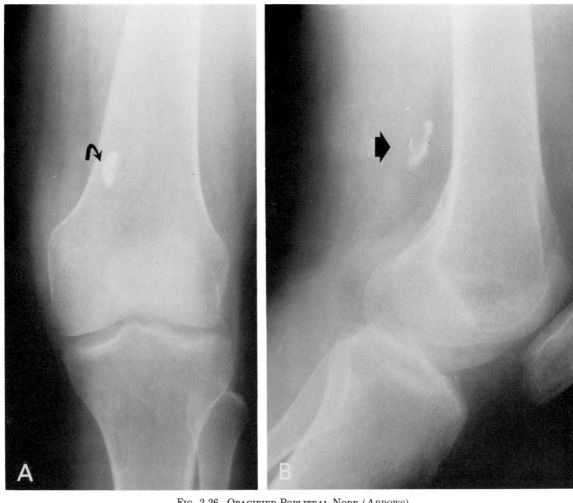

FIG. 2.26. OPACIFIED POPLITEAL NODE (*ARROWS*)
Frontal (*A*) and lateral (*B*) projections.

duct deviates toward the left. At the sixth thoracic vertebra body level, the duct crosses the left mainstem bronchus. It then courses anteriorly to travel just posterior and to the left but parallel with the trachea.

Continuation of the thoracic duct into the cervical segment is somewhat more dramatic. It rises 3–4 cm above the medial edge of the clavicle then sharply arches anteriorly and inferiorly as it merges into the wall of the junction of the left internal jugular and subclavian veins as a

bulbous structure. In this region, the valves are markedly accentuated.

The most frequent variation of the thoracic duct is some form of reduplication (Davis, 1915; Fuchs, 1969; Rosenberger and Abrams, 1971; Wirth and Frommhold, 1970). Fortuitous filling of multiple intrathoracic, supraclavicular, cervical, and even axillary nodes occurs under normal circumstances. Knowledge of these variations are of obvious significance in the management of patients with malignancies.

UPPER EXTREMITY

Clinical indications for lymphography of the upper extremity and cervical lymphatics include confirmation of lymphedema, primary or secondary, or delineation of the extent of lymphedema in the upper extremity (Browse, 1972b;

Kuisk, 1971) (see Chapter 6 on lymphedema). For oncologic purposes the clinical rewards for overcoming the technical difficulties of performing upper extremity lymphography are insignificant. Malignancies that affect lymph nodes in

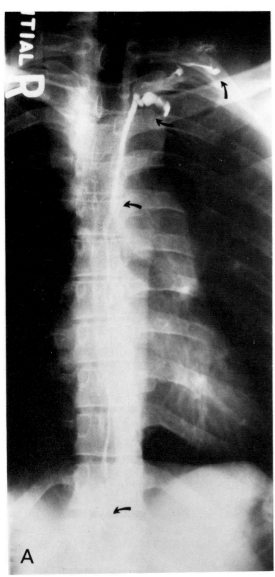
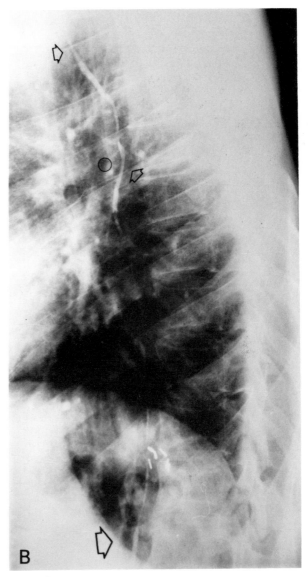

FIG. 2.27. THORACIC DUCT

On frontal projection, *A* displays the morphology of the usual adult thoracic duct. From its origin (cisterna chyli) to its termination (venous system on the left), all segments are visualized. *B*: The course of the thoracic duct on a lateral view is shown. Note the posterior course taken until reaching the level of the bronchus (*circle*). Further ascent through the thorax is parallel with the trachea (*open arrow* at *top*). *C*: The most common thoracic duct anomaly is some form of duplication. One form of duplication (*arrow*) is illustrated.

the axillary, supraclavicular, or cervical regions are often accessible to palpation. Also the natural history of malignant lymphomas, particularly Hodgkin's disease, is such that all of these nodal groups are included in treatment planning if either group has confirmed involvement. Additionally, interpretation of the lymphographic features of the majority of the nodes in these regions is extremely complex and most often misleading (Kuisk, 1971; Fisch, 1968).

Forearm and Arm

The anatomic and lymphographic description of this section is based primarily on the comprehensive work of Rouviere (1938) and Fisch (1968). As in the lower extremities, the upper extremity is drained by superficial and deep lymphatics. Multiple superficial plexuses drain the digits and the volar aspect of the palm. These plexuses drain into somewhat larger ves-

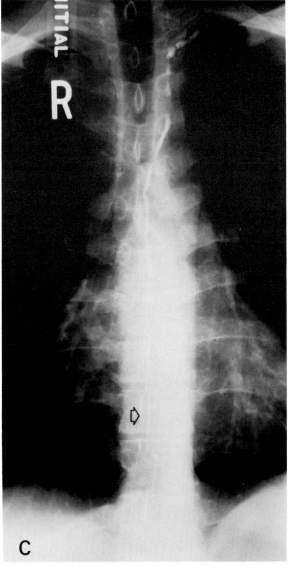

Fig. 2.27C

sels that merge dorsally. These vessels eventually anastomose with the major superficial lymphatics of the forearm.

The lateral and medial lymphatics ascend the upper extremity. The lateral group courses the forearm laterally and accompanies the cephalic vein. The medial group courses medially and accompanies the basilic vein. Some of the ascending medial channels pass through the epitrochlear nodes at the elbow, but most continue superiorly to the lateral axillary nodes. Many of the lymphatics of the lateral group become medially directed at the elbow and continue superiorly with the medial group. Those channels that persist laterally with the cephalic vein pass through the deltoidopectoral nodes. From these nodes efferent vessels then course to the sub-

clavicular axillary nodes or the inferior cervical nodes.

The vessels of the deep system ascend in juxtaposition to the arteries of the upper extremity. Some terminate in nodes along the brachial artery, but most continue to empty into the lateral group of axillary nodes. Fewer vessels are in the deep system than the superficial. Some communication exists between the superficial and deep systems.

Axilla

Almost all of the hand, forearm, arm, and thoracic wall lymphatics drain into the axillary lymph nodes. Similar to the nodes in the inguinal region, these nodes vary in size and number. Generally they are somewhat larger than more centrally located nodes and range between 20 and 30 in number. Anatomically, these nodes are subgrouped into (1) lateral group, (2) anterior or pectoral group, (3) posterior or subscapular group, (4) central or intermediate group, and (5) medial or subclavicular group (apical). The nodes in the apex of the axilla (medial or subclavicular) are separated from the more inferiorly positioned subgroups by the pectoralis minor tendon.

Lateral Group. This subgroup is composed of four to six nodes that are positioned medially and posteriorly to the axillary vein. Afferent vessels originate from the arm and efferent vessels empty into the central, subclavicular (apical), and inferior deep cervical nodes.

Anterior Group. This subgroup consists of four to six nodes along the lower border of the pectoralis major muscle. Afferent vessels emanate from the anterior-lateral thoracic cage and the lateral and central portions of the mammary gland. Efferent vessels empty into the central and subclavicular (apical) nodes.

Posterior Group. Nodes of this subgroup are somewhat small. It usually consists of six to seven nodes positioned on the inner wall of the axilla, along the course of the dorsal thoracic artery. Afferent vessels drain the lateral thoracic wall and efferent vessels drain into the nodes of the central group.

Central Group. These nodes are somewhat larger, more inferiorly positioned along the axillary artery, and three to five in number. Afferent vessels empty into the subclavicular (apical) nodes.

Medial (Subclavicular or Apical) Group. These nodes are positioned in the apex of the axillary fossa. There are 6–12 nodes in this subgroup and afferents emanate from all other more inferior axillary nodes. Efferent vessels unite to form the subclavian trunk which empties directly into the junction of the internal jugular and subclavian vein or into the jugular trunk. The subclavian trunk may empy into the thoracic duct.

Lymphography demonstrates the axillary nodes unpredictably but most often very poorly. Complete contrast filling of these nodes is not achieved by usual clinical lymphographic methods (Kuisk, 1971; Fuchs, 1969).

CERVICAL LYMPHOGRAPHY

Cervical lymphography has limited clinical utility. As with upper extremity and axillary lymphography, cervical lymphography is difficult to perform and currently is incapable of producing reliable information as to true extent of malignant disease. Hence, the reward for overcoming the technical difficulties is insignificant (Kuisk, 1971; Fisch, 1968).

Topographic Anatomy

Cervical lymph nodes broadly include Waldeyer's tonsillar ring, lymph nodes at the transition between the head and neck regions, and the true cervical nodes (Rouviere, 1938; Fisch, 1968). Waldeyer's ring is formed by a circular arrangement of lymph nodes. In the pharynx, this arrangement consists of the posterior lingual, palatine, tubal, and pharyngeal tonsils. Nodes at the transition region of the head and neck are arranged in a circular configuration and include occipital, retroauricular, parotidean, submandibular, submental, retropharyn-

geal, and sublingual lymph nodes. These nodes are both superficial and deep to the superficial fascia. Except for the retropharyngeal and sublingual groups, these nodal groups form a chain in the region of the transition between the head and neck.

The retropharyngeal and sublingual groups are incorporated in the chain as well, but they are also positioned in the vicinity of the pharyngeal wall and tongue, respectively. The nodes superficial to the superficial fascia drain the posterior aspect of the face, scalp, ears, posterior aspect of the head, and upper neck region. Efferent drainage is to the deep cervical nodes.

True cervical nodes are anatomically divided into the medial and lateral groups. These divisions are further subdivided into superficial and deep groups.

Acknowledgment: The author would like to thank Ms. Elaine James for her invaluable assistance in preparing the manuscript to this chapter.

REFERENCES

Abrams, H. L., Takahashi, M. and Adams, D. F.: Usefulness and accuracy of lymphangiography in lymphoma. Cancer Chemother. Rep., *52:* 157, 1968.

Baltaxe, H. A. and Constable, W. C.: Mediastinal lymph node visualization in absence of intrathoracic disease. Radiology, *90:* 94, 1968.

Baum, S., Bron, K. M., Wexler, L. and Abrams, H. L.: Lymphangiography, cavography, and urography. Comparative accuracy in the diagnosis of pelvic and abdominal metastases. Radiology, *81:* 207, 1963.

Bloom, W. and Fawcett, D. W.: The lymphatic system. In *A Textbook of Histology,* p. 291. W. B. Saunders, Co., Philadelphia, 1962.

Brash, J. C.: Blood-vascular and lymphatic systems. In *Cunningham's Textbook of Anatomy,* 8th ed., edited by J. C. Brash and E. B. Jamieson, p. 1177. Oxford University Press, New York, 1943.

Bron, K. M., Baum, S. and Abrams, H. L.: Oil embolism in lymphangiography. Radiology, *80:* 194, 1963.

Browse, N. L.: Normal lymphographic appearances: lower limb and pelvis. In *The Lymphatics: Diseases, Lymphography and Surgery,* edited by J. B. Kinmonth, p. 20. The Williams & Wilkins Co., Baltimore, 1972a.

Browse, N. L.: Normal lymphographic appearances of the lower limb and axilla. In *The Lymphatics: Diseases, Lymphography and Surgery,* edited by J. B. Kinmonth, p. 70. The Williams & Wilkins Co., Baltimore,

1972b.

Busch, F. M. and Sayegh, E. S.: Roentgenographic visualization of human testicular lymphatics: a preliminary report. J. Urol., *89:* 106, 1963.

Busch, F. M., Sayegh, E. S. and Chenault, O. W., Jr.: Some uses of lymphangiography in the management of testicular tumors. J. Urol., *93:* 490, 1965.

Butler, J. J.: Non-neoplastic lesions of lymph nodes of man to be differentiated from lymphomas. Natl. Cancer Inst. Monogr., *32:* 233, 1969.

Casley-Smith, J. R.: The functioning of the lymphatic system under normal and pathological conditions: its dependence on the fine structures and permeability of the vessels. In *Progress in Lymphology,* edited by A. Rüttimann, p. 348. Hafner Publishing Co., New York, 1967.

Castellino, R. A.: Observations on "reactive (follicular) hyperplasia" as encountered in repeat lymphography in the lymphomas. Cancer, *34:* 2042, 1974.

Castellino, R. A.: The role of lymphography in apparently localized "prostatic" carcinoma. Lymphology, *8:* 16, 1975.

Castellino, R. A., Bellani, F. F., Gasparini, M., Terno, G. and Musumeci, R.: Lymphography in childhood: six years experience with 242 cases. Lymphology, *8:* 74, 1975.

Castellino, R. A., Billingham, M. and Dorfman, R. F.:

Lymphographic accuracy in Hodgkin's disease and malignant lymphoma with a note on the "reactive" lymph node as a cause of most false-positive lymphograms. Invest. Radiol., 9: 155, 1974.

Castellino, R. A., Ray, G., Blank, N., Govan, D. and Bagshaw, M.: Lymphangiography in prostatic carcinoma. Preliminary observations. J.A.M.A., 223: 877, 1973.

Chavez, C. M.: Lymphatic drainage of the testicle. In Progress in Lymphology, edited by A. Rüttimann, p. 191. Hafner Publishing Co., New York, 1967.

Chiappa, S., Uslenghi, C., Bonadonna, G., Marano, P. and Ravasi, G.: Combined testicular and foot lymphangiography in testicular carcinomas. Surg. Gynecol. Obstet., 123: 10, 1966.

Clark, E. R.: The lymphatic system. Section VII In Morris' Human Anatomy: A Complete Systematic Treatise, 10th ed., edited by J. P. Schaeffer, p. 786. The Blakiston Co., Philadelphia, 1942.

Cox, S. J. and Kinmonth, J. B.: Lymphography of the thoracic duct. J. Cardiovasc. Surg., 16: 120, 1975.

Cutler, S. J., Myers, M. H. and Green, S. B.: Trends in survival rates of patients with cancer. N. Engl. J. Med., 293: 122, 1975.

Davis, H. K.: A statistical study of the thoracic duct in man. Am. J. Anat., 17: 211, 1915.

Drinker, C. K. and Yoffey, J. M.: Lymphatics, Lymph and Lymphoid Tissue: Their Physiological and Clinical Significance. Harvard University Press, Cambridge, 1941.

Dumont, A. E.: Lymph flow in the regulation of circulatory congestion and pancreatic interstitial pressure. In Progress in Lymphology, edited by A. Rüttimann, p. 91. Hafner Publishing Co., New York, 1967.

Fisch, U.: Lymphography of the Cervical Lymphatic System. W. B. Saunders, Co., Philadelphia, 1968.

Fischer, H. W., Lawrence, M. S. and Thornbury, J. R.: Lymphography of the normal adult male. Radiology, 78: 399, 1962.

Fischer, H. W. and Zimmerman, G.: Roentgenographic visualization of lymph nodes and lymphatic channels. Am. J. Roentgenol. Radium Ther. Nucl. Med., 81: 517, 1959.

Fuchs, W. A.: Normal anatomy. In Lymphography in Cancer, edited by W. A. Fuchs, J. W. Davidson and H. W. Fischer, p. 42. Springer-Verlag, Inc., New York, 1969.

Fuchs, W. A.: Neoplasms of epithelial origin. In Angiography, 2nd ed., Vol. II, edited by H. L. Abrams, p. 1369. Little, Brown & Co., Boston, 1971a.

Fuchs, W. A.: Normal anatomy of the lymphatics. In Angiography, 2nd ed., Vol. II, edited by H. L. Abrams, p.1337. Little, Brown & Co., Boston, 1971b.

Fuchs, W. A.: Technique and complications of lymphangiography. In Angiography, 2nd ed., Vol. II, edited by H. L. Abrams, p. 1325. Little, Brown & Co., Boston, 1971c.

Göthlin, J., Dahlbäck, O., Dencker, H., Håkansson, C.-H. and Lunderquist, A.: Retrograde angiography of the human thoracic duct. Am. J. Roentgenol. Radium Ther. Nucl. Med., 124: 472, 1975.

Gowans, J. L.: The recirculation of lymphocytes from blood to lymph in the rat. J. Physiol. (Lond.), 146: 54, 1959.

Gray, H.: The lymphatic system. In Anatomy of the Human Body, 27th ed., edited by C. M. Goss, p. 775. Lea & Febiger, Philadelphia, 1959.

Greening, R. R. and Wallace, S.: Further observations in lymphangiography. Radiol. Clin. North Am., 1: 157, 1963.

Ham, A. W. and Leeson, T. S.: Hemopoietic tissue. In Histology, 4th ed., chs. 17 and 18, p. 361. J. B. Lippincott Co., Philadelphia, 1961.

Hays, D. M.: The staging of Hodgkin's disease in children reviewed. Cancer, 35: 973, 1975.

Herman, P. G., Benninghoff, D. L., Nelson, J. H. and Mellins, H. Z.: Roentgen anatomy of the ilio-pelvic-aortic lymphatic system. Radiology, 80: 182, 1963.

Howett, M. and Greenburg, A. J.: Direct lymphangioadenography of the uterine cervix. Obstet. Gynecol., 27: 392, 1966.

Huntington, G. S. and McClure, C. F. W.: The development of the main lymphatic system channels of the cat and their relation to the venous system. Anat. Rec., 1: 36, 1906-1907.

Jackson, B. T.: Normal lymphographic appearances: lumbar region. In The Lymphatics: Diseases, Lymphography and Surgery, edited by J. B. Kinmonth, p. 44. The Williams & Wilkins Co., Baltimore, 1972.

Jackson, B. T. and Kinmonth, J. B.: Lumbar lymphatic crossover. Clin. Radiol., 25: 187, 1974a.

Jackson, B. T. and Kinmonth, J. B.: The normal lymphographic appearances of the lumbar lymphatics. Clin. Radiol., 25: 175, 1974b.

Jacobsson, S. and Johansson, S.: Normal roentgen anatomy of the lymph vessels of upper and lower extremities. Acta Radiol. [Diagn.] (Stockh.), 51: 321, 1959.

Kampmier, O. F.: The development of the thoracic duct in the pig. Am. J. Anat., 13: 401, 1912.

Kaplan, H. S., Dorfman, R. F., Nelsen, T. S. and Rosenberg, S. A.: Staging laparotomy and splenectomy in Hodgkin's disease: analysis of indications and patterns of involvement in 285 consecutive, unselected patients. Natl. Cancer Inst. Monogr., 36: 291, 1973.

Kinmonth, J. B.: Lymphangiography in man. A method of outlining lymphatic trunks at operation. Clin. Sci., 11: 13, 1952.

Kinmonth, J. B.: The Lymphatics: Diseases, Lymphography and Surgery. Williams & Wilkins Co., Baltimore, 1972.

Kinmonth, J. B., Harper, R. K. and Taylor, G. W.: Lymphangiography by radiological methods. J. Fac. Radiologists, 2: 217, 1955a.

Kinmonth, J. B., Taylor, G. W. and Harper, R. K.: Lymphangiography: a technique for its clinical use in the lower limb. Br. Med. J., 1: 940, 1955b.

Kirschner, R. H., Abt, A. B., O'Connell, M. J., Sklansky, B. D., Greene, W. H. and Wiernik, P. H.: Vascular invasion and hematogenous dissemination of Hodgkin's disease. Cancer, 34: 1159, 1974.

Kubik, I., Töndury, G., Rüttimann, A. and Wirth, W.: Nomenclature of the lymph nodes of the retroperitoneum, the pelvis, and the lower extremity. In Progress in Lymphology, edited by A. Rüttimann, p. 52. Hafner Publishing Co., New York, 1967.

Kuisk, H.: Technique of Lymphography and Principles of Interpretation. Warren H. Green, Inc., St. Louis, 1971.

Larson, D. L. and Lewis, S. R.: Deep lymphatic system of the lower extremity. Am. J. Surg., 113: 217, 1967.

Lemeh, C. N.: A study of the development and structural relationship of the testis and gubernaculum. Surg. Gynecol. Obstet., 110: 164, 1960.

Malek, P., Belan, A. and Kocandrle, V. L.: The superficial and deep lymphatic system of the lower extremities and their mutual relationship under physiological and pathological conditions. J. Cardiovasc. Surg., 5: 686, 1964.

Malek, P., Kolc, J. and Belan, A.: Lymphography of the deep lymphatic system of the thigh. Acta. Radiol. [Diagn.] (Stockh.), 51: 422, 1959.

Negus, D., Edwards, J. M. and Kinmonth, J. B.: Filling of cervical and mediastinal nodes from the thoracic duct and the physiology of Virchow's node-studies by lymphography. Br. J. Surg., *57:* 267, 1970.

Ngu, V. A.: The lymphatic drainage of the leg and its implications. Clin. Radiol., *15:* 197, 1964.

Nusbaum, M., Baum, S., Hedges, R. C. and Blakemore, W. S.: Roentgenographic and direct visualization of the thoracic duct. Arch. Surg., *88:* 105, 1964.

Pappenheimer, J. R., Renkin, E. M. and Borrero, L. M.: Filtration, diffusion and molecular sieving through peripheral capillary membranes. A contribution to the pore theory of capillary permeability. Am. J. Physiol., *167:* 13, 1951.

Parker, B. R., Blank, N. and Castellino, R. A.: Lymphographic appearance of benign conditions simulating lymphoma. Radiology, *111:* 267, 1974a.

Parker, B. R., Castellino, R. A., Fuks, Z. Y. and Bagshaw, M. A.: The role of lymphography in patients with ovarian cancer. Cancer, *34:* 100, 1974b.

Pomerantz, M., Herdt, J. R. L., Rockoff, S. D. and Ketcham, A. S.: Evaluation of the functional anatomy of the thoracic duct by lymphangiography. J. Thorac. Cardiovasc. Surg., *46:* 568, 1963.

Reiffenstuhl, G.: *The Lymphatics of the Female Genital Organs,* translated by L. D. Ekvall. J. B. Lippincott Co., Philadelphia, 1964.

Rosenberg, S. A.: Contribution of lymphangiography to our understanding of lymphoma. Cancer Chemother. Rep., *52:* 213, 1968.

Rosenberg, S. A. and Kaplan, H. S.: Clinical trials in the non-Hodgkin's lymphomata at Stanford University. Experimental design and preliminary results. Br. J. Cancer, *31:* 456, 1975.

Rosenberger, A. and Abrams, H. L.: The thoracic duct. In *Angiography,* 2nd ed., Vol. II, edited by H. L. Abrams, p. 1351. Little, Brown & Co., Boston, 1971.

Rouviere, H.: *Anatomy of the Human Lymphatic System,* a compendium translated from the original by M. J. Tobias. Edwards Brother, Inc., Ann Arbor, 1938.

Rusznyak, I., Földi, M. and Szabo, G.: *Lymphatics and Lymph Circulation. Physiology and Pathology,* 2nd ed. Pergamon Press, Inc., New York, 1967.

Rüttimann, A., ed.: Panel discussion IV. In *Progress in Lymphology,* p. 158. Hafner Publishing Co., New York, 1967.

Safer, M. L., Green, J. P., Crews, Q. E., Jr. and Hill, D. R.: Lymphangiographic accuracy in the staging of testicular tumors. Cancer, *35:* 1603, 1975.

Shieber, W.: The demonstration of thoracic duct abnormalities by lymphangiography. Angiography, *25:* 73, 1974.

Takahashi, M. and Abrams, H. L.: The accuracy of lymphangiographic diagnosis in malignant lymphoma. Radiology, *89:* 448, 1967.

Tjernberg, B.: The histology of the lymph node. In *Progress in Lymphology,* edited by A. Rüttimann, p. 71. Hafner Publishing Co., New York, 1967.

Töndury, G.: Embryology and topographic anatomy of the lymphatic system. In *Progress in Lymphology,* edited by A. Rüttimann, p. 10. Hafner Publishing Co., New York, 1967.

Twito, D. I. and Kennedy, B. J.: Treatment of testicular cancer. Ann. Rev. Med., *26:* 235, 1975.

Viamonte, M., Jr., Altman, D., Parks, R., Blum, E., Bevilacqua, M. and Recher, L.: Radiographic-pathologic correlation in the interpretation of lymphangioadenograms. Radiology, *80:* 903, 1963.

Von Keiser, D.: Testicular tumors. In *Progress in Lymphology,* edited by A. Rüttimann, p. 190. Hafner Publishing Co., New York, 1967.

Wahlqvist, L., Hulten, L. and Rosencrantz, M.: Normal lymphatic drainage of the testis studied by funicular lymphography. Acta Chir. Scand., *132:* 454, 1966.

Wallace, S.: Dynamics of normal and abnormal lymphatic systems as studied with contrast media. Cancer Chemother. Rep., *52:* 31, 1968.

Wallace, S. and Jackson, L.: Diagnostic criteria for lymphangiographic interpretation of malignant neoplasia. Cancer Chemother. Rep., *52:* 125, 1968.

Wallace, S., Jackson, L. and Greening, R. R.: Clinical applications of lymphangiography. Am. J. Roentgenol. Radium Ther. Nucl. Med., *88:* 97, 1962.

Wallace, S., Jackson, L., Schaffer, B., Gould, J., Greening, R. R., Weiss, A. and Kramer, S.: Lymphangiograms: their diagnostic and therapeutic potential. Radiology, *76:* 179, 1961.

Wiljasalo, M.: Lymphographic differential diagnosis of neoplastic disease. Acta Radiol. Suppl., 247, 1965.

Wirth, W. and Frommhold, H.: Lymphography. The normal thoracic duct and its variations: comparative anatomical-lymphographic study. In *Progress in Lymphology II,* edited by M. Viamonte, P. R. Koehler, M. Witte and C. Witte, p. 186. Georg Thieme Verlag, Stuttgart, 1970.

Yee, L., Llewellyn, G. A., Williams, P. A., May, I. A. and Dugan, D. J.: Scalene lymph node dissection. A study of 354 consecutive dissections. Am. J. Surg., *118:* 596, 1969.

3

Physiology—Lymph Formation, Function, Circulation

MELVIN E. CLOUSE, M.D.

The classic concept of the lymphatic system limits it morphologically to the endothelial lined pathways which transport fluid from the blood—lymphatic capillary interface centripetally into the venous system. The lymphatic capillary network is extensive and is located in all of the absorbing surfaces of the body and viscera. It also permeates the parenchyma of the organ musculoskeletal system as well as the endothelial lined pathways close to the arteries and veins.

Phylogenetically the lymphatic system is the most recent. Huntington and McClure (1906–1907) claim that the lymphatic trunks form by fusion of perivenous mesodermal clefts. Originally, these clefts have no communication with the veins but later establish it at certain points. A later article by these authors (1908) noted that the jugular lymphatic sacs arise from the capillary network of the embryonic anterior and posterior cardinal veins. The rest of the lymphatic system is formed according to their original theory. Huntington and McClure (1908), studying sections of cat embryos, confirmed this theory. They also found that the thoracic duct appeared as symmetric lymphatic channels. Later the left duct becomes the thoracic duct. The right duct drains the anterior mediastinum and empties into the right jugular sac. Lymphography has shown a number of anatomic variations in the upper thoracic duct. It may empty into both the right and left jugular areas by multiple channels as well as communicate with the mediastinal lymphatics.

An essential function of the lymphatic system is the absorption of large molecular particles, primarily protein, from the interstitial connective tissue spaces of organs, the body's potential cavities (such as the pleura, peritoneum, and pericardium), and the perivascular, perineural,

and subadventitial spaces. These absorbing areas are extensive and are all important in understanding lymphatic formation, resorption, and circulation. Approximately 15% of the body weight is extracellular fluid in the connective tissues (Gamble, 1952). This fluid is in direct contact with the capillaries and mingles with the capillary filtrate. Its absorption into the lymphatic capillaries produces lymph.

Virchow thought the connective tissue and intercellular space were incapable of function because they contained few cells. Hueck (1920) saw the connective tissue as a medium for the passage of water and dissolved substance between the blood stream and cells. Subsequently Rusznyak et al. (1967) recognized that fluid escapes from the blood capillaries, bathes the connective tissue cellular elements, and then passes into the lymphatic capillaries. The function of the ground substance discovered by Clark and Clark (1933) is still not completely clear. The ground substance is a hydrophilic colloid in a nonaqueous phase. It forms a continuous layer over the surface of connective tissue fibers and the fibrils, cementing them together. Day in 1952 and later with Eaves in 1953 suggested that the protein acts as a net in the ground substance and that a polysaccharide chain is situated in the net. This network acts as a sieve for the macromolecules filtered from the blood capillaries. The net is normally sealed by hyaluronic acid and other similar mucopolysaccharides. In abnormal conditions hyaluronidase decomposes the polysaccharide, leaving room for other macromolecules and increasing the permeability of connective tissue.

The mechanism of absorption of colloid, water, and other particles into the lymphatic capillaries after passing through the connective tissue remains elusive. Some authors postulated the existence of temporary stomata or pores, but this theory was contested by Drinker et al. (1933, 1934).

Bartels (1909) suggested that the lymphatic capillary membrane was permeable to colloid, water, and other particles because the wall consisted of a single layer of cells with large interlocking, serrated interdigitations cemented together by wide interendothelial cement. There is no basement membrane. Electron microscopic studies by Casley-Smith (1972) show overlapping endothelial cells with open junctions or pores (Pappenheimer, 1953) between the cells which act as passageways for colloid and other particles (see Chapter 1). Smaller molecules pass directly through endothelial cytoplasm (Casley-Smith, 1972). The endothelial cells are interlocked to fine microfibrils that are cemented to the interstitial connective tissues. Flow in the lymphatic vessel is produced by muscular contraction driving interstitial fluid into the lymphatic capillaries. At rest there is no flow (Genersich, 1871; Drinker and Field, 1933). Retrograde flow is prevented by valves. When the muscle relaxes and movement stops, fluid again collects in the interstitial space.

The absorption of lymph into capillaries from serosal surfaces such as the peritoneum is not clear. According to Rusznyak et al. (1967), the more likely explanation for absorption of fluid from the peritoneal cavity is via small holes which act like suction organs on the diaphragmatic surface of the peritoneum, but no genuine opening has been identified anatomically. Theoretically these holes are covered by a layer of mesothelial cells and are in close contact with the pleural cavity and the lymphatic system. According to Bizzozero and Salvioli (1878), the holes become wider and longer when the diaphragm contracts, decreasing the pressure and enabling them to aspirate fluid from the peritoneal cavity. When expiration occurs the holes are compressed and pressure increases; the substance is then squeezed into the lymphatics. Casley-Smith (1972) has not defined these pores; however, carbon particles can be seen passing through narrow intercellular junctions into the lumen of the lymphatic capillaries of the mouse diaphragm.

The serous cavities and connective tissue spaces cannot be regarded as part of the lymphatic system because there is no direct communication between them. These areas should more likely be regarded as absorbing surfaces and possibly reservoirs for fluid.

The relationship of the blood vascular system, the connective tissues, and the absorbing surfaces and lymphatic system can best be illustrated in diseases which result in insufficiency of the lymphatic system. In constrictive pericarditis and congestive failure, there is a generalized increase in venous pressure with a concomitant rise in the thoracic duct pressure and decrease in lymph flow. As the system is overwhelmed with more lymph than it can transport, fluid builds up in cavities lined by serosa and connective tissue, producing edema. When pericardial constriction is removed or when diuretics or digitalis is given, the fluid is excreted by the kidneys. The venous pressure decreases, the lymph flow returns to normal, and the fluid deposits are mobilized.

Starling (1909) first suggested that high venous pressure prevented the flow of lymph into the venous angle. Foldi and Papp (1961) and Wégria et al. (1963) supported this theory with data showing decreased flow in the thoracic duct during high venous pressure states. Dumont and Mulholland (1962) suggested that overloading the lymphatic system results in functional insufficiency because of increased lymph formation by elevated venous pressure and increased flow rate in the thoracic duct. Their data were based on measurements from a decompressed cannulated thoracic duct in patients with congestive heart failure and cirrhosis. Those investigators supporting decreased flow based their theory on a closed system.

The mechanism of fluid retention and edema in hepatic cirrhosis may be related to a renolymphatic shunt (Foldi, 1964). By this mechanism large amounts of sodium chloride and water may be shunted from the urinary tract to the renal lymphatic system and into the thoracic duct. In addition to fluid retention, lymph production by the liver is markedly increased and undoubtedly contributes to lymphatic decompensation, i.e., functional insufficiency with ascites and edema. Child in 1954 observed dilated lymphatics on the surface of the liver in patients suffering from cirrhosis, and in 1951 both Bollman and Volwiler noted a marked increase in hepatic lymph production in cirrhosis.

REFERENCES

Bartels, P.: Dos Lymphefäss System. Hand-buch d. Anatomie d. Menschen. G. Fischer, Jena, 1909.

Bizzozero, G. and Salvioli, G.: Studi sulla struttura e sui linfatici delle serose umane. Arch. Sci. Med., 2: 247, 1878.

Bollman, J. L.: Liver lymph and intestinal lymph in experimental cirrhosis and ascites. J.A.M.A., *145:* 1173, 1951.

Casley-Smith, J. R.: The role of the endothelial intercellular junctions in the functioning of the initial lymphatics. Angiologia, *9:* 106, 1972.

Child, C. G.: *The Hepatic Circulation and Portal Hypertension.* W. B. Saunders Co., Philadelphia, 1954.

Clark, E. R. and Clark, E. L.: Further observations on living lymphatic vessels in the transparent chamber in the rabbit's ear—their relation to tissue spaces. Am. J. Anat., *52:* 273, 1933.

Day, T.: The permeability of interstitial connective tissue and the nature of the interfibrillary substance. J. Physiol. (Lond.), *117:* 1, 1952.

Day, T. and Eaves, G.: Electron microscope observations on the ground substance of interstitial connective tissue. Biochim. Biophys. Acta, *10:* 203, 1953.

Drinker, C. K. and Field, M. E.: *Lymphatic, Lymph and Lymphoid Tissue.* The Williams & Wilkins Co., Baltimore, 1933.

Drinker, C. K., Field, M. E. and Homans, J.: The experimental production of edema—elephantiasis as a result of lymphatic obstruction. Am. J. Physiol., *108:* 509, 1934.

Dumont, A. E. and Mulholland, J. H.: Alterations in thoracic duct lymph flow in hepatic cirrhosis: significance in portal hypertension. Am. Surg., *156:* 668, 1962.

Foldi, M.: Some problems in renal lymph flow. Orv. Hetil., *105:* 104, 1964.

Foldi, M. and Papp, M.: The role of lymph circulation in congestive heart failure. Jap. Circ. J., *25:* 703, 1961.

Gamble, J. L.: *Chemistry, Anatomy, Physiology and Pathology of Extracellular Fluid.* Harvard University Press, Cambridge, 1952.

Genersich, K.: Die Aufnahme der Lymphe durch die Schnen und Fascien der Skelettmuskeln. Arb. Physiol. Anst. Leipzig, *5:* 53, 1871.

Hueck, W.: Uber das Mesenchym. Die Bedeutung seiner Entwicklung und seines Baues für die Pathologie. Beitr. Pathol. Anat., *6:* 330, 1920.

Huntington, G. S. and McClure, C. F. W.: The development of the main lymphatic channels of the cat and their relation to the venous system. Anat. Rec., *1:* 36, 1906–1907.

Huntington, G. S. and McClure, C. F. W.: The anatomy and development of the jugular lymph sacs in the domestic cat. Am. J. Anat., *2:* 1, 1908.

Pappenheimer, J. R.: The passage of molecules through capillary walls. Physiol. Rev., *33:* 387, 1953.

Rusznyak I., Foldi, M. and Szabo, G.: *Lymphatics and Lymph Circulation,* 2nd ed. Pergamon Press, New York, 1967.

Starling, E. J.: *The Fluids of the Body. The Herter Lectures.* W. T. Keener, Chicago, 1909.

Volwiler, W.: The relation of certain mechanical factors to the production of ascites. In *Liver Disease.* CIBA Foundation Symposium, London, 1951.

Wégria, R., Zekert, H., Walter, K. E., Entrup, R. W., De Schryver, C., Kennedy, W. and Paiewonsky, D.: The effect of systemic venous pressure on drainage of lymph from thoracic duct. Am. J. Physiol., *204:* 284, 1963.

4

Technique

MELVIN E. CLOUSE, M.D.

The steps in lymphography are visualization of the lymphatics by vital dyes, surgical exposure of the vessel, direct cannulation, injection of contrast material, and roentgenographic imaging of the vessels immediately after completion of the injection and 24 hours later for lymph node detail.

The technique generally used was developed by the British surgeon J. B. Kinmonth (1952). Dr. Kinmonth extended the technique of Hudack and McMaster (1933), who had used 11% patent blue violet dye to study the dermal lymphatics.

The first step in the procedure is examination of the patient and review of the chart to be certain that the procedure is indicated and that there are no contraindications. The major contraindications are cardiovascular or pulmonary disease (i.e., heart failure, angina, interstitial fibrosis, emphysema, or previous radiotherapy to the lung). Radiotherapy to the lung opens arteriovenous shunts and predisposes to systemic emboli (Davidson, 1969). The patient must also be quizzed for allergies to local anesthesia, vital dyes, and contrast material.

Lymphography may be performed on an outpatient basis, but it is better to observe the patient in the hospital for 24 hr. This may be accomplished through an observation unit or receiving ward.

The procedure is explained to the patient with special attention to local blue skin discoloration that may last several months and generalized light blue staining of the skin that will return to normal in 10–12 hr (if chronic renal disease or obstructive uropathy does not exist). The urine will be dark blue because the dye is almost completely excreted by the kidneys.

Premedication is adjusted according to the patient's weight and age. For an average 70-kg patient a combined injection of atropine 0.4 mg, Demerol 75 mg, and Nembutal 100 mg is given intramuscularly 30 min before the procedure is begun. For small patients or those over 60 years of age, adequate premedication can be achieved with atropine 0.4 mg alone or in combination with Demerol 75 mg.

The feet are shaved in the radiology department, prepared with Betadine surgical scrub, and cleansed with alcohol. The feet are then draped with sterile sheets. A lymphangiogram tray is used (Fig. 4.1).

---

6 towels
16 4 × 3 sponges
1 swab
1 20-cc vial Xylocaine 1% plain
1 medicine glass
1 6" basin
2 smooth sponge forceps
1 Adson smoothed forceps
1 Miltex 3-C
1 suture scissors
1 small needle holder
3 curved mosquitoes
1 #3 knife handle with #15 blade
2 straight mosquitoes
1 10-cc ring Luer-loc syringe (for Xylocaine)
2 10-cc Luer-loc syringes
3 #26 disposable needles

Available:
    4–0 silk suture
    sterile sheets
    11% patent blue violet dye
    Harvard apparatus injector
    proper surgical light
    Steri-Strip tape
    Ethiodol 2 10-ml vials

FIG. 4.1. LYMPHANGIOGRAM TRAY CONTENTS

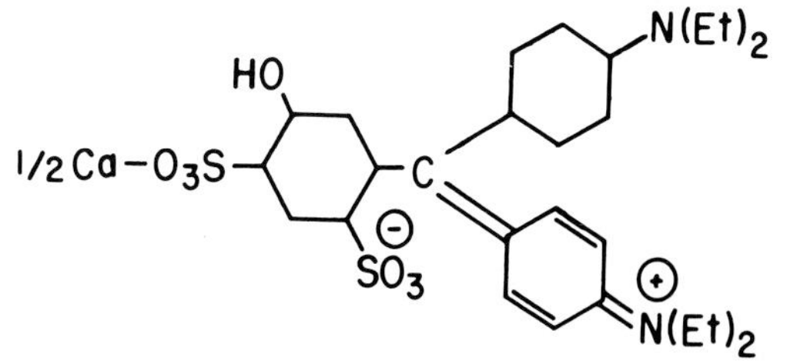

FIG. 4.2. MOLECULAR STRUCTURE, PATENT BLUE VIOLET
MCB Manufacturing Chemists, Norwood, Ohio 45212.

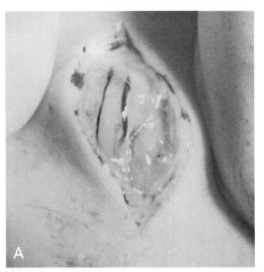

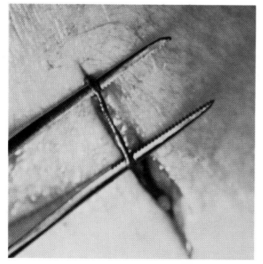

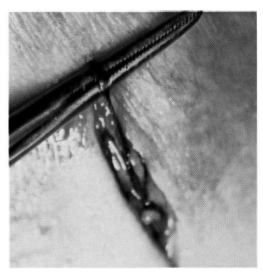

FIG. 4.3. EXPOSURE OF LYMPHATIC VESSEL

A: Longitudinal incision over lymphatic. *B:* Lymphatic elevated by probing under it with the 3-C Miltex forcep. *C:* Exposed lymphatic before the soft tissue has been removed.

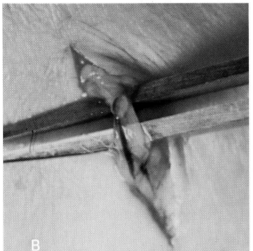

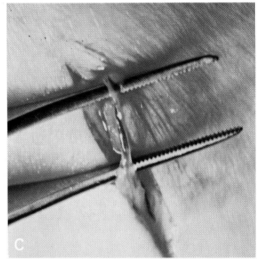

FIG. 4.4. EXPOSED LYMPHATIC AFTER THE SOFT TISSUE HAS BEEN REMOVED READY FOR CANNULATION

FIG. 4.5. EXPOSED LYMPHATIC TEMPORARILY OBSTRUCTED BY ADSON FORCEP

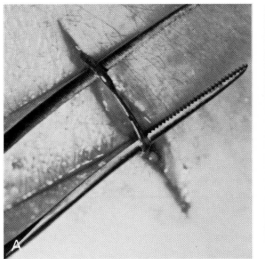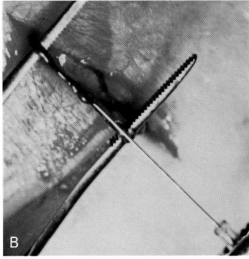

FIG. 4.6. LYMPHATIC CANNULATION TECHNIQUE

A: Taut, semidistended lymphatic ready for cannulation. *B:* Lymphatic immediately after needle has punctured lymphatic; needle is on a plane parallel to the lymphatic. When the lymphatic has been punctured, a small amount of contrast material is injected to further distend the vessel and the needle is advanced 2–3 mm.

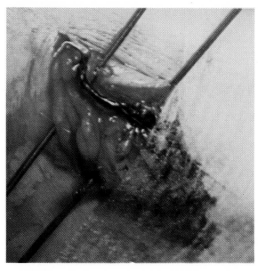

FIG. 4.7. NEEDLE IN LYMPHATIC SECURED WITH STERI- STRIP TAPE   The lymphatic is distended because the injection has begun. The needles in the subcutaneous tissue beneath the lymphatic elevate it to the skin surface.

Vital Dyes

Various indicator dyes such as direct sky blue, trypan blue, niagara sky blue, and methylene blue have been used for lymphography (Threefoot, 1960; Hreschyshyn et al., 1961; Riveros et al., 1967). The vital dyes are large molecular compounds that facilitate their absorption into the initial lymphatics rather than small molecular crystalloids that are absorbed into the blood vascular capillaries (Fig. 4.2). Patent blue violet 11% (MCB Manufacturing Chemists, 2809 Highland Avenue, Norwood, Ohio 45212) is a triphenylmethane dye which was eventually selected by Hudack and McMasters (1933) for outlining skin lymphatics. It is most widely used because it is rapidly absorbed in the lymphatics, slowly diffuses into the adventitia, and is rapidly excreted in the urine because it is not bound to plasma protein (Threefoot, 1960).

A mixture of 0.5 ml of 1% Xylocaine and 2 ml of 11% patent blue violet dye is used. When an examination of the deep lymphatics of the leg is desired, the vital dye is injected into the tissues below the lateral malleolus. For examination of the arm and axillary lymphatics, the vital dye is injected on the dorsal aspect between the fingers of the hand. For the cervical lymphatics, the posterior auricular area is injected.

It is easier to expose and cannulate the lymphatic before patent blue dye has extravasated into the surrounding tissue and stained the skin. It is therefore imperative to identify the lymphatic immediately after it has just filled with dye. This can be accomplished by focusing a bright light on the dorsum of the foot after injecting the dye. The blood can be compressed from the small veins by stretching and compressing the skin and making it taut. The lymphatics can then be seen as light blue streaks underneath the skin. The lymphatics cannot be visualized in this manner in dark skinned patients.

Sigurjonsson (1974) localizes pedal lymphatics without the aid of indicator dyes because of the considerable incidence of allergic reactions reported by Mortazavi and Burrows (1971). He reported no difference in failure rate or operation time with or without the use of indicator dyes.

Exposure of the Lymphatics

The site on the foot chosen to expose and cannulate a lymphatic is very important. The vessels near the toes are very small, and the patient may dislodge the needle from this site by slight movement of his foot or toes. It is best to select a vessel on the lateral aspect of the dorsum of the foot or just lateral to the base of the first metatarsal. It is much easier to expose and cannulate a single lymphatic. Occasionally there may be two very small lymphatics parallel to each other or the examiner may make the original incision at a bifurcation. The incision must then be extended in the direction of the largest trunk. If the first attempt is unsuccessful, a vessel higher up near the ankle may be chosen.

Xylocaine 1% is injected into the dermal and subcutaneous tissues on either side of the lymphatic. Injecting into the subcutaneous tissues helps dissect and free the lymphatic vessel from the surrounding tissues, elevates the skin, and reduces the chance of laceration of the lymphatic when the initial incision is made. A longitudinal incision is made over the lymphatic. When the vessel is exposed under direct vision, the incision is carried down into the subcutaneous tissues on either side of the vessel. The vessel is elevated by probing underneath it with a sharp pointed fine 3-C, Miltex forcep (Miltex

Instrument Co., 300 Park Avenue South, New York, NY 10010) (Fig. 4.3) and held exposed by passing a smooth Adson forcep (Codman Instrument Co., Randolph, MA 02054) underneath the lymph vessel with the opposite hand. Fat and loose areolar tissue are stripped off the lymphatic for a distance of 1–2 cm with the fine Miltex forcep (Fig. 4.4).

Although it is usually easy to differentiate lymphatics from veins, it may at times be difficult. It is for this reason that the foot is fluoroscoped immediately after the injection has begun. The wall of the small veins is usually thicker and denser when compressed while the lymphatic vessel is clear and more transparent when it is collapsed and the vital dye milked from the vessel.

Cannulation

Various modifications of the Kinmonth technique have been described. Jing (1966), Iriarte et al. (1964), Lee et al. (1969), Kropholler et al. (1968), and Tong (1969) have described techniques of directly inserting a fine polyethylene catheter into the lymph vessel. There have also been a proliferation of instruments designed to make cannulation easier and for securing the needle in the vessel once it has been cannulated. Damascelli et al. (1969) described a special forcep for removing loose connective tissue around the vessel. Special cannulas have been designed by Viamonte and Stevens (1966), Howland (1972), DeRoo (1966), and Tegtmeyer (1974). Turner (1966), Youker (1966), and DeRoo have all described special clamps for holding the needle in place once the vessel has been cannulated.

Over the years we have found that the easiest method of cannulation is one that avoids the need for special equipment. As an example we do not use ligatures to temporarily obstruct and distend the vessel for cannulation. This is best accomplished with the smooth Adson forcep. The proximal portion of the lymph vessel is temporarily obstructed (Fig. 4.5). The vessel is distended by massaging the tissues and milking the lymph up from the toes. The forcep is spread making the vessel taut and semidistended (Fig. 4.6A). The lymphatic set (Randall Faichney Co., Avon, MA 02322) with a 27- or 30-gauge needle is grasped with a large sponge forcep and the lymphatic vessel punctured. In making the approach into the lymphatic vessel, the needle must be on a plane parallel to and just above the vessel so that the posterior wall of the lymphatic is not punctured (Fig. 4.6B).

A small amount of contrast material is injected manually by the assistant from a 10-ml syringe attached to the lymphatic set to further distend the vessel. The needle is then advanced 2-3 mm into the lumen. It is much easier to visualize small air bubbles alternating with the column of contrast material indicating free passage into the lymphatic lumen than a solid column of contrast material. For this reason small air bubbles are trapped in the lymphography set tubing near the needle before cannulation is attempted.

The lymphatic needle is stabilized with the index finger. The catheter and needle are secured with strips of Steri-Strip (Minnesota Mining and Manufacturing Co., St. Paul, MN) tape that have previously been peeled from the heavy paper backing and taped to the surrounding drapes (Fig. 4.7). The heavy paper backing should remain on the corner to prevent the tape sticking to the examiner's glove. As the lymphographer gains experience and anticipates the procedure, assistance is only needed for contrast injection to distend the lymph vessel at the initial puncture.

Occasionally contrast material may leak from the puncture site even when the needle is securely in the vessel. In these instances a 4-0 silk ligature may be placed around the vessel distal to the needle tip but proximal to the puncture site by passing a fine Miltex forcep underneath the needle and vessel, grasping the suture, and pulling it underneath without disturbing the needle.

It is preferable to use a different vessel when a second puncture must be made because leakage of lymph and dye prevents vessel distention thus making the second puncture more difficult. If this is not possible the second puncture must be made proximal to the first to prevent leakage of contrast material during the injection.

The tubing is securely taped to the patient's foot. The patient remains supine during the procedure but may be given fluids and additional medication if necessary. The patient must never be left unobserved during the procedure.

Contrast Material

The standard contrast material used for lymphography is Ethiodol (Savage Laboratories, Inc., Missouri City, TX 77459), an iodinated ethyl ester of the fatty acids of poppy seed oil. Ethiodol is obtained by transesterification of Lipiodol. It is mainly composed of ethyl diiodostereate, monoiodostereate, and moniodinated ethyl stereate (Guerbet Laboratories, 16–24 rue Jean-Chaptal, 93 Aulnaysouse, Boise, France). Ethiodol has completely replaced other oily contrast materials such as Iodopin used by Bruun and Engeset (1956) and Lipiodol used by Zheutlin and Shanbrom (1958). Zheutlin and Shanbrom found that Ethiodol produced good opacification of the nodes and was easier than Lipiodol to inject because it is less viscous. Ethiodol also provides excellent opacification of the lymph vessels and nodes because it does not diffuse through the vessel wall like water-soluble contrast media. It remains in the nodes for months and sometimes years, allowing one to evaluate the effects of treatment or progression of disease. The single disadvantage of Ethiodol is that it is not completely inert. It produces an inflammatory reaction in the lymph nodes and lungs that does not cause permanent damage and is not clinically significant.

The viscosity of Ethiodol at 15°C is 0.5–1.0 poise compared to 20.0 poise for Lipiodol. Ethiodol is a clear, light amber oily fluid. If exposed to oxygen or sunlight, it will decompose (liberating iodine) and turn a dark brown color. It should not be used in this condition.

The biologic fate of Ethiodol has been reported by Fischer (1959a,b), Koehler et al. (1964), and Threefoot (1968). The contrast material that is not held within the nodes enters the venous system via the thoracic duct of lymphovenous communications. When normal doses of Ethiodol (7 ml in each extremity) are used, the excess is largely filtered by the lungs. If excessive doses are given, there is spill-over from the lungs into other organs.

Koehler et al. (1964) have shown that after 3 days an average of 25% of radioactively tagged [131]I Ethiodol (30 Ci/gm) remained in the lymph nodes of the dog while an average of 50% was cleared from the lungs. The remainder of an injected dose of 0.16 gm/kg was distributed fairly evenly throughout the remaining body organs. The amount of contrast material entering the systemic circulation in humans should be considerably less because the usual dose is lower (0.2 ml/kg) and there are more iliac and para-aortic nodes to retain contrast material. The fate of the lipid molecule is unknown, but presumably it is degraded by beta oxidation (Koehler, 1968).

Iodine is stripped from the lipid molecule by esterases. Threefoot (1968) has shown that the lipid form of ^{131}I-labelled Ethiodol gradually decreases to insignificant amounts. By 9 days nearly all of the iodine is in the aqueous phase

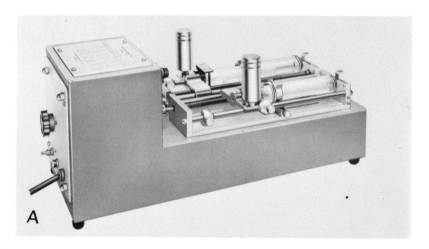

HARVARD APPARATUS

Infusion/Withdrawal Pump

Rates in ml/minute per Syringe

SERIES 900, 930, 940, 950, 954
Syringe Sizes

50 ml.	30 ml.	20 ml.	10 ml.	5 ml.	2 ml.
114.0	74.1	58.2	30.9	20.4	11.8
45.9	29.7	23.3	12.4	8.16	4.71
22.9	14.8	11.6	6.18	4.08	2.36
11.5	7.41	5.82	3.09	2.04	1.18
5.73	3.69	2.91	1.53	1.02	0.591
2.29	1.48	1.16	0.618	0.408	0.237
1.15	0.741	0.582	0.309	0.204	0.118
0.573	0.369	0.291	0.153	0.102	0.0591
0.229	0.148	0.116	0.0518	0.0408	0.0237
0.115	0.0741	0.0582	0.0309	0.0204	0.0118
0.057	0.0369	0.0291	0.0153	0.0102	0.00591
0.0229	0.0148	0.0116	0.00618	0.00408	0.00237

B

FIG. 4.8. INJECTORS
A: Harvard apparatus injector pump. B: Injection rates (ml/min/syringe).

and is excreted by the kidneys in the iodide form.

Dosage

To evaluate the inguinal, iliac, and para-aortic nodes and the thoracic duct by pedal lymphography in a 70-kg patient, 6-7 ml of Ethiodol are injected into the lymphatics of each extremity. The rate of injection is 0.0618–0.153 ml/min depending upon the size of the lymphatic. Too rapid a rate of injection will rupture the lymphatic.

For lymphography in the upper arm, 2–5 ml of Ethiodol are used. The injection is discontinued when the axillary nodes fill. The injection rate is 0.0618 ml/min.

Injectors

The various types of injectors described for lymphography all offer a slow steady rate of injection. Wallace et al. (1961) described a manually operated C-clamp. Gilchrist (1965), Jing (1966), Arts (1967), and Cusick and Panning (1967) use gravity types of injectors. Various automatic injectors have been used by DeRoo (1966), Clementz and Olin (1961), and Viamonte (1964).

We use a Harvard apparatus, Model 941 Automatic Injector (Harvard Apparatus Co., Inc., Millis, MA 02054) (Fig. 4.8). The Harvard apparatus injector is similar to that described by Clementz and Olin (1961). It operates on a screw-driven mechanism with a gear box, is simple to operate, and is very accurate at all rates of injection.

Roentgenographic Technique

The foot and lower leg are fluoroscoped after the injection has begun to be certain that the needle is in the lymphatic and there are no peripheral lymphovenous communications (see Fig. 6.21). After approximately 4 ml have been injected, an anteroposterior film of the pelvis is taken to check for obstruction or lymphovenous communications in the pelvis (see Figs. 6.19 and 6.20).

A supine film of the abdomen is taken after 6–7 ml of Ethiodol have been injected. If the injection rate has been 0.153 ml/min, the total injection time will be just over 45 min. The cisterna chyli may not have filled, and it will be necessary to delay the complete film series for 15–30 min to allow for complete filling of the para-aortic vessels and cisterna chyli.

Seven views are routinely taken after the injection has been terminated and repeated 24 hr later for lymph node detail: an anteroposterior view of the abdomen; an anteroposterior view of the pelvis; right and left posterior oblique views of the abdomen including the iliac and inguinal areas; lateral view of abdomen using lumbar spine technique; and posteroanterior and lateral views of the chest and thoracic duct to evaluate the presence of drainage into paratracheal nodes and the amount of embolized oil.

High quality films and short exposure times to prevent motion unsharpness are most important. High or low kilovoltage may be used for filming depending upon the preference of the examiner.

The technical factors are 40-inch target-to-film distance, regular screens (Kodak X-omatic), and Kodak RPL film (Table 4.1). We have found that multiple views and on occasion 2× magnification are more helpful than stereoscopy (Mannila and Wiljasalo, 1965) and tomography (DeRoo et al., 1965). The vessel phase must be compared to the node films to determine whether filling defects represent metastases or lymph node hila.

In addition localized obstruction of one or more vessels by a node completely replaced by tumor may be demonstrated only in the vessel phase. Significant amounts of contrast material remaining in the vessels after 24 hr and collateral circulation indicate obstruction.

Direct 2× magnification is especially helpful for evaluating a conglomerate of nodes high in the para-aortic and iliac areas. The presence of multiple small superimposed nodes prevents one from clearly determining the boundary of each node. In addition to enlargement, magnification changes the spatial relationship of the node images to each other and thereby sharply delineates the node boundaries and the intranodal architecture. Questionable nodes at first examination will become clearly normal or abnor-

TABLE 4.1

	mA	kVp
Chest		
Posteroanterior	6	110
Lateral	20	120
Abdomen		
Anteroposterior	75	78
RPO-LPO	75	84
Lateral	150	100
Pelvis		
Anteroposterior	50	88

mal with magnification. Magnification is least helpful when there is no node superimposition.

Direct magnification has been used by Ditchek and Scanlon (1967). In order to use direct 2× magnification, a focal spot of 0.3 mm is needed. The advertised 0.3-mm focal spot may actually increase to 0.5-mm or become distorted at conventional milliamperage and kilovoltage. Special nonbiased tubes for 0.3-mm and under focal spots may be purchased, but they are expensive and not absolutely essential for lymphography.

Follow-Up

The needles are removed after the injection has been terminated. The wound is thoroughly cleansed with a saline scrub, sutured with 4-0 silk, and covered with band-aids. The sutures are removed after 12 days by the patient's physician or radiologist.

Follow-up films of the abdomen are made to evaluate progress of treatment or recurrent disease until the node contains insufficient amounts of contrast material for evaluation.

BREAST LYMPHOGRAPHY

Kett et al. (1970) have performed direct lymphography of the breast on 88 patients by injecting 0.2 ml of an equal mixture of 11% patent blue violet dye and 1% Xylocaine into the region of the mammary areola. The exposure is similar to pedal lymphography, but cannulation is much more difficult because of deep small fragile lymphatics and chest movement. After cannulation, 2 ml of Ethiodol are injected. The authors found direct lymphography useful for differentiating lymph node metastases from breast cancer. Because the procedure is time-consuming and somewhat difficult, it has not gained wide acceptance.

THYROID LYMPHOGRAPHY

Gruart et al. (1967) attempted to outline the cervical lymph nodes by injecting 8 ml of Ethiodol into the muscles at the base of the tongue and having the patient chew. Matoba and Kikuchi (1969) described a method of injecting Lipiodol ultrafluid directly into the thyroid gland. This outlines the gland and its nodules by spreading throughout the periacinar tissues. Later the external thyroid lymphatics and nodes fill. Beales et al. (1971), Sachdeva et al. (1974), Compana et al. (1974), and Pelu et al. (1974) have also found this method to be successful. The method appears to be extremely safe and trouble-free. It appears to add considerably to the knowledge of thyroid disease, but as a clinical pathologic examination, little physiologic information is gained. It has been found reliable for diagnosis of multinodular goiter, solitary nodule, and carcinoma. The cervical nodes were visualized in 28 of 40 cases (70%) reported by Sachdeva et al. (1974) and mediastinal nodes in 4 cases (10%). Detection of nodal metastases was disappointing.

PERCUTANEOUS LYMPH NODE ASPIRATION NEEDLE BIOPSY

Percutaneous lymph node aspiration needle biopsy is a logical extension of the concept of aspiration needle biopsies of the pancreas or lung and should be performed by the lymphographer (Arnesjo et al., 1972; Christoffersen and Pall, 1970; Forsgren and Orell, 1973; Tylen, 1974). It can be performed with little or no risk to the patient and is no more difficult to perform than aspiration needle biopsies of lung nodules. It is more precise than pancreatic needle biopsies because the lymph nodes are much smaller.

The guidelines for premedication are the same as for the initial lymphography. In addition 5 mg of Valium may be given intravenously if necessary for a very apprehensive patient.

The patient is placed under an image intensifier in the supine position. A biplane image intensifier is preferable; however, the lymph node may be localized by a single plane fluoroscope. The skin over the lymph node is infiltrated with 3 or 4 cc of 1% Xylocaine. A 15-cm (23 gauge) needle inserted through a 3.8-cm

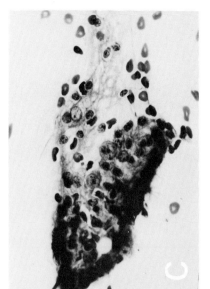

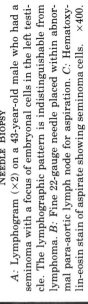

FIG. 4.9. PERCUTANEOUS LYMPH NODE ASPIRATION NEEDLE BIOPSY

A: Lymphogram (×2) on a 43-year-old male who had a seminoma with a focus of embryonal cells in the left testicle. The lymphographic pattern is indistinguishable from lymphoma. *B:* Fine 22-gauge needle placed within abnormal para-aortic lymph node for aspiration. *C:* Hematoxylin-eosin stain of aspirate showing seminoma cells. ×400.

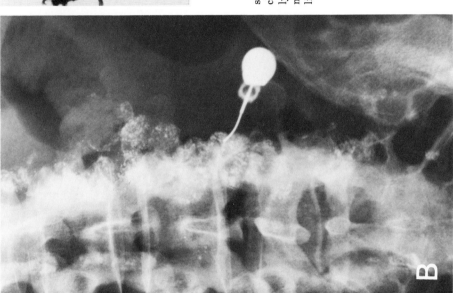

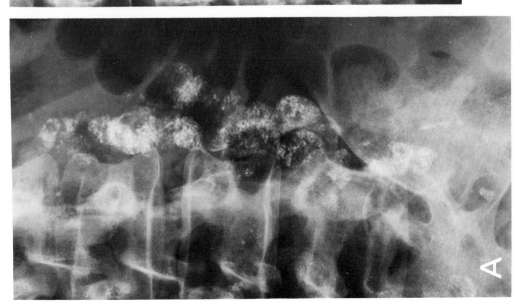

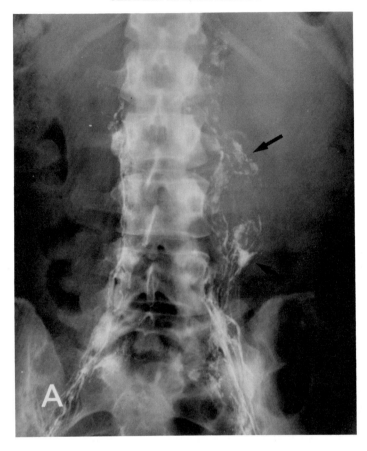

FIG. 4.10. NODE DISEASE WITH ULTRASOUND

Displacment of (A) left para-aortic channels (*arrows*) and (B) abnormal nodes (*arrows*). C: Ultrasound shows large mass of nodes (N) extending out from the base of the mesentery.

disposable thin-walled (18 gauge) needle is placed in a vertical position under the intensifier fluoroscope directly over the lymph node to be biopsied. The 18-gauge needle is advanced through the abdominal wall and directed toward the lymph node. The 23-gauge needle is then advanced through the 18-gauge needle. This guidance is essential because the long 23-gauge needle is very flexible and can easily be deflected from the path of the lymph node as it passes through the abdominal wall. The 23-gauge needle is advanced into the node and aspirated with a 10-cc syringe attached to an aspirating mechanism similar to that described by Forsgren and Orell (1973). The syringe pistol allows one to easily create a tremendous vacuum and aspirate cells from the node.

The needle is moved rapidly back and forth a few millimeters during maximal aspiration. It is withdrawn and the contents flushed onto a microscopic slide. Maximal aspiration should be discontinued as the needle is withdrawn from the node because any blood mixed with the tumor cells may be aspirated into the syringe. The node aspirate is then more difficult to flush from the syringe and one may get false negative results. A thin smear is made and immediately dropped into a 10% zinc alcohol formalin solution. It is imperative to immerse the slide in the alcohol solution before the smear dries as drying destroys cellular morphology. The slide can then be stained with hematoxylin-eosin and the results available in a few hours.

Overlying structures are penetrated during the procedure as when aspirates are made of the pancreas; complications have not occurred in the few reported cases (Wallace, 1975; Göthlin, 1976; Zornoza, 1976). A bloody aspirate does impair the efficacy of the aspirate but does not render it useless: acinar cells can be evaluated for tumor even when large amounts of blood are present (Fig. 4.9).

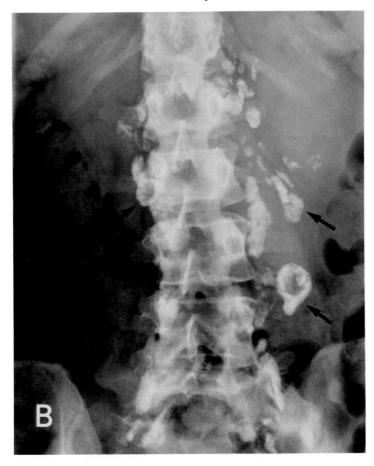

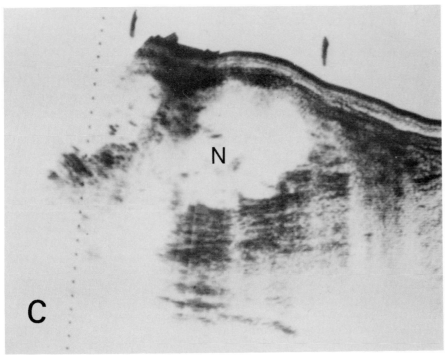

FIG. 4.10 B and C

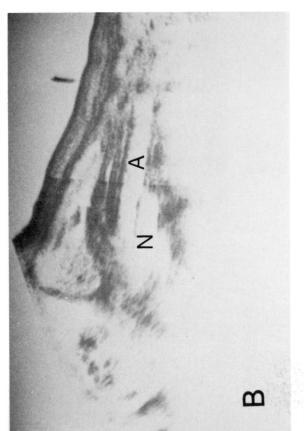

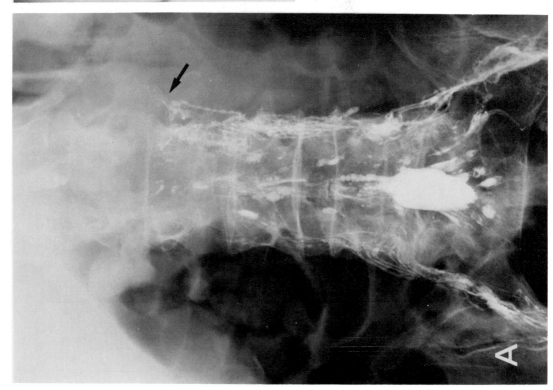

FIG. 4.11. RECURRENT HODGKIN'S DISEASE

A: The more cephalad lymphatic channels are draped around the lower margin of a retroperitoneal mass (arrow). B: Ultrasound demonstrates a large mass of retroaortic nodes. N, Nodes; A, aorta.

LYMPHOGRAPHY AND ULTRASOUND

Lymphography was a definite major advance in detecting abnormal nodes. It was the major probe into the retroperitoneal and iliac area until the advent of computed tomography and ultrasound. Kreel (1976) using computed tomography detected nodal disease that was not demonstrated by lymphography. This would be expected because all of the para-aortic nodes do not fill during pedal lymphography. In addition, celiac and mesenteric nodes and the primary drainage nodes from the testis do not fill via pedal lymphography.

We are currently comparing the results of lymphography and ultrasound for detecting node disease in the mesenteric, celiac, and ret-

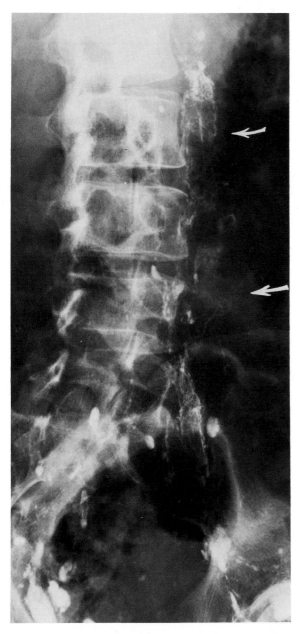

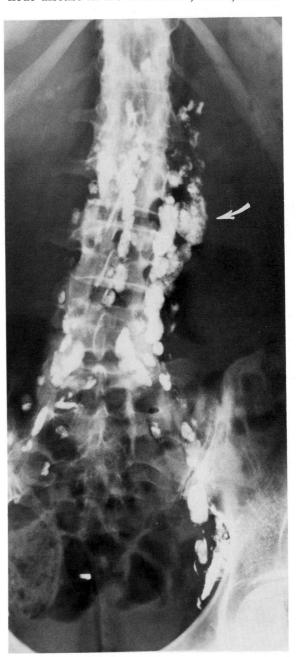

FIG. 4.12. HODGKIN'S DISEASE
Lymphogram with positive nodes in left para-aortic (*arrows*) area not demonstrated by ultrasound.

FIG. 4.13. HODGKIN'S DISEASE
Abnormal left para-aortic nodes (*arrows*) not demonstrated by ultrasound.

roperitoneal area. Preliminary results indicate a 90% correlation of ultrasound and lymphography. It would appear that ultrasound can replace cavography for evaluating node disease above the cisterna, i.e., mesenteric and celiac nodes. Frequently, node disease is much more pronounced by ultrasound (Figs. 4.10 and 4.11).

The limitations of ultrasound are large patients who do not have a large amount of bulky disease (Figs. 4.12 and 4.13).

REFERENCES

Arnesjo, B., Stormby, N. and Ackerman, M.: Cytodiagnosis of pancreatic lesions by means of fine-needle biopsy during operation. Acta Chir. Scand., *138:* 363, 1972.

Arts, V.: An injection apparatus for lymphangiography. Am. J. Roentgenol. Radium Ther. Nucl. Med., *100:* 466, 1967.

Beales, J. S., Nundy, S. and Taylor, S.: Thyroid lymphography. Br. J. Surg., *58:* 168, 1971.

Bruun, S. and Engeset, A.: Lymphadenography. Acta Radiol., *45:* 389, 1956.

Christoffersen, P. and Pall, P.: Preoperative pancreatic aspiration biopsies. Acta Pathol. Microbiol. Scand [B], *112:* 28, 1970.

Clementz, B. and Olin, T.: Apparatus for controlled infusion of saline in angiography and contrast medium in lymphography. Acta Radiol., *55:* 109, 1961.

Compana, F. P., DeAntoni, E., Cordone, M. N. and DiMatteo, G.: Thyrolymphadenography and thyroid scintigraphy. A diagnostic comparison. Minerva Chir., *29:* 335, 1974.

Cusick, H. and Panning, W. P.: A simple practical technique of lymphography. Radiology, *88:* 576, 1967.

Damascelli, B., Musumeci, R. and Uslenghi, C.: Instruments for lymphography. Lymphology, *2:* 166, 1969.

Davidson, J. W.: Lipid embolism to the brain following lymphography. Am. J. Roentgenol. Radium Ther. Nucl. Med., *105:* 763, 1969.

DeRoo, T.: An improved, simple technique of lymphography. Am. J. Roentgenol. Radium Ther. Nucl. Med., *98:* 948, 1966.

DeRoo, T., Thomas, P. and Kropholler, R. W.: The importance of tomography for the interpretation of lymphographic picture of lymph node metastases. Am. J. Roentgenol. Radium Ther. Nucl. Med., *94:* 924, 1965.

Ditchek, T. and Scanlon, G. T.: Direct magnification lymphography. J.A.M.A., *199:* 654, 1967.

Fischer, H. W.: Lymphangiography and lymphadenography with various contrast agents. Ann. N.Y. Acad. Sci., *78:* 799, 1959a.

Fischer, H. W.: A critique of experimental lymphography. Acta Radiol., *52:* 448, 1959b.

Forsgren, L. and Orell, S.: Aspiration cytology in carcinoma of the pancreas. Surgery, *73:* 38, 1973.

Franzen, S., Giertz, G. and Zajicek, J.: Cytological diagnosis of prostatic tumors by transrectal aspiration biopsy: a preliminary report. Br. J. Urol, *32:* 193, 1960.

Gilchrist, M. R.: Lymphangiography. A local evaluation. Minn. Med., *48:* 1000, 1965.

Göthlin, J. H.: Post-lymphographic percutaneous fine needle biopsy of lymph nodes guided by fluoroscopy. Radiology, *120:* 205-207, 1976.

Gruart, F. J., Yoel, J. and Wagner, A. M.: Value of perilingual lymphography in cancer of the head and neck. A means of exploration of the lymphatic system of the neck. Am. J. Surg., *114:* 520, 1967.

Howland, W. J.: A cannula method for lymphography. Am. J. Roentgenol. Radium Ther. Nucl. Med., *114:* 830, 1972.

Hreschyshyn, M. M., Sheehan, F. and Holland, J. F.: Visualization of retroperitoneal lymph nodes. Lymphangiography as an aid in the measurement of tumor growth. Cancer, *14:* 205, 1961.

Hudak, S. and McMaster, P. D.: The lymphatic participation in human cutaneous phenomenon. A study of the minute lymphatics of the living skin. J. Exp. Med. *57:* 751, 1933.

Iriarte, P., Jagasia, H. and Thurman, W. G.: Lymphangiography for malignant disease in children. J.A.M.A., *188:* 501, 1964.

Jing, B. S.: Improved technique of lymphangiography. Am. J. Roentgenol. Radium Ther. Nucl. Med., *98:* 952, 1966.

Kett, K., Varga, G. and Lukac, S.: Direct lymphography of the breast. Lymphology, *1:* 3, 1970.

Kinmonth, J. B.: Lymphangiography in man: a method of outlining lymphatic trunks at operation. Clin. Sci., *11:* 13, 1952.

Koehler, R. P.: Discussion: Pulmonary hazards of lymphography (Threefoot, S. A.). Cancer Chemother. Rep., *52:* 110, 1968.

Koehler, R. P., Meyers, W. A., Skelley, J. F. and Schaffer, B.: Body distribution of Ethiodol following lymphangiography. Radiology, *82:* 866, 1964.

Kreel, L.: The EMI whole body scanner in the demonstration of lymph node enlargement. Clin. Radiol., *27:* 421, 1976.

Kropholler, R. W., Blom J. M. H. and Irto, I.: Lymfografie met behulp van een polytheencatheter. Ned. Tijdschr. Geneeskd., *112:* 696, 1968.

Lee, K. F., Roy, W. M. and Hodes, P. J.: Improved techniques of lymphography: reliable isolation and cannulation method. J. Can. Assoc. Radiol., *20:* 48, 1969.

Mannila, T. and Wiljasalo, M.: Stereolymphography. Ann. Med. Intern. Fenniae, *54:* 139, 1965.

Matoba, N. and Kikuchi, T.: Thyroidolymphography. Radiology, *92:* 239, 1969.

Mortazavi, S. H. and Burrows, B. D.: Allergic reactions to patent blue dye in lymphangiography. Clin. Radiol, *22:* 389, 1971.

Pelu, G., Modigliani, V., Dal Pozzo, G. and Carini, L.: Thyroid adenolymphography. Minerva Chir., *29:* 261, 1974.

Riveros, M., Garcia, R. and Cabanas, R.: Lymphadenography of the dorsal lymphatics of the penis. Technique and results. Cancer, *20:* 2026, 1967.

Sachdeva, H. S., Chowdhary, G. C., Bose, S. M., Gupta, B. B. and Wig, J. D.: Thyroid lymphography. Arch. Surg., *109:* 385, 1974.

Sigurjonsson, K.: Lymphography without the aid of vital dyes. Lymphology, *7:* 121, 1974.

Tegtmeyer, J.: A new technique for cannulating lymphatic vessels: experience in 140 extremities. Lymphology, *7:* 116, 1974.

Threefoot, S. A.: Some chemical, physical and biological characteristics of dyes used to visualize lymphatics. J. Appl. Physiol., *15:* 925, 1960.

Threefoot, S. A.: Pulmonary hazards of lymphography.

Cancer Chemother. Rep., *52:* 107, 1968.

Tong, E. C. K.: Improved technique of lymphatic cannulation for lymphography. Experience with 300 cases.
Am. J. Roentgenol. Radium Ther. Nucl. Med., *107:*
877, 1969.

Turner, A. F.: Lymphangiographic needle clamp. Am. J.
Roentgenol. Radium Ther. Nucl. Med., *96:* 1053, 1966.

Tylen, U.: Personal communication, 1974.

Viamonte, M.: Advances in lymphangioadenography. Acta
Radiol. [Diagn.] (Stockh.), *2:* 394, 1964.

Viamonte, M. and Stevens, R. C.: A new tracer for lymphatic cannulation. Radiology, *86:* 934, 1966.

Wallace, S.: Personal communication, 1975.

Wallace, S., Jackson, L., Schaffer, B., Gould, J., Greening, R., Weiss, A. and Kramer S.: Lymphangiograms:
their diagnostic and therapeutic potential. Radiology,
76: 179, 1961.

Youker, J. E.: A clamp to facilitate lymphangiography. Br.
J. Radiol., *39:* 556, 1966.

Zheutlin, N. and Shanbrom, E.: Contrast visualization of
lymph nodes. Radiology, *71:* 702, 1958.

Zornoza, J., Wallace, S., Goldstein, H. M., Lukeman, J.
M. and Jing, B. S.: Transperitoneal percutaneous retroperitoneal lymph node aspiration biopsy. Radiology,
122: 111–115, 1976.

5

Interpretation

SIDNEY WALLACE, M.D., BAO-SHAN JING, M.D., MELVIN E. CLOUSE, M.D., AND DEWEY A. HARRISON, M.D.

Interpretation of the spectrum of lymphographic findings in clinical oncology has two major expectations. The first is to determine if nodes are abnormal and if so, the extent of dissemination of the disease or its stage.

A technically adequate bilateral pedal lymphangiogram consists of opacification of lymphatics and nodes of the inguinal, pelvic, and lumbar regions to the thoracic duct. This can be accomplished in adults by the use of 7 ml of contrast medium injected into a lymphatic in each lower extremity. When this is inadequate to visualize the lymphatic channels to the thoracic duct, a complete series of roentgenograms are done and then repeated after 15–30 min of ambulation. The contrast media will move from the lower extremities to fill lumbar lymphatics and the thoracic duct.

In analyzing lymphographic characteristics, the most difficult decision of the lymphographer is determining the presence or absence of malignancy in nodes. This can be perplexing when evaluating lymph node changes for lymphoma or solid tumors. The lymphographer must keep in mind the nonspecific response of lymph nodes to a variety of stimuli (Butler, 1968; Viamonte et al., 1963; Wallace and Greening, 1963; Parker et al., 1974; Castellino et al., 1974) and consider the lymphatic system as a functional unit.

Interpretation of the lymphangiogram depends upon the careful scrutiny of both the lymphatic and node phases. The lymphatic phase is especially important when evaluating metastases from solid tumors. Under normal circumstances the skeletal lymphatics from the lower extremities run a course paralleling the arteries and veins to empty eventually into the venous angle in the neck. A primary function of the lymphatic system is transporting fluid; continuity of the vessel through the nodes must be seen in the vessel phase. With aging, distortion of the lymphatic channels is secondary to dilatation and tortuosity of the adjacent blood vascular tree. The normal emptying time varies but is usually less than 4 hr after the end of the injection, depending upon the patient's activity.

Stasis of contrast material in lymphatics may be associated with obstruction. Frequently, however, the specific etiologic agent is not apparent. Most often stasis is not a clinically significant finding but usually a technical artifact.

Extravasation of contrast material is usually due to increased intralymphatic pressure either as the result of obstruction or the overzealous pressure of injection. If the obstructive process is not obvious, extravasation is also most frequently a technical artifact.

The nodal phase presents a fairly even distribution of the contrast material within the nodes which has been described as a reticular or granular pattern (Fig. 5.1). The margin of the node is well defined with the hilar area usually demarcated by a smooth indentation. *Lymphatic channels seen on the lymphatic phase must traverse this defect in order to consider the filling defect the hilum of the node.* Under normal circumstances there is an inverse relationship between the size and number of nodes: the larger the nodes, the fewer the number. The size varies in that the inguinal nodes are larger than the pelvic nodes which in turn are slightly larger than the lumbar nodes. A reversal of this relationship bears further investigation. The shape of the node is usually an elongated oval or kidney-shaped. Alterations in size, number, contour, and architecture occur in disease states. An increase in size and number is frequently seen as an abnormal finding as is the presence of a more rounded contour, but these are nonspecific. Architectural changes are most important.

The afferent, endothelium-lined lymphatics

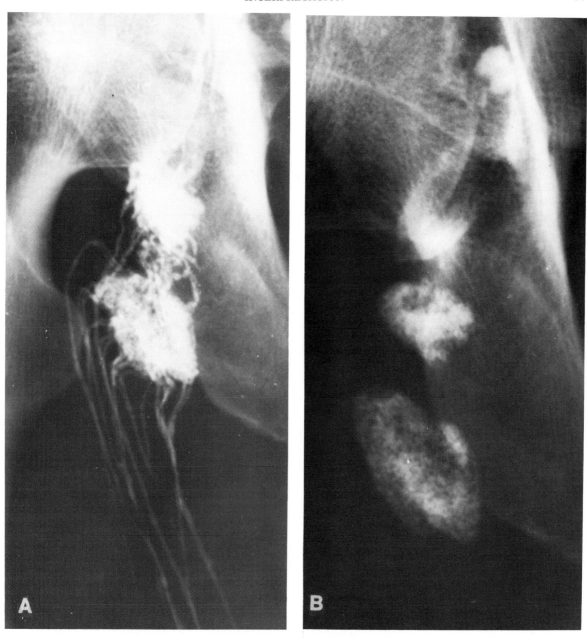

FIG. 5.1. NORMAL LYMPH NODES

A: Lymphatic phase. The afferent lymphatics enter at the marginal sinus. The efferent lymphatics exit at the hilus. *B:* Nodal phase. The defect in the node at the hilus must be confirmed by comparison with the lymphatic phase. The internal architectural pattern is granular and fairly homogeneous.

enter the node at the periphery and are continuous with the partially endothelium-lined sinusoids of the node. The efferent channels, completely lined by endothelium, emerge from the hilum of the node. In order to delineate individually the opacified lymphatics and nodes, it is essential to view each by multiple projections to obtain a three-dimensional evaluation. Magnification techniques and tomography are em-

ployed to enhance the presentation of this information.

Each lymphangiogram must be considered either positive or negative for nodal metastases, for equivocal interpretations are of little value in the management of the patient. If there is any doubt, the examination should be considered negative and the patient examined with follow-up films and, when necessary, a second lym-

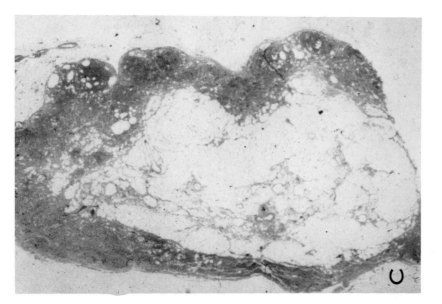

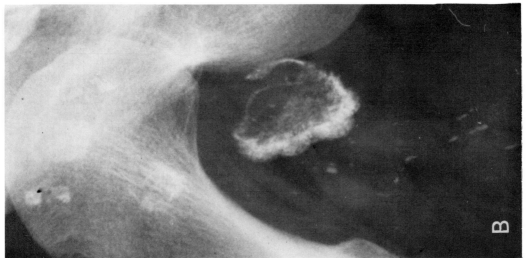

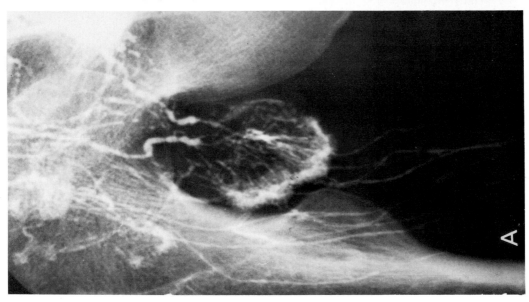

FIG. 5.2. FATTY REPLACEMENT

A: Lymphatic phase. The efferent lymphatics traverse the defect in the node. *B*: Nodal phase. The defect in the node must be further evaluated by comparison with the lymphatic phase. *C*: Specimen. There is deposition of fat in the hilus. The fat is traversed by the lymphatics.

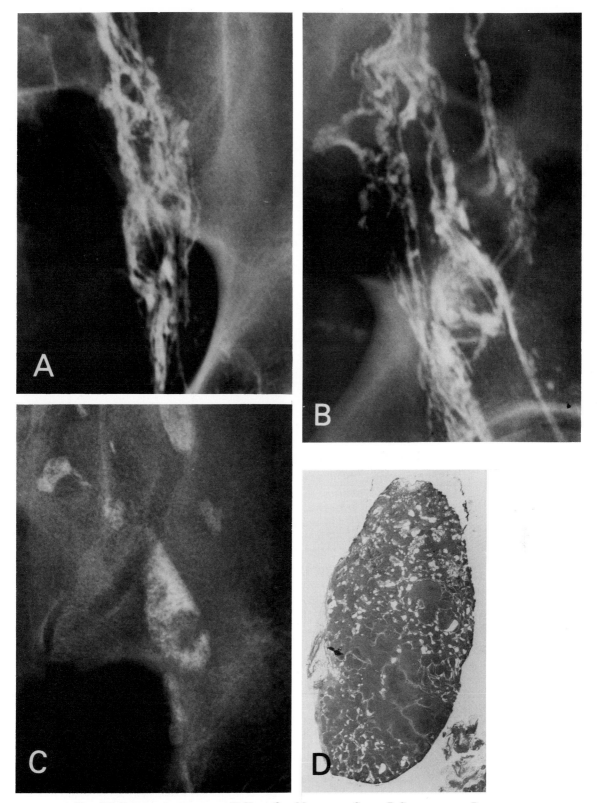

FIG. 5.3. LYMPHANGIOGRAM ON 55-YEAR-OLD MALE WITH STAGE B CARCINOMA OF PROSTATE
A: Lymphangiogram frontal view, nodes superimposed over unobstructed lymphatics. *B:* Left posterior oblique view. *C:* Lymph node shows filling defects. (2× magnification.) *D:* Microscopy. The filling defect was produced by reactive follicular hyperplasia. There is absence of contrast media in the sinusoids. (4× magnification.)

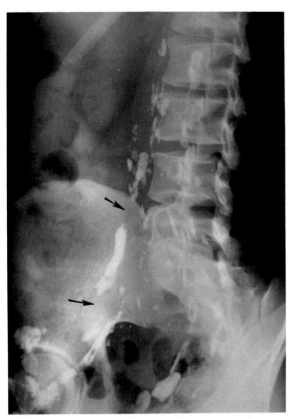

FIG. 5.4. 23-YEAR-OLD MALE WITH EMBRYONAL CELL
CARCINOMA OF RIGHT TESTIS

Two nodes in the right common iliac region (*arrows*) were completely replaced with tumor. The lymphatics did not show evidence of obstruction. Abnormal nodes could not be identified.

phangiogram. On the other hand, a definite diagnosis of metastatic disease must have a high degree of accuracy since its influence on patient management is great.

False positive interpretation of lymph node metastases has provoked considerable adverse criticism of lymphangiography. A proper evaluation must have a three-dimensional display since a false impression of a nodal defect may be due to superimposition of nodes. As previously stated, each node may exhibit a hilar defect which can be properly identified by reviewing the lymphatic phase. Of particular interest is an understanding of the problems that arise in the evaluation of the inguinal nodes. These nodes must be carefully scrutinized when they function as the primary site of drainage from neoplasms involving the lower extremities, perineum, and at times from the pelvic viscera. False positive findings have been reported in the inguinal area because of fatty replacement of nodal parenchyma (Fig. 5.2). False positive findings also occur in the iliac nodes but are

extremely rare (Fig. 5.3). Fibrosis is relatively rare and may occur as the result of repeated insults from minor infection or injuries to the lower extremities. In general these defects will be traversed by lymphatic channels which may be identified in the lymphatic phase (Fig. 5.2). Because of the difficulty of interpreting the inguinal nodes, the para-aortic nodes assume a position of unquestioned importance and value to the lymphographer; these nodes are more constant and the changes less variable with infrequent filling defects from fat or fibrosis (Abrams et al., 1968; Castellino, 1974; Fuchs, 1971; Kuisk, 1971; Jackson and Kinmonth, 1974; Viamonte et al., 1963).

A false positive interpretation may also be the result of inflammation. Acute inflammation is usually depicted by enlargement of the node with maintenance of the architecture. The acute reaction to the oil-based contrast material may produce temporary generalized enlargement of

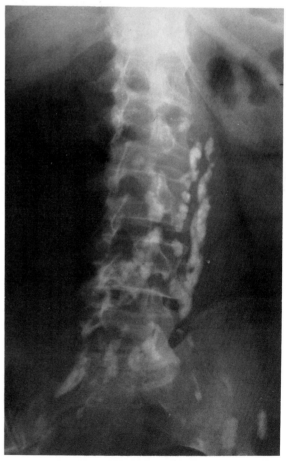

FIG. 5.5. 55-YEAR-OLD MALE WITH HODGKIN'S DISEASE IN
SUPRACLAVICULAR NODE

Lymphogram A and B negative. At laparotomy staging small positive celiac and splenic nodes were found.

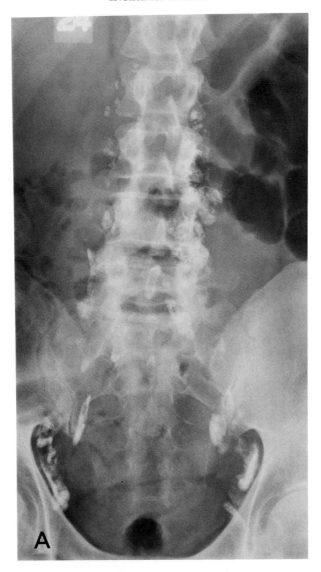

FIG. 5.6. SEMINOMA OF LEFT TESTICLE

A: The nodes in the left para-aortic area are foamy and indistinguishable from lymphoma secondary to reactive changes to seminoma metastases. The nodes in the left external iliac area show acute reactive changes from the orchiectomy. The iliac nodes on the right are normal.

Microscopy: *B* (400× magnification) shows areas of pure seminoma cells with little or no reaction, progressing to a histiocytic response (*C*, 400× magnification). With eventual destruction of the seminoma cells (*D*), there are complete caseation necrosis (*E*, 40× magnification) and giant cell formation (*F*, 400× magnification). The giant cells do not represent tumor giant cells.

the lymph nodes. The nodes will spontaneously decrease to normal size within a few months (Steckel and Cameron, 1966). Local defects such as small abscesses may also simulate carcinoma.

False negative interpretation has also invoked criticism of lymphography and may occur when microscopic metastases are present but not visible lymphographically. Small nodes, when completely replaced by tumor, may obstruct channels in lower order nodes without

evidence of collateral flow (Fig. 5.4). In addition, nodes may contain tumors that are not in drainage areas normally filled by pedal lymphography. This can occur with carcinoma of the testicle that drains to lateral lumbar nodes. In malignant lymphoma, disease may be present in lumbar, celiac, or splenic nodes that do not fill with contrast material (Fig. 5.5).

Another problem for the lymphographer is differentiating malignant lymphoma, leukemia, and solid tumor metastases from reactive

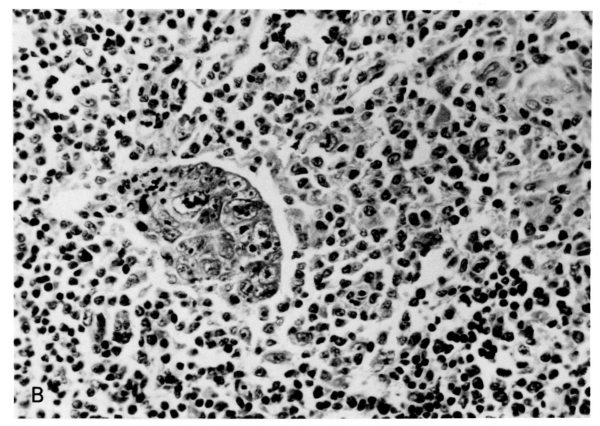

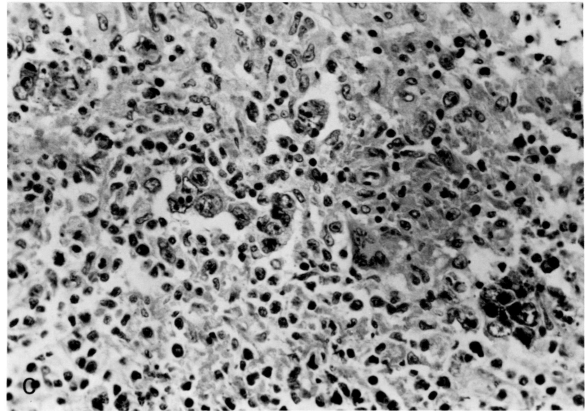

FIG. 5.6 B AND C

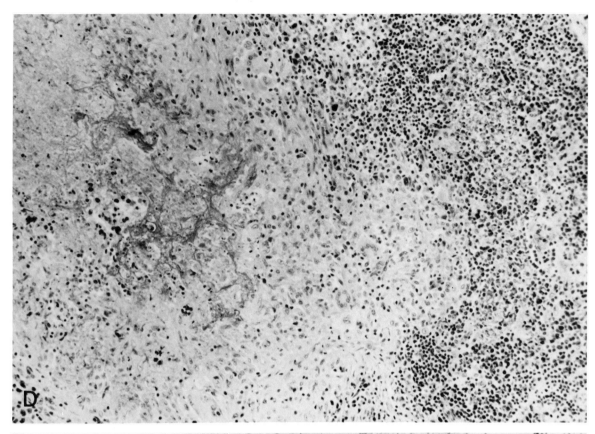

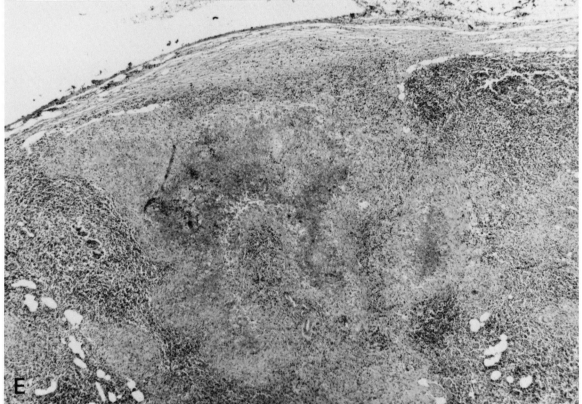

Fig. 5.6 D and E

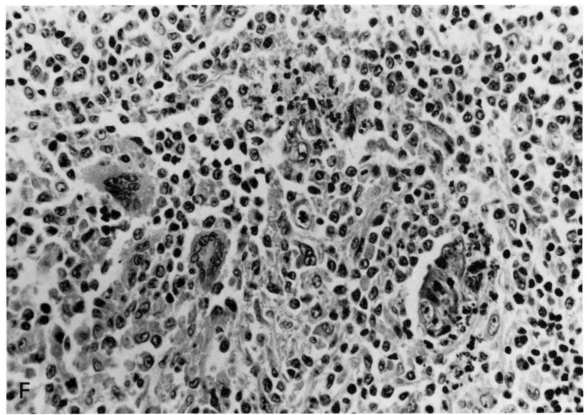

FIG. 5.6F

hyperplasia and other benign diseases affecting the lymph nodes (Akisada et al., 1969; Bergstrom and Navin, 1973; Kuisk, 1971; Viamonte et al., 1963; Parker et al., 1974; Raasch et al., 1969; Rauste, 1972; Renner et al., 1971; Wolfel and Smalley, 1971; Walter et al., 1975). Parker et al. indicate that malignant lymphoma can be differentiated from reactive hyperplasia. They believe that in reactive hyperplasia the nodes in every region are involved to the same degree whereas lymphomatous nodes usually exhibit gradations of involvement (even though the nodes in all areas may be diseased). The mechanism for the dissemination of reactive hyperplasia in patients with lymphoma may be different from that seen with solid tumors because generalized reactive changes are consistent with generalized inflammatory processes. Reactive hyperplasia associated with solid tumors is more local than in Hodgkin's disease. It begins and is more pronounced in the primary echelon drainage nodes. The nodes downstream from the tumor show reactive changes while those upstream have normal architecture. As an example, carcinoma of the bladder may produce reactive hyperplasia in iliac and para-aortic nodes while the inguinal nodes remain normal (see Fig. 7.2A and B). The same is true for carcinoma of the testicle (Fig. 5.6). The primary testicular drainage nodes in the aortic area are large and foamy (pseudolymphoma appearance) with reactive changes from seminoma metastases. The nodes of the left iliac and inguinal areas have minimal reactive changes from the orchiectomy. The reactive response in the inguinal and iliac areas after operation is almost always present.

Lymphoid hyperplasia associated with many infections or collagen diseases presents a picture similar to that seen with leukemia. Granulomatous diseases would naturally cause confusion as they do microscopically (i.e., sarcoidosis, tuberculosis, etc.). Hodgkin's disease, especially of the nodular sclerosing variety, and histiocytic lymphoma (reticulum cell sarcoma) may result in similar abnormal architectural patterns.

Tuberculosis with cavitation and destruction of a portion of the node (Fig. 5.7) and Hodgkin's disease or histiocytic lymphoma with partial replacement of the lymph nodes at times are difficult to differentiate from carcinoma. Despite these problems, considerable valuable in-

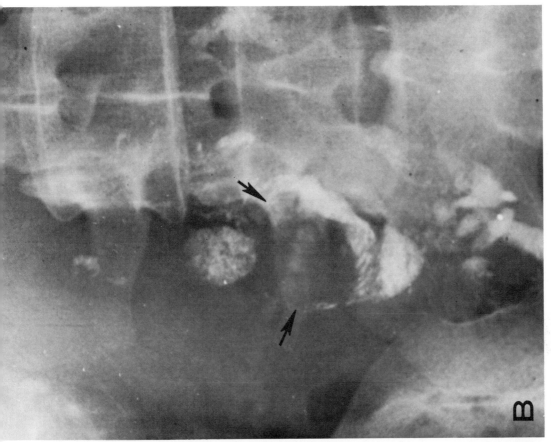

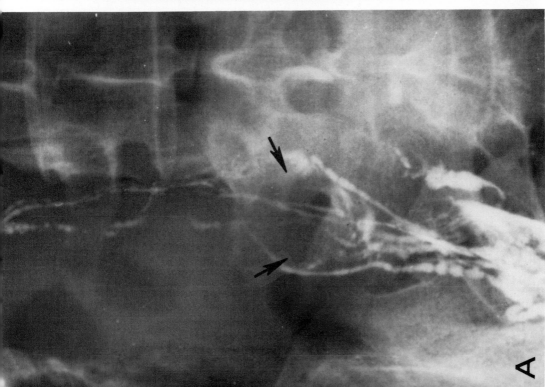

FIG. 5.7. SIMULATING CARCINOMA PATTERN

A and B: Tuberculosis. Caseation necrosis produces destruction of a portion of the node (*arrows*). The lymphatics do not traverse the area of caseation. C and D: Hodgkin's disease, mixed cellularity. The area of involvement was not traversed by lymphatics (*arrows*). Six months later the more classical pattern was obvious in this and the surrounding nodes. E: Histiocytic lymphoma (*arrow*) may mimic carcinoma.

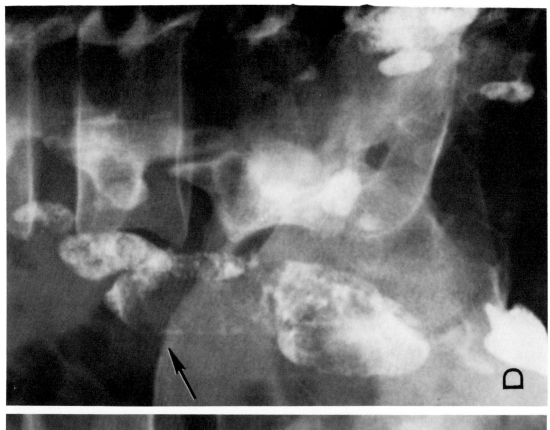

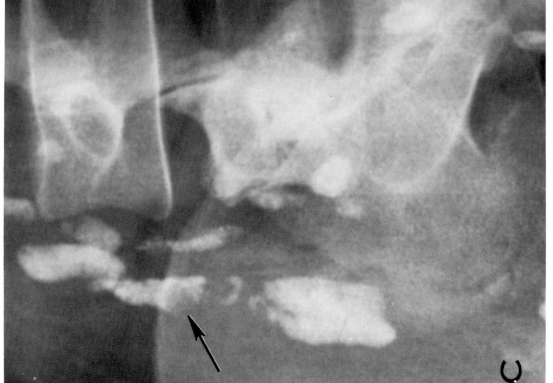

FIG. 5.7 C AND D

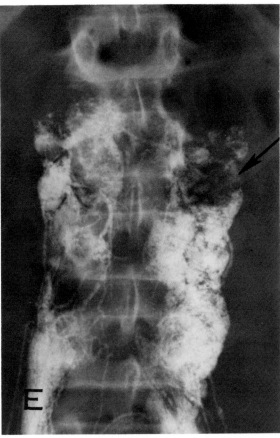

FIG. 5.7E

formation is offered by lymphangiography in assisting in the formulation of the differential diagnosis and the localization of grossly abnormal lymph nodes. In the presence of a known malignancy, lymphangiography has considerable value in determining the extent of involvement.

REFERENCES

Abrams, H. L., Takahashi, M. and Adams, D. F.: Usefulness and accuracy of lymphangiography in lymphoma. Cancer Chemother. Rep., 52: 157, 1968.

Akisada, M., Tasaka, A. and Mikami, R.: Lymphography in sarcoidosis: comparison with roentgen findings in the chest. Radiology, 93: 1273, 1969.

Bergstrom, J. F. and Navin, J. J.; Luetic lymphadenitis: lymphographic manifestations simulating lymphoma. Report of a case. Radiology, 106: 287, 1973.

Butler, J. H.: Nonneoplastic lesions of lymph nodes of man to be differentiated from lymphoma. Natl. Cancer Inst. Monogr., 32: 233, 1968.

Castellino, R. A.: Lymphographic-histologic correlation in patients with Hodgkin's disease and non-Hodgkin's lymphoma undergoing staging laparotomy. Lymphology, 7: 153, 1974.

Castellino, R. A., Billingham, M. and Dorfman, R. F.: Lymphographic accuracy in Hodgkin's disease and malignant lymphoma with a note on the "reactive" lymph node as a cause of most false positive lymphograms. Invest. Radiol., 9: 155, 1974.

Fuchs, W. A.: Neoplasms of epithelial origin. In Angiography, ch. 79, edited by H. L. Abrams. Boston, Little, Brown & Co., 1971.

Jackson, B. T. and Kinmonth, J. B.: The normal lymphographic appearances of the lumbar lymphatics. Clin. Radiol., 25: 175, 1974.

Kuisk, H.: Technique of Lymphography and Principles of Interpretation, pp. 275–278. Green, St. Louis, 1971.

Parker, B. R., Blank, N. and Castellino, R. A.: Lymphographic appearances of benign conditions simulating lymphoma. Radiology, 111: 267, 1974.

Raasch, F. O., Cahill, K. M. and Hanna, L. K.: Histologic and lymphangiographic studies in patient with clinical lepromatous leprosy. Int. J. Lepr., 37: 382, 1969.

Rauste, J.: Lymphographic findings in granulomatous inflammations and connective tissue diseases. Differential diagnosis between those diseases and lymphomas.

Acta Radiol. Suppl., *317:* 1, 1972.

Renner, R. R., Nelson, D. A. and Lozner, E. L.: Roentgeno-logic manifestations of primary macroglobulinemia (Waldenstrom). Am. J. Roentgenol. Radium Ther. Nucl. Med., *113:* 499, 1971.

Steckel, R. J. and Cameron, T. P.: Changes in lymph node size induced by lymphangiography. Radiology, *87:* 753, 1966.

Viamonte, M., Altman, D., Parks, R., Blum, E., Bevilac-qua, M. and Recher, L.: Radiographic-pathologic cor-relation in the interpretation of lymphangioadeno-

grams. Radiology, *80:* 903, 1963.

Wallace, S. and Greening, R.: Further observations in lymphangiography. Radiol. Clin. North Am., *1:* 157, 1963.

Walter, J. F., Soderman, T. M., Cooperstock, M. S., Book-stein, J. J. and Whitehouse, W. M.: Lymphangio-graphic findings in histoplasmosis. Radiology, *114:* 65, 1975.

Wolfel, D. A. and Smalley, R. H.: "Lipoplastic" lymphade-nopathy. Am. J. Roentgenol. Radium Ther. Nucl. Med., *112:* 610, 1971.

6

Abnormal Lymphatics

THE LYMPHEDEMAS

THOMAS F. O'DONNELL, JR., M.D.

Most investigators have accepted the basic classification of lymphedema into primary and secondary forms as set forth by Allen et al. (1946). Secondary lymphedema is usually acquired, while primary lymphedema is related to in utero developmental defects. Kinmonth et al. (1957) have further subdivided the primary lymphedemas by age of onset: congenital, present at birth; praecox, present before age 35; and tarda, occurring after age 35. The utility of this later classification rests in its applicability to the clinical diagnosis and management of lymphedema. This subdivision also recognizes the concept that developmental defects in the lymphatic system are present at birth but may express themselves later in life (praecox or tarda). After the development of clinical lymphography, Kinmonth (1969) proposed another form of subdividing the primary lymphedemas by lymphographic pattern. Not only did this method permit further classification along anatomic lines, but it also provided an approach to investigation of the etiology of primary lymphedema.

On the basis of lymphography the lymphedemas are divided into aplasia, no demonstrable lymphatic vessels; hypoplasia, a decreased number of vessels; and hyperplasia, an increased number of lymphatic vessels. Lymphography determines whether the process is indeed lymphatic in origin, has important prognostic value (e.g., hyperplasia may be associated with lesser degrees of lymphedema and may be more frequently bilateral than hypoplasia), and assesses the feasibility of potential surgical therapy (e.g., whether a lymphovenous shunt is possible).

Etiology

Primary Lymphedema

Primary lymphedema is probably due to a developmental defect in the lymphatic system. In this regard lymphedema resembles the other vascular dysplasias. Lymphatic abnormalities are often associated with arterial and venous dysplasia in the same limb (O'Donnell et al., 1976a) as well as other congenital anomalies. Lymphographic examinations of a few congenital cases of lymphedema have demonstrated aplasia or severe hypoplasia. Why some forms of lymphedema are delayed in their clinical expression is less clear. Certainly, other factors must influence the appearance of the functional abnormality. Bilateral lymphography of clinically unilateral lymphedema frequently demonstrates hypoplastic lymphatics in the clinically normal leg. The predilection for the left lower extremity, female preponderance, and peak incidence at puberty suggest that hormonal changes may be associated with the appearance of clinical lymphedema. In contrast, the development of lymphedema after minor surgery or trauma implicates damage to functioning collateral pathways.

Two groups have favored an acquired cause of primary lymphedema. Olszewski and his colleagues (1972b) suggested that inflammatory changes within the lymphatic vessels or lymph nodes may result in primary lymphedema. Biopsy specimens from 30 patients with primary lymphedema demonstrated that all layers of the wall were normally developed but that the lumen was obstructed by a thickened intima. In addition, 50% of their patients, who had a hypoplastic lymphographic pattern, exhibited lymph stasis changes similar to those observed in postinflammatory states. Based on these histologic and radiologic findings, Olszewski and his colleagues felt that inflammation, most likely related to infection, caused progressive obliteration of the lymphatic vessel to hypoplasia. By contrast the hyperplastic form had different histologic findings characterized by a hypertrophied muscular layer with an unobstructed vessel lumen. On cinelymphography, increased contractility was observed. These investigations offered a different explanation for the hyperplastic type of primary lymphedema, i.e., that it was a consequence of obstruction.

An alternate acquired theory has been forwarded by Calnan (1968). He challenged the belief that alterations in the lymphatics were the basic cause of primary lymphedema. Since lymphedema has its highest incidence of onset during puberty with many cases presenting later, an acquired cause seemed more likely. The preponderance of females affected and the predilection for involvement of the left leg suggested that an anatomic defect was responsible. Subsequent experiments conducted by Calnan and Kountz (1965) and by Burn (1968) demonstrated that structural and functional lymphatic abnormalities resulting in lymphedema could develop after venous obstruction. Calnan proposed that the left iliac vein was compressed by the right iliac artery and that the resultant obstruction led to increased venous pressure and subsequent lymphatic abnormalities. This theory gained support from the observations of Rigas et al. (1971) that femoral vein pressure increased in several patients with primary lymphedema. Unfortunately, the venous obstruction theory could not be substantiated by other investigators. Negus et al. (1969) disproved two links in the chain of events. In a series of 12 patients with primary lymphedema, he found normal femoral vein pressures. Both

in acrylic injection casts of the left iliac vein and on femoral venograms, Negus and associates noted indentation of the vein but no true obstruction. Moreover, the fundamental weakness of the venous obstruction theory is that it is difficult to rationalize hypoplasia, the most common (90%) pattern of lymphography, as a result of obstruction.

In view of the evidence to date, primary lymphedema, particularly of the hypoplastic type, would appear to be due to a developmental defect. Factors which can be construed as secondary may modify its expression.

Secondary Lymphedema

Although the causes of secondary lymphedema are varied (Table 6.1), interruption of lymphatic continuity by obstruction or by extirpation is the usual cause. This may occur either at the nodal or truncal level. For example, removal of the major lymphatic trunks and regional nodes of the arm may be followed by significant limb swelling in 10–30% of cases. Other factors such as secondary infection or radiation modify the incidence of lymphedema. In an experimental preparation of secondary lymphedema (Olszewski, 1973), removal of skin, subcutaneous tissue, and lymphatics is followed by transient edema within the first month in all animals (acute surgical lymphedema). This edema resolved by 6 weeks, but 35% of the animals had significant lymphedema at 2 years and 55% at 5 years. Serial lymphograms revealed progressive dilatation of lymph vessels and numerical hyperplasia. Lymph protein content was increased two-fold.

Following cancer surgery, especially radical mastectomy, several factors other than removal of lymph nodes and trunks have been suggested as responsible for secondary lymphedema. Trauma to the axillary vein with subsequent perivenous fibrosis and obstruction, postoperative infection leading to destruction of lymphatic collaterals, and radiotherapy with result-

TABLE 6.1

Cause	Pathophysiology	Lymphographic Pattern
Malignant disease	Obstruction	Obstruction with collateral circulation
Radiation	Obstruction of lymphatic trunks by extrensic fibrosis at lymph node level	Obstruction
Surgical or traumatic excision	Obstruction	Obstruction with collateral circulation
Filariasis	Obstruction at lymph node level	Obstruction – widened varicose lymphatics with reflux
Pyogenic infection	Obliteration of lymphatic trunks	Hypoplasia

ant fibrosis of collaterals have all been incriminated in the development of secondary lymphedema.

Many authors have focused on the role of venous obstruction in relation to secondary lymphedema. In Hughes and Patel's 1966 study of 19 women with postmastectomy edema, all had partial or complete obstruction of the axillary vein as well as valvular damage, while 50% showed concomitant damage of their cephalic veins. Larson and Crampton (1973) emphasized that the venogram should be performed in 90% adduction, because 34% of normal limbs will show a positional obstruction. His series revealed obstruction or nonvisualization of the axillary vein in 8 of 14 patients evaluated for secondary lymphedema. Arnulf (1973) found similar venographic changes on 8 of 13 cases evaluated following radical mastectomy. In contrast to these abnormalities in venous *anatomy*, we were able to demonstrate significant venous hemodynamic changes in only 2 of 14 patients evaluated for problematic (<2 cm) secondary lymphedema (O'Donnell et al., 1976b; Raines et al., 1977). Maximal venous outflow examinations, which assess venous flow and therefore the presence of obstruction, were normal in the other 12 patients. It is evident that venous obstruction is not the sole cause of secondary lymphedema. Collateral lymphatic vessels must develop to bridge the deficit caused by surgery.

In postmastectomy patients Kreel and George (1966) have shown by lymphography that this collateral flow may re-establish across the mastectomy site by 1–2 months and even drain to the opposite axilla. Kinmonth and Taylor (1954) had previously emphasized the importance of collateral pathways to the supraclavicular nodes, parasternal nodes, and across the operative site. Failure of these collateral pathways to develop, early destruction by infection, or late obliteration by radiotherapy or lymphangitis

may be responsible for the development of lymphedema. In our experience hemodynamically significant venous obstruction can aggravate edema caused by lymphatic abnormalities, while venous insufficiency alone can cause edema, much as it does in the lower extremity.

Filarial infection, an uncommon cause of secondary lymphedema in the United States, is related to the obstruction of the node or lymph trunk by the adult worm. That this infection is directly lymphatic and not blood-borne has been suggested by Gooneratne (1969). He linked the site of inoculation by the mosquito to the regional area eventually involved by lymphedema.

Although infection or inflammation is less a cause than a sequela of lymphedema, in patients with dermatitis or chronic venous insufficiency recurrent infection may lead eventually to secondary lymphedema. In several patients with post-thrombotic syndrome, we have shown obliteration of the superficial lymphatics. Vitek and Kaspar (1973) revealed obliteration of the *deep* lymphatic in 3 of 16 patients undergoing lymphograms of the deep lymphatic system for post-thrombotic syndrome.

Clinical Considerations

Symptoms. Since many of the symptoms and physical findings are similar in primary and secondary lymphedema, they will be discussed together (Table 6.2). In the initial or less advanced cases of lymphedema, the patient usually calls attention to the cosmetic defect produced by limb swelling. The edema generally involves the ankle or hand first, is worse at the end of the day, and resolves somewhat with elevation of the limb. As the degree of edema increases and involves more of the limb, it may not diminish with simple elevation. This lack of fluctuation with elevation or with simple compressive measures correlates well with the development of subcutaneous fibrosis. As the de-

TABLE 6.2
CLINICAL DIAGNOSIS OF LYMPHEDEMA

Symptoms	Physical Findings	Helpful Concomitant Physical Findings	Methods of Evaluation
Limb swelling	Edema of limb	Hyperplastic form	Lymphography
Heaviness	Dorsal buffalo hump	Distichiasis	Measurement of limb circumference
Recurrent lymphangitis	Elephantine distribution	Pedal angiomata	
Skin changes	Pinkish-red skin color	Amelogenosis imperfecta	Volume displacement
Fungal infections	Lichenification, peau d'orange	Congenital cardiac deformities	Xeroradiography radioactive albumin disappearance curves
	Subcutaneous tissue has lack of resilience	Gonadal dysgenesis	
		Pes cavus	
		Changes in long bones	

gree of lymphedema increases, the patient may experience a sensation of heaviness. The additional weight of fluid-filled tissue may actually encourage the patient to drag his foot or to avoid use of the upper limb in the performance of daily tasks. Mild aching discomfort or fatigue is common. By contrast, intense or severe pain is unusual in lymphedema and signifies a rapid increase in the degree of edema or massive swelling. The patient often describes the pain as bursting, "my leg feels like it is going to blow up." Lymphangitis, a frequent complication of lymphedema, also may produce a painful limb, but it is described as "prickly" and localized to the skin.

Physical Findings. With further progression of the disease process, the patient may observe skin changes such as thickening, lichenification, and pruritus (Table 6.2). These changes are aggravated by fungal, bacterial, or viral infections common to lymphedema. The development of these infections may be favored by pruritus-induced excoriation of the skin. The patient's scratching may lead to linear shallow areas of skin breakdown, but it is unusual for the patient with lymphedema to present with a frank ulcer.

The dimension and shape of the lymphedematous limb may be surprisingly characteristic (Fig. 6.1). The dorsum of the forefoot demonstrates a pathognomonic increase in the tissue contour. This distribution of edema is like a

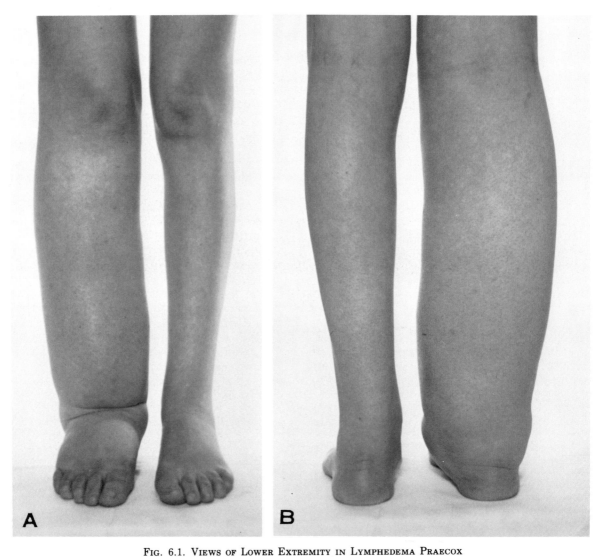

FIG. 6.1. VIEWS OF LOWER EXTREMITY IN LYMPHEDEMA PRAECOX
Right leg shows marked increase in subcutaneous tissue, producing a tree-trunk shape. Crease across ankle joint should be noted. The skin is relatively free of complications.

"buffalo hump" because the anterior margin of the ankle joint may be spared out of proportion to the degree of edema. There is usually a crease across the ankle joint and less edema distally at the metatarsal-phalangeal joint line. Both areas of sparing create a humping-up of tissue over the dorsum when viewed from the side (Fig. 6.2). The lower limb may be shaped like a tree trunk in a roughly cylindrical shape (Fig. 6.1). This contrasts with the distribution of edema in congestive heart failure or in venous insufficiency, where the edema is most severe in dependent or ankle areas. To take issue with an old clinical axiom, lymphedema, especially in the early stages, will pit. It is only when the degree of subcutaneous fibrosis becomes markedly increased that diminished tissue compliance prevents pitting (Young et al., 1976).

The type of skin changes observed in a lymphedematous limb mayu be helpfu in differential diagnosis as well as in grading the severity of the process. In mild lymphedema the skin is near normal in texture and in color (Fig. 6.3). Digital pressure will show pitting and yield a doughy sensation. A peau d'orange effect may be observed. Moderate lymphedema is associated with skin thickening, definite peau d'orange, and episodic bouts of cutaneous erythema (Fig. 6.2). The latter is due to lymphangitic attacks. Mild lichenification may be pres-

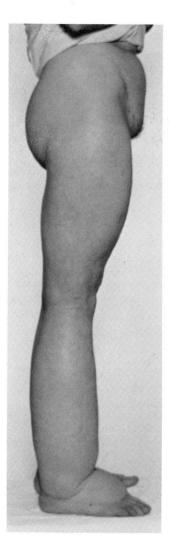

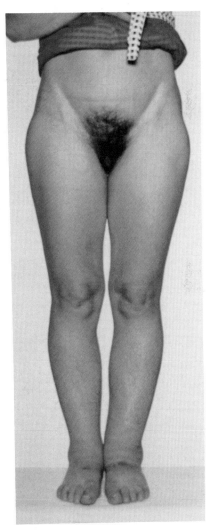

FIG. 6.2. LATERAL VIEW OF PATIENT WITH MODERATE LYMPHEDEMA PRAECOX
"Buffalo hump" effect can be seen on the dorsum of the right foot.

FIG. 6.3. YOUNG FEMALE PATIENT WITH MILD LYMPHEDEMA OF LEFT LOWER EXTREMITY
Edema is principally above and about the ankle joint. Dermal backflow is apparent at the interdigital clefts, where patent blue dye has been injected.

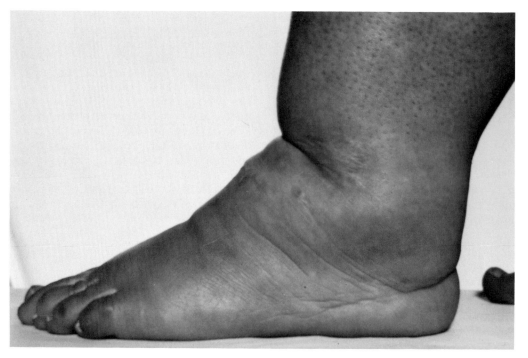

FIG. 6.4. LATERAL VIEW OF FOOT IN SEVERE LYMPHEDEMA
This demonstrates metatarsal-phalangeal joint sparing and "buffalo hump."

ent, and fungal infection may be observed in the interdigital clefts. More resiliency in the subcutaneous tissue indicates fibrosis. In severe lymphedema (Fig. 6.4) hyperkeratosis, lichenification, and fissures are observed in the skin. The subcutaneous tissue is firm. The skin may be discolored pinkish-red due to indolent cellulitis.

Distichiasis (reduplication of the eyelashes) and blotchy angiomata frequently accompany hyperplastic lymphedema. Amelogenesis imperfecta may also be present. A variety of cardiac lesions including pulmonic stenosis, atrial septal defect and patent ductus arteriosus have been associated with lymphedema. Careful auscultation of the heart should rule out previously unrecognized cardiac disease in patients with primary lymphedema. In Kinmonth's 1972 series 7% had gonadal dysgenesis in association with hypoplastic lymphatics. Four patients had the chromosomal pattern of Turner's syndrome and the characteristic webbed neck and increased carrying angle of the arms. In addition, pes cavus (Jackson and Kinmonth, 1970) and

abnormalities of the long bones of the lower leg have been described in association with primary lymphedema.

Milroy (1892) described a type of hereditary lymphedema characterized by its "congenital origin." Unfortunately, in practice Milroy's disease has become a synonym for any form of primary lymphedema. The term should be reserved for those rare cases of primary lymphedema (2% of 100 cases studied by Kinmonth, 1972) which are congenital, familial, and usually involve the lower limb. Kinmonth has reviewed the sex incidence of patients and their affected relatives and described a ratio of 48 males to 49 females. The genetics of Milroy's disease have not been fully elucidated, but an autosomal dominant mode of transmission has been favored. Esterly (1965) ruled out a different mode of inheritance. In Kinmonth's series (1972) lymphography revealed aplasia in the majority of cases. Two cases, however, showed severe hypoplasia. The degree of lymphedema is progressive and usually extends to involve the entire limb.

METHODS OF EVALUATION

The purposes of any investigation in lymphedema are three-fold: to establish the diagnosis, to assess lymphatic function, and to document the degree of lymphedema and its change with therapy. Lymphography is perhaps the most widely accepted form of evaluation (Table 6.3).

Some information can be obtained from the preparatory phase of the procedure, immediately following dye injection of patent blue dye into the dermis. In the normal limb a blue wheal is formed without any spidery streaming from the central hub. By contrast in lymphedema filamentous strands of dye-stained dermal lymphatics (dermal backflow) are observed. "Dermal backflow" may be more widespread in the obstructive or hyperplastic forms of lymphedema.

Lymphographic Patterns

Primary Lymphedema

Patients may exhibit aplasia, hypoplasia, or hyperplasia. Eustace and Kinmonth (1976) carried out a detailed analysis of 68 normal lymphangiograms (Fig. 6.5). In this study they described: (1) the mean number of lymphatic vessels; (2) the number of lymph nodes, i.e., h (1 mm $\pm$ 0.23); and (3) inguinal lymph node area of 88.35 mm^2 $\pm$ 418 mm^2. These data provide a unique reference point for objectively reviewing any lymphangiogram (Table 6.3).

Employing this method we (O'Donnell et al.,

TABLE 6.3
RESULTS OF LYMPHOGRAPHY IN PRIMARY LYMPHEDEMA

Series	No. of Cases	Aplasia	Hypoplasia	Hyperplasia	Normal
Buonocore and Young, 1965	20	7	13	–	–
Thompson, 1970	50	11	36	3	–
			(17 prox.*)		
Chilvers and Kinmonth, 1975	100	5	87	8	–
Olszewski et al., 1972a	120	46	65	9	–
			(24 prox.*)		
Saijo et al., 1975b	12	7	–	5	–

* Proximal hypoplasia with an obstruction.

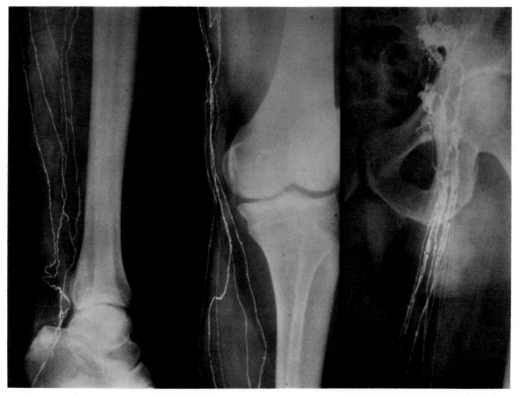

FIG. 6.5. NORMAL LYMPHANGIOGRAM OF THE LOWER EXTREMITY WITH VIEWS OF CALF AND THIGH
At the tibial plateau 4–5 beaded lymphatic trunks can be seen while 5–15 normal-calibered lymphatic trunks are visible in the inguinal region. This series of lymphangiograms provides a reference for the abnormal lymphangiograms.

1976a) have reviewed 20 lymphangiograms on patients with lymphedema associated with mixed vascular deformities. In this series 7 patients showed hypoplasia with 2.1 ± 0.8 vessels with a width of 0.63 mm ± 0.24 mm, 7 had hyperplasia with 18.5 ± 3.5 vessels with a width of 1.73 mm ± 0.53 mm, and 3 patients were normal. It is apparent that hypo- or hyperplasia can be described on the basis of number of trunks, their width, or both. This is less a problem than it appears. In general, lymphedema has been classified by the number of trunks. Hypoplasia is a decreased number of lymphatic trunks at a specific point—leg, thigh, inguinal, lumbar. Vessel width is usually decreased in addition or at the upper limits of normal (Fig. 6.6). Occasionally, as in proximal hypoplasia with distal hyperplasia, the width of the numerically hypoplastic trunk may be wider than usual (Figs. 6.7 and 6.8). By contrast, hyperplasia is defined by an increased number of trunks and may take one of two forms. In unilateral

megalymphatics, the more common form, the vessels are increased both in number and in width (Fig. 6.9) and are valveless. They resemble varicose veins. Megalymphatics may be associated with arterial and venous dysplasia, usually an arteriovenous fistula, capillary angiomata, chylous reflux, early presentation of edema, and an equal sex distribution without a family history of edema.

The second form of hyperplasia, which is frequently bilateral, has a striking increase in the *number* of lymphatic trunks (Fig. 6.10). Their width may be normal or only slightly increased. Besides mild bilateral edema, this group has several other unifying clinical findings. They demonstrate blotchy angiomata along the sides of the feet, distichiasis, and other congenital deformities; a family history of edema is common.

Table 6.3 compares the lymphographic findings in Kinmonth's series to other well known series. Hypoplasia is the most common abnor-

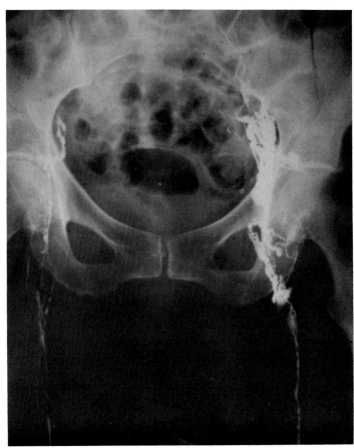

FIG. 6.6. LYMPHANGIOGRAM ILLUSTRATING HYPOPLASTIC PATTERN IN LOWER EXTREMITY DUE TO PRIMARY LYMPHEDEMA

There is numerical hypoplasia and a suggestion of decreased lymphatic caliber.

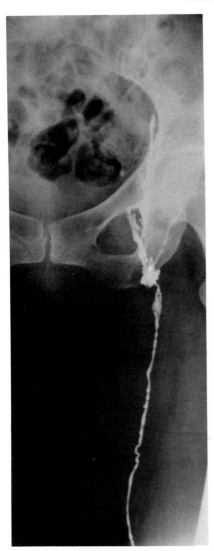

FIG. 6.7. ANOTHER FORM OF HYPOPLASIA (NUMERICAL TYPE) WITH NORMAL CALIBER LYMPHATIC VESSEL Valves are visibly intact in this vessel.

mality demonstrated on lymphography. The incidence of aplasia, which Kinmonth feels is a severe variant of hypoplasia, usually directly reflects the persistence and patience of the lymphographer.

Secondary Lymphedema

The pathogenesis of acquired lymphedema and the concomitant changes in the lymphogram are discussed in the section on obstruction (Table 6.3). The pattern which develops in patients with clinical lymphedema after cancer surgery is characterized by a progressive increase in the width and number of lymphatic trunks. Kreel and George (1966) demonstrated

this pattern of hyperplasia and marked dermal backflow in 8 patients following radical mastectomy. Hughes and Patel (1966) showed similar lymphographic changes.

In filariasis, widened varicose lymphatics are opacified with numerical hyperplasia. Cinelymphography reveals incompetence of lymphatic valves. By contrast lymphedema due to recurrent lymphangitis or cellulitis results in fibrosis and narrowing of the lymphatic vessels (hypoplasia), while the regional nodes are usually hyperplastic. Lymphography demonstrates small caliber, wispy lymphatic vessels.

Deep Lymphatics

Since most investigations have focused on the superficial or subcutaneous lymphatics, there is little data on the deep system in lymphedema. Kinmonth (1972) felt that they were deficient in primary lymphedema, much like the superficial system, and was unable to identify any trunks after injection of patent blue. Vitek and Kaspar (1973) carried out lymphography of the deep system in 12 patients with lymphedema. Two of 8 patients with primary lymphedema exhibited obliteration of their deep lymphatics with anastomosis to a defective superficial system. One of the 4 patients with secondary lymphedema showed a similar pattern. The remaining 9 patients had normal deep lymphatic systems.

Lymphatic Function

For clinical purposes transit time and radioactive albumin disappearance curves are the only two techniques which have enjoyed widespread use in the evaluation of lymphedema. Although the measurement of the time taken by a column of contrast media to reach a specific spot is crude and subject to many variables, a standardized technique does afford the opportunity to quantitate lymphatic function. Lipiodol injected into the pedal lymphatics at a rate of 0.142 ml per min will reach the inguinal nodes in 5 min and the sacroiliac joint in 35 min in a normal lymphatic system. Lymphatic stasis due to decreased vessel caliber (hypoplasia) or increased capacitance (numerical hyperplasia) may slow the transit time. The transit time may be the only evidence of lymphatic malfunction in some patients with mild edema and normal lymphatic anatomy by lymphography (Kinmonth, 1972)

One of the main functions of the lymphatic tree is to clear protein from the extravascular extracellular fluid space and return it to the intravascular space. The rate at which labeled

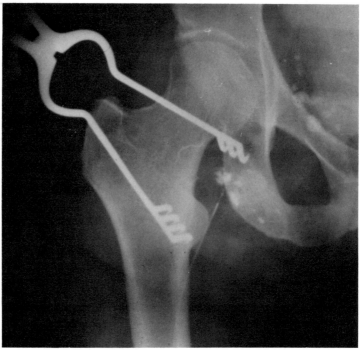

FIG. 6.8. NODOGRAM SHOWING SEVERE BILATERAL HYPOPLASIA

No lymphatic vessels could be found under microscopic examination of the foot, calf, and thigh. Injection of contrast material into a solitary inguinal lymph node demonstrates a thin wispy lymphatic vessel winding over the neck of the femur.

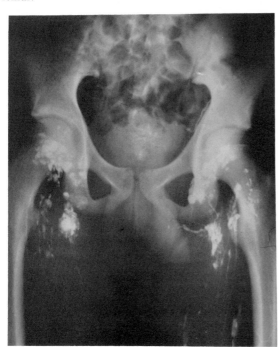

FIG. 6.9. LOWER LIMB LYMPHANGIOGRAM IN
LYMPHEDEMA OF RIGHT EXTREMITY
WITH HYPERPLASIA

There is persistence of contrast material within the abnormal lymphatic vessels. The vessels are increased in number and in width. There is an increased number of nodes.

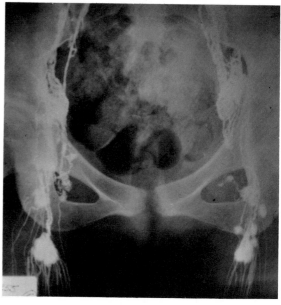

FIG. 6.10. LYMPHANGIOGRAM FROM PATIENT WITH
NUMERICAL HYPERPLASIA

The number of afferent lymphatic trunks is increased in the inguinal area.

albumin is cleared from this site should assess lymphatic function. Indeed, ^{131}I-albumin disappearance curves are prolonged in the lymphedematous limb. This delayed clearance may be related to pooling of albumin ("trapping") or to reversal of the normal subcutaneous tissue to muscle compartment pressure ratio. In lymphedema, interstitial fluid protein concentration is elevated and subcutaneous pressure is higher than muscle compartment pressure. Despite this attractive physiologic rationale, however, measurements of disappearance curves are of little value in the initial assessment of lymphedema (Emmett et al., 1967). This technique has found its greatest use in determining the effects of various surgical procedures on lymphedema (Thompson, 1970).

Degree of Lymphedema

The two standard methods for assessing the degree of lymphedema are measurement of limb circumference at specific anatomic sites and measurement of limb volume by water displacement. The *amount* of lymphedematous tissue is represented by the abnormal minus the normal dimension (Δ), while the *degree* of lymphedema is related to the Δ(abnormal-normal)/normal. Since there are no tables of normal values applicable to a wide range of limb dimensions, most clinicians use the contralateral limb as the control or normal value. These techniques are hampered by variation of technique, observer error from measurement to measurement, difference in "normal" limb size (especially in upper limbs), and lack of reproducibility.

To obviate this lack of consistency we have employed xeroradiography to assess the response to therapy. Skin and subcutaneous widths are measured by a standardized radiographic technique in millimeters at the midshaft of the radius or tibia. In a series of 11 patients with secondary lymphedema, we have demonstrated a four-fold increase in skin thickness and a two-fold increase in subcutaneous thickness (O'Donnell et al., 1976b). In addition to tissue widths, xeroradiography reflects the degree of subcutaneous fibrosis, which is related to tissue compliance on compressibility.

TREATMENT

Nonsurgical

The goals of nonoperative therapy are to decrease limb size, to preserve skin quality (if not to improve it), to minimize attack of lymphangitis, and to soften subcutaneous tissue (Table 6.4). Reduction in the degree of edema is accomplished by improving the function of remaining lymphatics and by utilizing alternative pathways for fluid transport. In addition to simple elevation, which reduces hydrostatic pressure, compressive therapy of some form is fundamental to accomplishing this end. Massage of the edematous limb and specially fitted elastic sleeves or hose are associated with reduction of limb girth. The effects of such a program are cumulative in my experience, but after a period the patient does reach a plateau. There is very little hard data on long term objective changes with this program. Zeissler et al. (1972) followed up 183 patients by questionnaire in a series of 385 patients with secondary lymphedema after mastectomy. Subjective improvement was noted by 123 patients, but unfortunately no objective measurements were carried out. This is a recurrent problem in evaluating results after the treatment of lymphedema. Despite the shortcomings of documentation in the literature, we have seen *objective* improvement on this program. Progressive skin changes appear to be minimized.

Greater reductions in limb size can be achieved by applying some form of intermittent compression to the limb. Molen and van der T'oth (1974) wind a soft rubber tube around the leg starting from the toes and progress proximally for compression, which they term "extubation." By developing a pressure of approxi-

TABLE 6.4
TREATMENT OF LYMPHEDEMA

Nonoperative	Operative	
	Physiologic	Excisional
Elevation	Buried dermal flap	Skin and subcutaneous tissue with split thickness skin graft coverage
Elastic compression	Lymphovenous shunt	
Massage	Full thickness skin bridge	Staged excision of subcutaneous tissue with vascularized local flaps
External pneumatic compression	Omental transposition	
Skin care	Subcutaneous tunnels	
Treatment of fungal and bacterial infections	Lysis of fibrotic venous obstruction	

mately 200–300 mm Hg, a rim of lymph was advanced up the leg proximal to the compressive force. They noted "good results." Terrier et al. (1973) also employed high pressure compression by applying 400 mm Hg to the limb with "successful" results. The possible trauma to arteries and other tissues from these high pressure forces is not yet clear.

We have employed external pneumatic compression, which is delivered at 60 mm Hg and at a rate of 12½ sec of compression alternating with 35 sec of rest. This pressure cycle is different from that of Allenby et al. (1973) (40 mm Hg pressure compression once per minute). Our pressure wave form is characterized by a fast upstroke and an even sharper downstroke. In a prospective study 11 patients were hospitalized to control pressure time and cycle. These patients showed a 51 ± 9% decrease in the degree of lymphedema as measured by hand circumference, 22 ± 6% by upper arm circumference, and 39 ± 5% by arm volume. Regression analysis demonstrated that greater changes in forearm circumference, 38 ± 8%, were observed with lesser degrees of subcutaneous fibrosis as documented by xeroradiography. Two patients with venous obstruction secondary to tumor were refractory to treatment. In our experience patients without significant venous obstruction and with lesser degrees of subcutaneous fibrosis appear to benefit the most from external pneumatic compression.

Besides compression, scrupulous skin care is essential in management of the lymphedematous limb. Foot hygiene with careful nail trimming and foot bathing with complete drying between the toes prevent the development of infection. Prompt treatment of fungal infection, which provides a beachhead for bacterial invasion, can decrease the frequency of lymphangitis. Although we have not advocated the prophylactic use of antibiotics in patients with lymphedema to prevent lymphangitis, we do recommend supplying the patient with the appropriate agents to treat fungal infections or early cellulitis. By early and aggressive treatment full-blown lymphangitis can be prevented.

Surgical Treatment

Indications for surgery are (1) *cosmetic,* to improve the shape and size of the limb and perhaps the psychological effect on the patient; (2) *functional,* to reduce limb weight and to improve skin texture; and (3) *preventative,* to minimize development of angiosarcoma, a lethal complication of lymphedema, or to decrease the incidence of lymphangitic attacks. We avoid surgery under the following circumstances: (1) minimal edema (i.e., when the difference in circumference between the two limbs is less than 3 cm); (2) gross obesity; (3) active progression of the disease (i.e., when the disease is not in a plateau stage); and (4) failure to establish a firm diagnosis of a lymphatic etiology. Kinmonth (1972) has divided the many forms of surgical treatment into two broad categories: physiologic and excisional (Table 6.4).

Physiologic Procedures (Table 6.4)

The essential purpose of these procedures is to promote drainage from deformed superficial lymphatics to normal lymphatics. The latter may be either deep lymphatics in the limb or lymphatic trunks more proximal to the abnormal. Although Kondoleon (1912) believed that excision of a wedge of deep fascia permitted superficial to deep lymphatic anastomosis, the changes in limb size were related more to removal of subcutaneous tissue than functional lymphatic anastomosis. Sistrunk (1918) further modified this procedure by excising a greater amount of subcutaneous tissue, which may explain the slightly better results.

Several surgeons have revived Handley's original operation (1908) in which subcutaneous tunnels are created by inserting a large silk thread from the hand to the shoulder area. The purpose of this procedure is to fashion a conduit to bypass fluids through the abnormal subcutaneous tissue and lymphatics to normal tissue. O'Reilly (1972) used nylon setons in postmastectomy edema with encouraging results in 2 patients, but no change in radioactive albumin studies. A recent series by Silver and Puckett (1977) showed that subcutaneous tunnels were "quite effective" in primary lymphedema. Perhaps the most attractive physiologic operation is the lymphovenous shunt first reported clinically by Nielubowicz and Olszewski (1968). In 4 patients with secondary lymphedema improvement in limb size was observed. Patency of the medulla and sinuses was demonstrated on postmortem examination in 1 patient who died from her primary disease, while lymphography showed a functioning lymphovenous anastomosis in the other 3 patients. A subsequent report of 16 patients with primary lymphedema (Politowski et al., 1969) observed from 6–18 months, however, revealed "good" results in only 8 patients, "fair" in 6, and "unsatisfactory" in 2. The lack of "very good" results is disappointing. Although the theoretical advantage of this technique is suggested by extensive animal experiments (Firica et al., 1972), lymphovenous shunt has not enjoyed widespread clinical use or success. This procedure appears ideally suited for an obstructive lymphedema with preservation of normal or near normal lymphatic vessels. Unfortunately, this is not the usual case.

The Thompson procedure (1962) or a variation thereof is presently the most widely used surgical procedure for lymphedema. The operation combines excision of subcutaneous tissue with fixation of the buried posterior flap to the deep fascia. Thompson felt this latter maneuver brought the subcutaneous and dermal lymphatics into contact with the deep lymphatics and muscle tissue so that spontaneous lymphatic or lymphovenous shunts could develop. Functional assessment with radioactive albumin disappearance curves has led to conflicting results. Thompson (1970) has demonstrated increased radioactive albumin clearance postoperatively. Sawney (1974), however, found a reduction in limb circumference and increased clearance only in the immediate postoperative period; these findings were not present in repeat follow-up studies several months later. Kinmonth (1972) has been unable to find any lymphatico-lymphatic or lymphovenous shunts on postprocedure lymphography. He feels that the improvement beyond what could be expected from simple removal of subcutaneous tissue is related to the compressive effect of the buried flap. Cinelymphography has shown traction and massaging of the abnormal lymphatics by the calf muscles. In addition the procedure may lead to normalization of the reversed subcutaneous to muscle compartment pressure ratio. Table 6.5 compares the results of several series for the Thompson procedure.

In an attempt to provide a pathway of normal lymphatics, Goldsmith (1974) employed omental transposition to bridge the area of lymphatic insufficiency. The long term results were disappointing. In 22 patients followed for 1–7 years, only 38% showed evidence of good results (by very liberal criteria), while 23% had fair results. He wisely suggests that the procedure be used by only a few surgeons experienced with this technique. Various surgeons have revised the original Gillies procedure, which employs a full thickness graft of tissue to bypass the lymphatic obstruction. Again this procedure depends on an area of localized blockage and relatively normal lymphatics below the block (Hirshowitz and Golden, 1971). In most cases this is not the anatomic finding. The various types of

TABLE 6.5

PHYSIOLOGIC OPERATIONS FOR LYMPHEDEMA

Series	Type of Procedure	No. Patients	Type	Results* Good	Results* Satisfactory (Fair)	Results* Poor	Criteria	Length of Follow-up (Years)
Thompson, 1970	Buried dermal flap	50	1°	29	17	4	Circumference, clearance studies	1–10
Thompson, 1969	Buried dermal flap	23	2°	14	8	1	Circumference, clearance studies	1–9
Sawney, 1974	Buried dermal flap	5	1°	No change	5		Circumference, clearance studies	>1
Bunchman and Lewis, 1974	Buried dermal flap	10	1°	2	4	4	Circumference, volume displacement	>1
Chilvers and Kinmonth, 1975	Buried dermal flap	79	1°	27%	56%	17%	Circumference, patient's and surgeon's evaluation	>1
Politowski et al., 1969	Lymphatic-venous fistula	16	1°	8	6	2	Circumference	1/2–1 1/2
Goldsmith, 1974	Omental transposition	22	Mixed	10	4	8	Size, function, frequency of cellulitis attacks	1–7

* Author's interpretation of varied criteria for each series.

physiologic procedures are further compared in Table 6.5.

Excisional Procedures (Table 6.4)

Charles (1912), working in an endemic area for tropical elephantiasis, developed a procedure consisting of removal of skin in addition to subcutaneous tissue. Split thickness skin grafts were applied to cover the exposed deep fascia. At present we restrict the Charles procedure to patients with severe skin changes that may prevent the use of vascularized skin flaps in the Thompson procedure. The thigh area must be tapered to avoid a "baseball pants" appearance. Late results are often complicated by the development of hyperkeratosis, recurrent sepsis, and condylomata.

Many surgeons now employ a variant of an excisional operation first described by Homans of Boston (1936). Subcutaneous tissue is excised in stages and well vascularized flaps are developed. Table 6.6 summarizes the results of various recent series which have used some form of subcutaneous lipectomy. In many instances the lack of uniform objective measurements or criteria for assessing the degree of lymphedema and its change with surgery limits meaningful interpretation of this data. With this procedure large volumes of subcutaneous tissue can be excised and the incidence of both flap necrosis and sinus formation are lower than with the buried dermal flap.

Special Procedures for Secondary Lymphedema

Both the lymphovenous shunt and the buried dermal flap have been employed in the treatment of secondary lymphedema. The lymphovenous shunt appears ideally suited for the obstructive form of lymphedema. In comparison to primary lymphedema, Thompson (1969) does not favor cosmesis as an indication for this procedure. The results of both the lymphovenous shunt and the Thompson procedure appear slightly better in secondary lymphedema than in primary lymphedema.

Whereas improvement of lymphatic function and removal of tissue bulk are the main targets of surgical intervention in primary lymphedema, relief of venous obstruction has been the focus of several procedures in secondary lymphedema. Hughes and Patel (1966) lysed the fibrotic encasement around the axillary vein with "good" results in 15 of 19 patients with postmastectomy lymphedema. More recently, Larson and Crampton (1973) described good results in 4 of 8 patients who underwent a similar procedure.

TABLE 6.6
EXCISIONAL OPERATIONS FOR LYMPHEDEMA

Series	Type of Procedure	No. of Patients	Type 1°	Type 2°	Results* Good	Results* Satisfactory (Fair)	Results* Poor	Criteria	Length of Follow-up (Years)
Fonkalsrud and Coulson, 1973	Subcutaneous lymphangiectomy	6	6	—	6	—	—	Cosmetic, functional	At least 1
Bunchman and Lewis, 1974	Charles (complete excision of subcutaneous tissue and skin)	14	14	—	14	(But undesirable pantaloon effect)	—		>5
Miller, 1975	Staged subcutaneous excision	14	6	8	—	←14→	—	Circumference	1/2–6 (6 for 4–6)
Bunchman and Lewis, 1974	Staged subcutaneous excision	5	5	—	5	—	—		1 1/2

* Author's interpretation of varied criteria for each series.

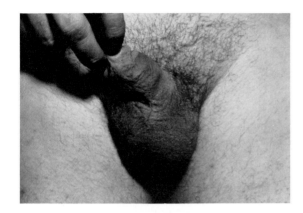

FIG. 6.11. VIEW OF SCROTAL AREA IN PATIENT
WITH CHYLOUS VESICLES

Other vesicles can be noted in the right anterior thigh area.

Genital Lymphedema

Genital lymphedema is the third most common form of lymphedema and its classification follows that used for the extremities. Genital lymphedema may be the sole clinical manifestation of lymphedema or associated with (1) involvement of adjacent tissue, (2) vesicle formation (Fig. 6.11), (3) skin changes, or (4) signs of sepsis (abscess, cellulitis, and inguinal adenopathy). Proximal hyplasia with arborization of the more distal subdermal lymphatics is demonstrated on lymphography, which differs from the pattern observed in secondary genital lymphedema. The acquired form is frequently due to filariasis, which lymphography shows as dilated incompetent lymphatics with reflux.

Indications for surgery in genital lymphedema are similar to those for lymphedema of the extremities: (1) gross swelling of the scrotum or penis and (2) recurrent fistula or sepsis. Concomitant reduction of the mons veneris may be required in women. At St. Thomas Hospital the procedures on male patients have ranged from excision of tissue (such as simple circumcision or partial excision of penile and scrotal tissue) to more extensive operations such as scrotal reduction. When the penile skin is severely lichenified, replacement with split thickness skin graft is favored. Good functional results have been obtained. In a series of 28 patients with genital lymphedema due to filariasis, 18 underwent partial or subtotal scrotectomy, while 7 had total scrotectomies with repair by skin graft or by inguinal replacement (Khamma, 1970). Nineteen required some form of penoplasty. Other than considerable lymphatic drainage in the early postoperative period, no other complications were noted and the later results were quite good.

CHYLOUS SYNDROMES

The anatomic locations of chylous disorders are varied and range from the peritoneal and thoracic cavities where chyle forms fluid collections to the neck, urinary tract, and genitalia where chyle may drain as a fistula. Chylous syndromes, like lymphedema, may be either primary (idiopathic) or secondary. As discussed in the preceding section, obstruction of the main lymphatic vessels by malignancy, infection, or trauma are the chief causes of the chylous syndromes. They are best discussed in detail according to their anatomic relationships.

Lower Extremities

The triad of lymphedema (commonly unilateral), cutaneous vesicles, and angiomata are characteristic of chylous syndromes involving the lower extremities. Lymphography demonstrates markedly dilated and capacious lymphatics—megalymphatics (Fig. 6.12). In a few patients with megalymphatics, Kinmonth (1972) visualized an abnormally functioning thoracic duct on cinelymphography. Obstruction of the thoracic duct was not, however, a consistent finding in all cases of megalymphatics studied by Kinmonth. Because of this inconsistency and the frequent finding of unilateral involvement, many have found it difficult to rationalize the mechanism on the basis of thoracic duct obstruction alone. As suggested by Kinmonth et al. (1964), the association of chylous diseases with other congenital anomalies such as angiomata make it utero developmental error the most likely cause. Ligation of the incompetent lymphatic trunks at the pelvic (Fig. 6.12) or inguinal level may prevent reflux and result in both subjective and objective improvement.

Chylous Ascites

The primary form may be of two types, fistulous or exudative. A rent in a large and dilated lymphatic vessel leads to the formation of a fistula which may be visualized on lymphography. In addition to a fistulous communication with the peritoneal cavity, large capacious megalymphatics are demonstrated by lymphography. Weichert and Jamieson (1970) have described 2 cases of chylous ascites that showed dilated lumbar lymphatics and lymphographic findings suggestive of thoracic duct obstruction.

In contrast the exudative type of chylous ascites is associated with a hypoplastic pattern on lymphography. No discrete site of lymphatic leakage is defined. Before undertaking treatment of chylous ascites, lymphography should be carried out to demonstrate whether it is of the fistulous or exudative type. The fistulous form may be corrected by closure of the defect in the lymphatic vessel, its level also being localized by lymphography. The exudative form may require a lymphovenous shunt or a mechanical peritoneal-atrial shunt. In general, chylous ascites secondary to a fistula responds better to therapy than the exudative form.

Acquired chylous ascites was four times more frequent than the primary type in Vasko and Tapper's (1967) extensive review of 126 cases of chylous ascites. Of these, 28 cases were due to an inflammatory process, 24 to neoplasm (lymphoma 6, pancreatic carcinoma 4), and 9 due to trauma. The authors emphasize the high mortality in the untreated cases, being 43% for adults and 29% for children. By contrast 16 of the 28 treated cases recovered.

Chylothorax

The causes of chylothorax are similar to chylous ascites: idiopathic, neoplasm, and trauma. The thoracic duct carries approximately 2400 ml/24 hr of lymph, rich in protein and fat. Continued loss of this fluid results in electrolyte and nutritional depletion. Lymphography not only assists in localizing the site of fistulous formation but also defines the anatomy of this highly variable (50%) structure. Therapy of chylothorax is difficult and is well discussed in a recent review of 15 cases by Selle and his colleagues (1973). The *congenital* or idiopathic cases appear to respond well to a more conservative regimen of multiple thoracenteses, which was advocated originally by Randolph and Gross (1957). When associated with *malignant* disease, chylothorax is usually indicative of widespread disease and a conservative approach is warranted. Those cases following trauma, which may be as varied as cardiac surgery, subclavian catheterization, scalene node biopsy, radical neck surgery, and gunshot wounds, require the most judgment. An initial nonoperative course is recommended with surgery reserved for (1) large chylous loss (1500 ml/24 hr); (2) no decrease in chyle drainage after 10–14 days; and (3) electrolyte or nutritional complica-

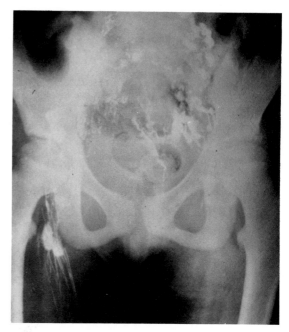

FIG. 6.12. LYMPHANGIOGRAM SHOWING CHYLOUS REFLUX
There is numerical hyperplasia in the right groin; large dilated and capacious lymph vessels are visible in the pelvic region.

tions. This latter problem is substantial, being the primary cause of death of one patient in Kinmonth's series (1972). This latter patient was apparently improved by a lymphovenous shunt, but died from the effects of preoperative depletion by the chylothorax.

Chyluria

Chyluria is an abnormal condition in which intestinal chyle appears in the urine because of a fistulous communication between the intestinal lymphatics and the urinary tract. Tropical chyluria is a widespread disease of the tropical and subtropical areas of Asia, Africa, Australia, and America, especially along the seacoast and neighboring islands. It is most commonly associated with the Filaria parasite, but other parasites have been found in patients with chyluria. Wücherer (1868) discovered the pathogen, and Lewis (1873) in Calcutta found the microfilaria in the blood and urine of a chyluric patient. Manson (1883) pointed to the mosquito as the intermediate host transmitting the larvae to humans. The larvae migrate into the large lymphatic vessels and nodes and mature. The filarial parasite causes a lymphangitis with lymphocytic and eosinophilic infiltration and fibroblastic proliferation (Cohen et al., 1961). Possibly the most serious damage occurs from the debris of dead parasites. O'Connor (1932) described a foreign body granulomatous reaction to the dead parasite with obstruction of the lymphatic vessel.

The nontropical form of chyluria is unusual and is frequently associated with conditions which obstruct the thoracic duct. Etiologies associated with this form include malignancy, especially those involving the retroperitoneum and chronic inflammatory disease such as tuberculosis.

Various theories have been advanced to explain the transit of chyle into the urine. Ackerman (1863) attributed it to obstruction of the lymphatics between the intestines and the thoracic duct, but 42 chyluric patients with completely normal thoracic ducts have been described elsewhere (Koehler et al., 1968; Rajaram, 1970). Nine others had mild abnormalities. In addition, experiments by Field and Drinker (1931a, b) and Blalock et al. (1937) make it apparent that simple obstruction of the lymphatics is difficult to obtain. In only 3 of Blalock's 52 animals could the lymphatics be completely obstructed. Field and Drinker did produce lymphedema by repeated injections of sclerosing material into the lymphatics and repeated ligations of lymphatic vessels.

The most likely explanation for the reflux of the chyle into the retroperitoneal lymphatics is

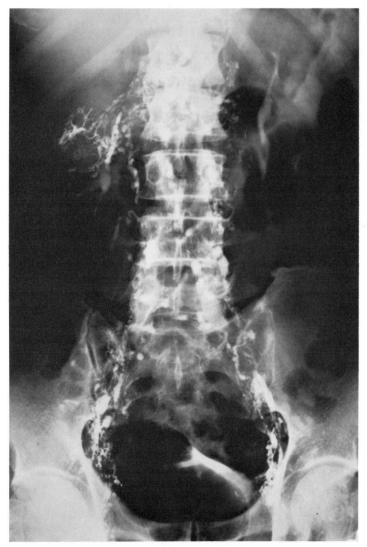

FIG. 6.13. PARASITIC CHYLURIA

Lymphangiogram shows large tortuous lymphatics in the iliac and para-aortic region with reflux of contrast material into dilated renal pedicle and tubular lymphatics. (Courtesy of Maria Zelia Silva, Rio de Janeiro, Brazil.)

obstructive fibrosis in the retroperitoneal lymph nodes with incompetence of the valves and lymphatic dilatation from increased pressure or endolymphatic inflammation.

The final escape of chyle and contrast material from the renal and tubular lymphatics into the collecting system has never been produced experimentally. Presumably, the tubular lymphatic ruptures with extravasation of contrast material from the lymphatic vessels into the interstitial space and then into the collecting tubules. Lee (1944) showed that fluid escapes through an intact lymphatic wall when the intralymphatic pressure is sufficiently elevated. The method of escape from the interstitial space into the collecting tubules, however, is far from clear.

Clinically, the onset of chyluria is sudden and may be associated with trauma or straining. Many patients experience back pain and weakness. Renal colic may occur, and there may be associated hematuria. The character of the urine is typical. Without associated hematuria, the urine is milky in color and clears dramatically by shaking the urine with ether or chloroform. Another simple test is the Sudan III fat stain. The duration of chyluria is rarely more than 2 weeks and in the majority of cases 1 week or less. There is loss of plasma protein and an increased susceptibility to infection. There is no correlation between an abnormal BUN or serum creatinine and chyluria. The disease is accompanied frequently by impaired renal function with decreasing glomerular filtration, especially when there is associated infection and pyuria.

The intravenous urogram is rarely abnormal. Hilar lymphatics may be seen on retrograde urography, but they are also seen occasionally in normal patients. The lymphographic findings are related to the degree of involvement. The pelvic and retroperitoneal vessels increase in size and number and may become tortuous. When there is elephantiasis, dilated tortuous vessels may be found in the leg, groin, and genitalia. Contrast material transit in the lymphatic vessels and various collateral lymphatics is prolonged. Contrast material may reflux into the renal and tubular lymphatics with demonstration of lymphaticourinary fistulae (Kittredge et al., 1963; Choi and Weidemer, 1964; Koehler et al., 1968; Rajaram, 1970) (Fig 6.13). Treatment is either by direct ligation of abnormal communicating lymphatics (Lloyd-Davies et al., 1967) or by injection of sclerosing solutions into the renal pelvis. The former is the favored approach.

NEOPLASMS OF THE LYMPHATIC VESSELS

The most common tumors arising from the lymphatic vessels are benign and are of three types (Kinmonth, 1972): (1) lymphangioma simplex, (2) cavernous lymphangioma, and (3) cystic hygroma.

Whether these abnormalities deserve the designation neoplasm is debated. They probably originate from sequestrated or poorly developed analages, rather than from actively proliferating neoplasms. By contrast angiosarcoma does represent a new growth, usually occurring in a limb with long-standing primary or secondary lymphedema.

Nearly 60% of lymphangiomata are present at birth as a mass or as an enlarging lesion (Saijo et al., 1975a). The head and neck region are the most common locations overall, especially for cystic and cavernous lymphangiomata. By contrast, simple lymphangiomata are most usually distributed on the trunk and chest wall (Fonkalsrud, 1974). In simple lymphangiomata lymphography demonstrates no communication with the superficial and deep lymphatic system, which is usually normal. Direct intralesional injection in cystic hygromas demonstrates a large dilated structure, distinct again from the lymphatic system. By contrast, cavernous lymphangiomata may communicate with the main lymphatic trunks. For example, we noted communication with the inguinal and pelvic lymph vessels in one 21-year-old male with a cavernous lymphangioma (Fig. 6.14).

The treatment of cystic hygromas and large cavernous lymphangiomata is usually excisional, but care must be taken to avoid injury to adjacent vital structures. Because of this threat, radiation and injection of sclerosing solutions have been advocated by some surgeons. Incomplete excision of the lesion is a common problem and may result in recurrence of the lymphangioma.

The appearance of reddish-brown nodules and plaques in a limb with chronic lymphedema may represent sarcomatous change. Angiosarcoma has been called Kaposi's sarcoma, but the latter is a distinct entity. Kaposi's sarcoma may

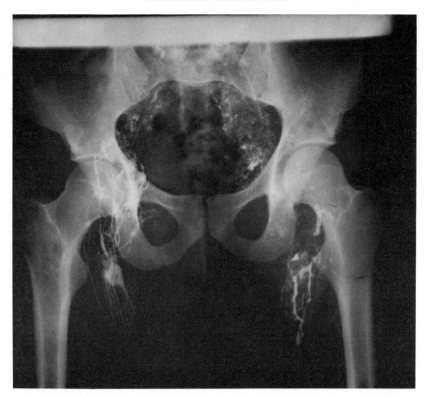

Fig. 6.14. Lymphangiogram from 21-Year-Old White Man with Lymphangioma of the Retroperitoneal Space
Lymphatic vessels are decreased in number in the left lower extremity. Multiple capacious primitive lymph capillaries are visible. Biopsy of this mass through a retroperitoneal space revealed recurrent lymphohemangioma.

arise in a nonedematous limb, is slow growing, and on histologic examination consists of spindle cells (Kinmonth, 1972). By contrast, angiosarcoma appears to be rapidly growing, especially when first clinically detected, and metastasizes widely. It is of endothelial cell origin. Despite radiation and surgical treatment, the outlook at present is bleak.

OBSTRUCTION AND COLLATERAL FLOW

MELVIN E. CLOUSE, M.D.

Obstruction of the lymphatics may not lead to edema if competent collateral pathways are available. Reichert (1926) completely transected the lymphatics and demonstrated a decrease in edema after the fourth preoperative day. This decrease correlated with regeneration and bridging of the superficial lymphatics at the incision site. Edema had cleared completely on the fifth postoperative day (after the bridging of the deep lymphatics at the incision). Blalock (1937) found patent collateral lymphatic pathways in the immediate vicinity of the obstruction after multiple attempts to completely ligate the thoracic duct, the right lymphatic duct, and the cisterna chyli.

In conventional foot lymphangiography, the contrast material is injected into the lymphatics draining into the superficial inguinal nodes. When these nodes are obstructed, the deep inguinal nodes fill. However, the deep nodes occasionally fill in normal subjects as well, so their filling alone cannot be considered abnormal. When the obstruction is more complete, collateral lymphatic channels in the thigh, perineum, external genitalia, and anterior abdominal wall may fill (Fig. 6.15). If the obstruction is higher in the iliac area, back flow may occur into the presacral, hypogastric, and lumbar areas (Fig. 6.16).

Obstruction and increased intralymphatic pressure result in the dilatation, stasis, and valvular insufficiency visible on the lymphangiogram (Yune and Klatte, 1969; Escobar-Prieto et al., 1971). Flow in the lymph vessel sometimes reverses in search of an alternate pathway (Figs. 6.15 and 6.17), and occasionally the vessels rupture with extravasation of lymph and contrast material into the interstitial spaces of the leg (Fig. 6.18) or the pleural and peritoneal cavities. Cunningham (1969) demonstrated extensive collateral lymphatic pathways and peritoneal extravasation of contrast material in a patient with malignant disease of the pelvis. Peritoneal extravasation has also been noted by Camiel et al. (1964), Cook et al. (1966), Craven et al. (1967), Fuchs and Zuppinger (1965), and Takahashi et al. (1968).

Dilatation and local extravasation may occur in normal lymphatic vessels after too rapid an injection during lymphangiography. Small droplets appear as beads along the lymphatic

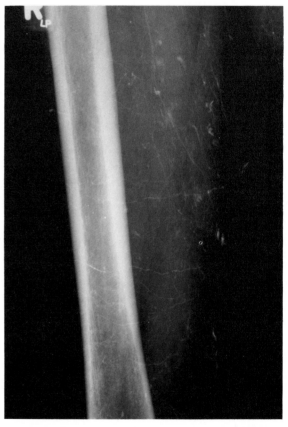

FIG. 6.15. OBSTRUCTION: INGUINAL LYMPHATICS
A 74-year-old man presented with right leg and scrotal edema. Urography showed a rigid area on the inferior and right lateral wall of the bladder that was a transitional cell carcinoma. Lymphangiography showed complete obstruction of the inguinal lymphatics with retrograde filling of superficial channels in the thigh and scrotum. The inguinal and iliac nodes showed central filling defects of metastatic tumor.

vessel. This should not be interpreted as obstruction in an otherwise normal lymphangiogram.

Backflow and drainage via the collateral cir-

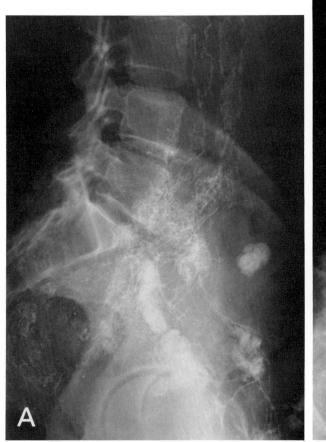

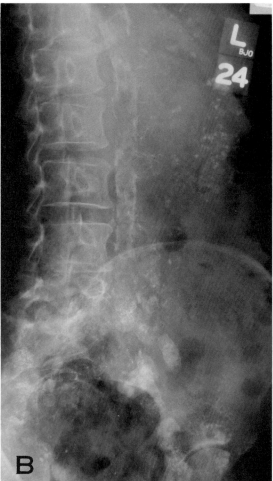

FIG. 6.16. OBSTRUCTION: PERIAORTIC LYMPHATICS

A 58-year-old woman noted swelling of her feet and ankles for 1 month. She had been treated 2 years previously for stage 2A Hodgkin's (lymphocyte depletion). *A*: Lymphangiogram showed almost complete obstruction above L5. Note calcium in the aorta. There is marked reflux of contrast material into the presacral and hypogastric lymphatics. *B*: Film at 24 hr shows contrast material in mesenteric lymph nodes.

culation are the final alternatives of the lymphatic system to bypass an obstruction. The pattern of collateral flow is unpredictable and not specific for any particular disease. There may be changes in the lymph nodes, however, which suggest a benign or malignant disease as the cause. Wallace (1968) and Wallace and Jing (1972) have shown that metastatic spread of carcinoma is not haphazard but rather an orderly response depending upon the development of collateral lymphatic flow.

Lymphaticovenous Communication

When the lymphatic system is overwhelmed and edema develops, there may be an attempt to decompress by lymphaticolymphatic and lymphaticovenous shunts. These routes are most often functional in chronic obstructive states such as neoplastic invasion of lymph nodes with complete obstruction, surgical resection, or certain benign conditions such as retroperitoneal fibrosis (Figs. 6.19 and 6.20). Most authors conclude that the lymphaticovenous communications are enlarged pathways normally present, which function only under stress from increased volume or pressure within the lymphatic system (Rusznyak et al., 1960; Yoffey and Courtice, 1956).

The communications between lymphatics and veins have been discussed periodically in the literature, but until the advent of clinical lymphography the concept was controversial. In 1834 Wutzer demonstrated communication between the thoracic duct and the azygous vein in

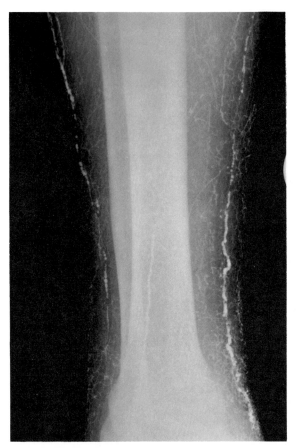

FIG. 6.17. OBSTRUCTION: DERMAL LYMPHATIC FILLING
Obstruction of inguinal lymphatics with marked reflux
of contrast material into dermal lymphatics in lower leg.

a woman whose thoracic duct was obstructed. Silvester (1911–1912) described openings of the lymphatic from the mesentery and lower limbs into the inferior vena cava near the renal vein in monkeys. Also in 1911, Baum declared the existence of lymphaticovenous communications in the sacral, jugular, and cephalic veins of the canine and bovine animals. Pressman et al. (1962) and Mayerson (1962) demonstrated communication between the lymphatic and venous systems within lymph nodes. Their findings provide one explanation for the observation that considerably more lymph is produced in the body than can be explained by measurement of total lymphatic flow from the thoracic and mediastinal trunks (Bollman et al., 1948; Kubik, 1952).

A number of authors have noted a marked decrease in circulating lymphocytes after ligation of the thoracic duct with return to normal levels within 4–6 days after establishment of collateral flow (Lee, 1922; Biedl and Decastello,

1901; Drinker and Yoffey, 1941). Threefoot et al. (1963), using plastic corrosion models of the lymphatic system, demonstrated lymphaticovenous and lymphaticolymphatic communications after prolonged ligation of the cisterna chyli. The venous channels involved were vena cava, renal, adrenal, iliac, and hemiazygous veins. Shanbrom and Zheutlin (1959) demonstrated accessory lymphatics draining directly into the jugular vein without traversing the lymph nodes. Bron et al. (1963) and Wallace et al. (1964) demonstrated these communications fluoroscopically while performing lymphography on clinical subjects. Wolfel (1965) demonstrated a direct communication between the

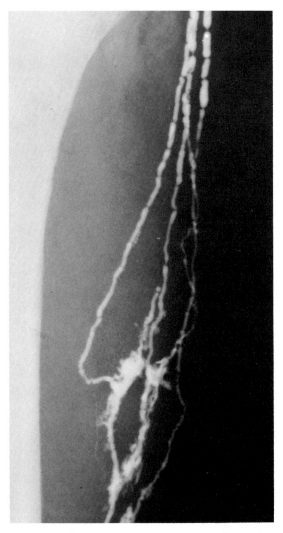

FIG. 6.18. OBSTRUCTION WITH LYMPHATIC RUPTURE
A 55-year-old man presented with metastatic sarcoma obstructing the inguinal lymphatics. The lymphangiogram shows dilatation of the lymphatic vessels and rupture with extravasation of contrast material.

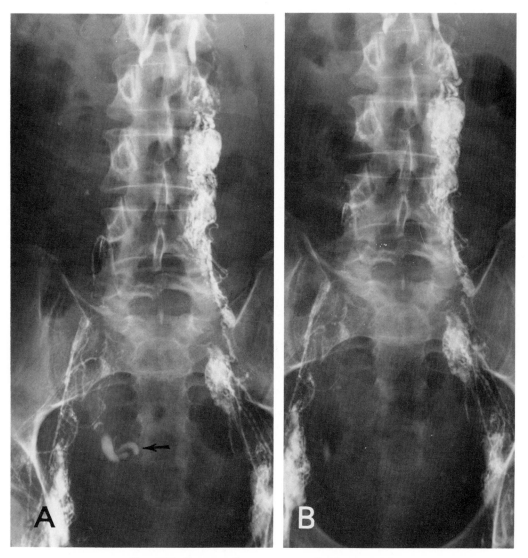

FIG. 6.19. SYSTEMIC LYMPHOVENOUS COMMUNICATION

A 60-year-old man had 6 months of progressive right leg edema and testicular pain after an acute episode of right flank and back pain. *A*: Lymphangiogram. There is complete obstruction of right iliac lymphatics. A lymphovenous communication fills a pelvic vein (*arrow*). The examination was terminated. *B*: A film 15 min later shows a second lymphovenous communication with venous filling. The venous collection of contrast material seen in *A* has passed centrally. Retroperitoneal fibrosis was found at operation.

para-aortic lymphatics and the inferior vena cava after complete obstruction of the retroperitoneal nodes by metastatic seminoma. Roentgenographically these communications are most frequently seen in the iliac and para-aortic areas. They may also occur peripherally when there is complete obstruction of the inguinal or axillary nodes (Fig. 6.21).

When performing lymphography, especially when obstruction is suspected, it is imperative to film frequently and possibly fluoroscope to demonstrate lymphaticovenous communica-tions and thus prevent extensive oil embolization. The flow in the vein is considerably more rapid than in the lymphatic vessel, and the contrast material appears as tiny droplets in the dependent portion of the vein. In a dependent vein or in the presence of venous stagnation, the contrast material may outline the entire vein (Fig. 6.20).

Perineural and Perivascular Spaces

Considerable controversy exists concerning the presence and functional significance of the

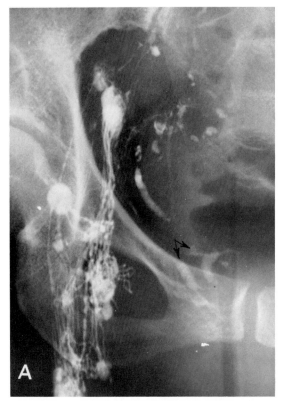 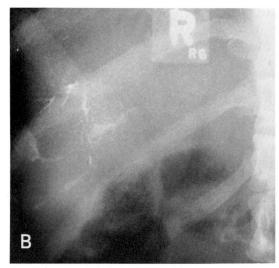

FIG. 6.20. PORTAL LYMPHOVENOUS COMMUNICATION

A 60-year-old woman with postradiation therapy for carcinoma of the cervix with recurrent disease. *A*: Lymphangiogram. Film after 5 ml of Ethiodol shows lymphovenous communication with the hemorrhoidal veins (*arrows*). The injection was terminated. *B*: Abdominal film 30 min later shows Ethiodol in right hepatic branch of the portal vein.

perivascular and perineural spaces. These potential spaces are soft tissue planes which surround the nerves and blood vessels and which have no endothelial lining. Included are the Virchow-Robbins space surrounding the cerebral blood vessels, perineural and perivascular spaces around nerves and blood vessels, and the intra-adventitial space surrounding branches of the pulmonary arterioles.

Larson et al. (1966) were unable to demonstrate any communication between the perineural space and the lymphatic system after injecting sky blue dye, vinyl acetate, and India ink into the soft tissue and nerves. There was no communication with the perineurium when contrast material was injected into the lymphatics. When contrast material was injected into the perineurium, it passed both proximally and distally in the nerve sheath without communication with the lymphatic vessels.

According to Sidney Wallace (1968) the concept of paralymphatics was proposed by Ottoviani. Wallace demonstrated contrast material in the perivascular space during lymphography.

These spaces are more frequently seen in patients with edema (Fig. 6.22), although they have been demonstrated in patients without lymphatic obstruction. The pattern of opacification follows the contour of the particular vessel and occasionally the nerve.

The perivascular space usually fills in an orthograde manner. The perivenous space is occasionally filled after the intradermal injection with patent blue violet dye during pedal lymphography, usually when there is a decrease in number of lymphatics. This may necessitate another incision to find a suitable lymphatic for cannulation.

Perivascular contrast material is rarely seen even in patients with lymphedema, and one must agree with Larson that tumor and lymph progress along tissue planes of least resistance. The lymphatic vessels lie in close proximity to the neurovascular bundle, and it is understandable that tumor enters the perineural and venous space by direct extension.

Wallace believes, however, that lymphographic findings are supportive of the concept of

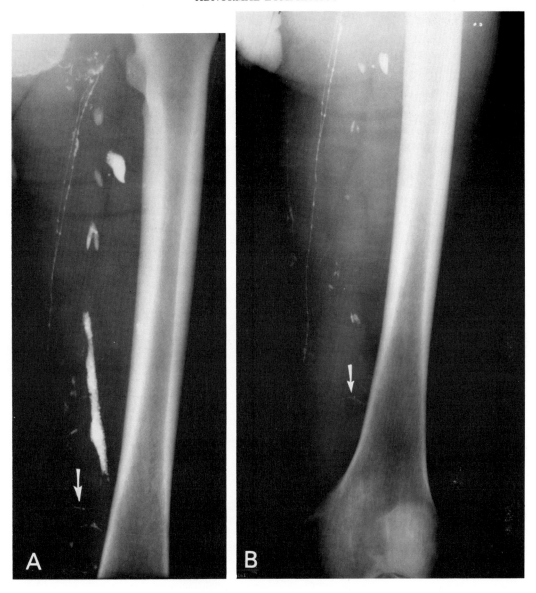

FIG. 6.21. PERIPHERAL LYMPHOVENOUS COMMUNICATION

This 56-year-old man had Kaposi's sarcoma and leg edema for 3 months. *A*: Lymphangiogram, left leg. Fluoroscopy was delayed on the left because of difficulty in cannulating right pedal lymphatics. Fluoroscopy after 4 ml of Ethiodol revealed complete obstruction of the inguinal lymphatics with a large amount of contrast material in the femoral vein. Contrast material could be seen passing from the lymphatic vessel transversely across the leg (*arrow*) to the femoral vein. *B*: Injection was discontinued. Contrast material remained in the communication (*arrow*). The contrast material in the vein passed centrally. Oil pneumonitis cleared in 1 week.

a functionally significant paralymphatic system even though contrast material may remain in these locations for 5 months (Kusick, 1971). These spaces may not be artifactual as suggested by Larson; however, the long term presence of contrast material and the findings of Larson indicate that the perivenous and perineural spaces have limited functional significance for transport of lymph and tumor cells.

The intra-adventitial spaces in the lung are those potential spaces surrounding the pulmonary arterioles. As with the perivascular and perineural spaces, there is no endothelial lining. They were first described by Ivanov (1936) and demonstrated by Foldi et al. (1954) in patients with pulmonary edema. These spaces contain the same edema fluid as the pulmonary lymphatics and alveoli. Ivanov's original con-

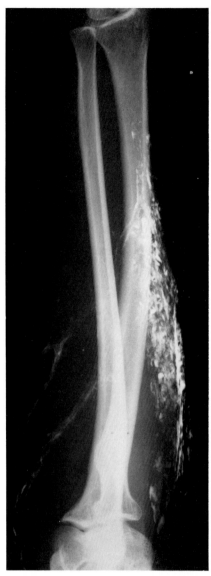

FIG. 6.22. PERIVENOUS LYMPHATICS
A 32-year-old woman developed edema of the arm after
surgical removal of a subcutaneous nodule on the forearm.
The lymphangiogram shows extensive perivenous contrast
material with extravasation into the soft tissue. (Courtesy
of W. G. Eklund, M.D., Portland, Oregon).

cept was that this space served as a communication between lymphoid slits (the connective tissue) and endothelium-lined lymphatic capillaries. Investigators to date have failed to demonstrate a connection between the lymph vessels
and the intra-adventitial space.

Lymphocele and Lymph Fistulae

Injury to lymphatic vessels, such as surgery
or blunt trauma, leads to passage of lymph into
soft tissues of body cavities. The lymph may be

confined and form a lymphocele or may exit
through an operative wound. The lymphocele
may be small such as those resulting from inguinal node biopsy (Fig. 6.23). After renal
transplantation, lymphoceles may be very
large, compressing the renal vein and requiring
drainage (Madura et al., 1970; Moreau et al.,
1973; Koehler and Kyaw, 1972; Sampson et al.,
1973; Rashid et al., 1974). Untreated, they may
lead to renal failure, venous thrombosis, and
pulmonary embolism (Lorimer et al., 1975).

Lymph fistulae may be insignificant with minor drainage from the incision site after scalene
node biopsy. Severe lymph fistulae with a large
amount of lymphatic drainage may follow thoracic duct injury due to radical chest surgery.
Storen et al. (1974) have demonstrated lymph
extravasation and fistulae in the lower leg after
arterial reconstructive surgery (Fig. 6.24).
Lymph fistulae may occur spontaneously when
tumor completely replaces the lymph nodes and
obstructs the lymph channels (Fig. 6.25).

Lymphatic damage is encountered frequently

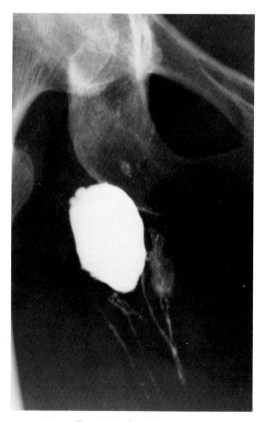

FIG. 6.23. LYMPHOCELE
This 63-year-old woman had a right inguinal node removed that proved to be Hodgkin's disease. Eight months
later she noted swelling in the same area. The lymphogram revealed a lymphocele that was subsequently excised.

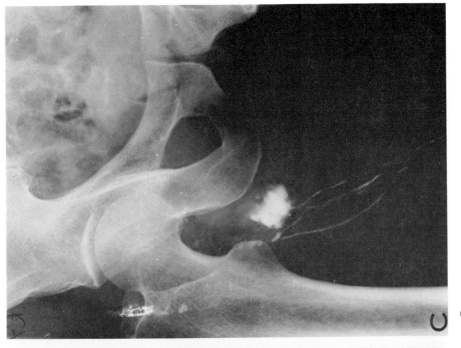

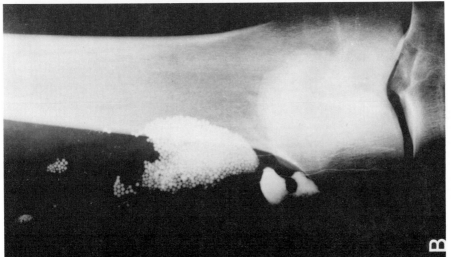

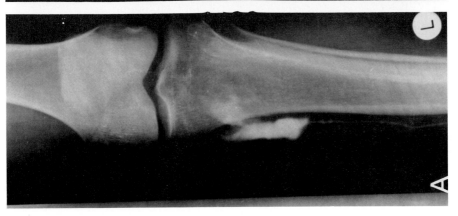

FIG. 6.24. LYMPH FISTULA AFTER ARTERIAL SURGERY

Lymphangiogram 2 weeks after arterial reconstruction of the lower limb shows interruption of lymphatic vessels and formation of lymphoceles at dissection sites. (Courtesy of Drs. E. J. Storen, H. O. Myhre, and G. Stiris, Oslo, Norway.)

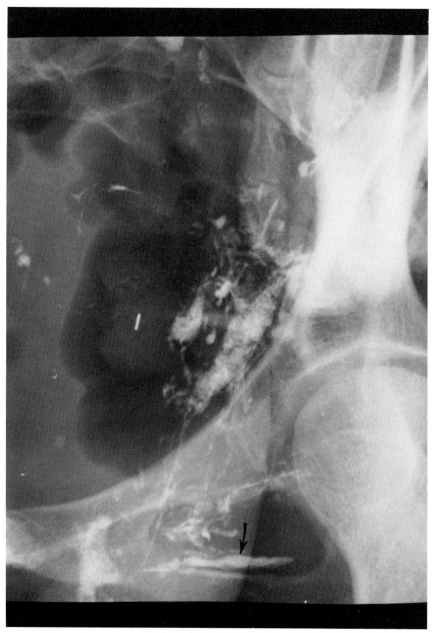

FIG. 6.25. LYMPH FISTULAE

A 55-year-old woman following postirradiation and surgery for carcinoma of the cervix with recurrent disease. Lymphangiogram demonstrated obstruction high in the external iliac nodes. There is extravasation of contrast material above the ischial tuberosity (*arrow*).

in the pelvic area after radical surgery for carcinoma of the cervix. The surgeon is faced with the dilemma when performing a radical node dissection. If all of the lymphatics are removed and ligated, there may be obstruction and postoperative edema in the lower leg. If dissection is not extensive, nodes may be left behind. Transection of lymphatic channels that are not ligated may result in considerable lymph escape into the peritoneal cavity. In these cases the degree of edema depends upon the number of lymphatic vessels ligated and the adequacy of the collateral circulation to bypass the interrupted channels.

PRIMARY INTESTINAL LYMPHANGIECTASIA

Intestinal lymphangiectasia is characterized by marked tortuosity and irregular dilatation of the mesenteric and mucosal lymphatics. Clinically an extreme loss of protein in the gastrointestinal tract results in hypoalbuminemia. Lymphocytopenia is an almost universal accompaniment of the syndrome. Mucosal jejunal biopsy shows dilated lymphatics in the mucosa.

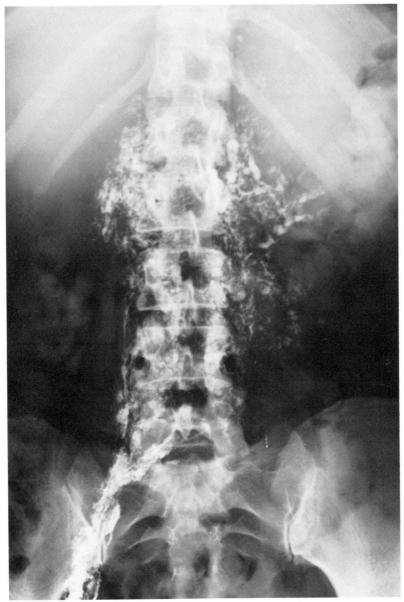

FIG. 6.26. INTESTINAL LYMPHANGIECTASIA WITH PROTEIN-LOSING GASTROENTEROPATHY
Lymphangiogram shows marked reflux into numerous dilated mesenteric lymphatic vessels. (Courtesy of Joseph J. Bookstein, M.D., Ann Arbor, Michigan.)

testinal tract results in hypoalbuminemia, hypogammaglobulinemia, edema, and pleural effusion. There appears to be a poor correlation between the extent of edema and severity of

The cause of hypoproteinemia in patients with intestinal lymphangiectasia appears to be rupture of dilated lymphatic vessels with loss of lymph into the bowel lumen or exudation through the lymphatic capillaries. Discharge of lymph into the intestinal lumen has been demonstrated by intestinal intubation (Stoelinga et al., 1963) and extravasation of contrast material into the intestinal lumen by pedal lymphography (Mistilis et al., 1965).

Intestinal lymphangiectasia may be part of a systemic lymphatic dysplasia (Stoelinga et al., 1963; Bookstein et al., 1965). Pomerantz and Waldmann (1963) demonstrated systemic lymphatic abnormalities in 4 patients with intestinal lymphangiectasia by lymphography. Studies of the arteries and veins in primary intestinal lymphangiectasia have not been reported.

Shimkin et al. (1970) analyzed nine pedal lymphangiograms of patients with intestinal lymphangiectasia. The findings included hypoplasia of lower extremity lymphatics, dermal backflow in the skin, possible thoracic duct obstruction with a tortuous and dilated thoracic duct, and a stippled appearance of the contrast material in the lymph nodes. Others have reported dilated and varicose lymphatics (Bookstein et al., 1965; Pomerantz and Waldmann, 1963) (Fig. 6.26).

Although the exact pathogenesis is obscure, lymphangiectasia is probably due to a congenital malformation with symptoms developing in childhood and a family history of hypoproteinemia with effusion. The associated protein-losing gastroenteropathy may also be seen in a number of acquired lesions (Waldmann, 1966), including constrictive pericarditis, congestive heart failure, retroperitoneal fibrosis, and conpancreatitis.

In constrictive pericarditis venous hypertension obstructs the flow of lymph into the venous angle, increasing intralymphatic pressure and decreasing lymphatic flow. Takashima and Takekoshi (1968) have reported hypoproteinemia and intestinal lymphangiectasia as a presenting symptom in a patient with constrictive pericarditis.

The mechanism of protein-losing enteropathy associated with congestive heart failure is not clear. Davidson et al. (1962) have suggested that it is caused by functional obstruction of the lymphatics by increased venous pressure (i.e., similar to constrictive pericarditis) (Petersen and Hastrup, 1963; Petersen and Ottosen, 1964). There is an increase in lymph production in congestive heart failure as well as a later increase in venous pressure; thus a combination of both factors may cause lymphatic hypertension.

In retroperitoneal fibrosis and pancreatitis there is obstruction of the lymphatic channels with dilatation and loss of lymph into the intestinal tract.

REFERENCES

Ackerman, T.: Ein Fall von Galacturia (urina chylosa). Deutsch. Klin., *15:* 221, 1863.

Allen, E. V., Barker, N. W. and Hines, E. A.: *Peripheral Vascular Diseases.* Philadelphia, W. B. Saunders, 1946.

Allenby, F., Calnan, J. S. and Pflug, J. J.: The use of pneumatic compression in the swollen leg. J. Physiol. (Lond.) *231:* 65, 1973.

Arnulf, G.: Lymphedema of the upper limb after Halstead's operations of radical mastectomy, lymphography and phlebography. Therapeutic consequences. Vasc. Surg., 7: 36, 1973.

Baum, H.: Können Lymphagefässe direkt in Venen einmünden? Anat. Anz., *39:* 593, 1911.

Biedl, A. and Decastello, A.: Über Änderungen des Blutbildes nach Unterbrechung des Lymph Zuflusses. Pflügers Arch. ges Physiol., *86:* 259, 1901.

Blalock, A., Robinson, C. S., Cunningham, R. S. and Gray, M. E.: Experimental studies on lymphatic blockage. Arch. Surg., *34:* 1049, 1937.

Bollman, J. L., Cain, J. C. and Grindlay, J. H.: Technique for collection of lymph from the liver, small intestine and thoracic duct of the rat. J. Lab. Clin. Med., *33:* 1349, 1948.

Bookstein, J. J., French, A. B. and Pollard, M. H.: Protein-losing gastroenteropathy: concepts derived from lymphangiography. Am. J. Dig. Dis., *10:* 573, 1965.

Bron, K. M., Baum, S. and Abrams, H. L.: Oil embolism in lymphangiography. Incidence, manifestation and mechanism. Radiology, *80:* 194, 1963.

Bunchman, M. M. and Lewis, S. R.: The treatment of lymphedema. Plast. Reconstr. Surg., *54:* 64, 1974.

Buonocore, E. and Young, J. R.: Lymphangiographic evaluation of lymphedema and lymphatic flow. Am. J. Roentgenol. Radium Ther. Nucl. Med., *95:* 751, 1965.

Burn, J. I.: Obstructive lymphopathy. Ann. R. Coll. Surg. Engl., *42:* 93, 1968.

Calnan, J.: Lymphoedema: the case for doubt. Br. J. Plast. Surg., *21:* 32, 1968.

Calnan, J. and Kountz, S. I.: Effect of venous obstruction on lymphatics. Br. J. Surg., *52:* 800, 1965.

Camiel, M. R., Benninghoff, D. L. and Herman, P. G.: Chylous ascites with lymphographic demonstration of lymph leakage into the peritoneal cavity. Gastroenterology, *47:* 188, 1964.

Charles, H.: In *A System of Treatment,* Vol. 3, edited by A. Latham. J. & A. Churchill, Ltd., London, 1912.

Chilvers, A. S. and Kinmonth, J. B.: Operation for lymphedema of the lower limbs. A study of the results in 108 operations using vascularized dermal flaps. J. Cardiovasc. Surg., *16:* 115, 1975.

Choi, J. K. and Weidemer, H. S.: Chyluria: lymphographic study and review of the literature. J. Urol., *92:* 723, 1964.

Cohen, L. B., Nelson, G., Wood, A. M., Manson-Bahr, P. E. and Bowen, R.: Lymphangiography in filarial lymphedema and elephantiasis. Am. J. Trop. Med. Hyg., *10:* 843, 1961.

Cook, P. L., Jelliffe, A. M., Kendall, B. and McLoughlin, M. J.: The role of lymphography in diagnosis and management of malignant reticulosis. Br. J. Radiol., 39: 561, 1966.

Craven, C. E. et al.: Congenital chylous ascites: lymphographic demonstration of obstruction of cisterna chylus reflux into peritoneal space and small intestines. J. Pediatr., 70: 340, 1967.

Cunningham, J. B.: The demonstration of an unusual combination of collateral channels during lymphography—a case report. J. Can. Assoc. Radiol., 20: 189, 1969.

Davidson, J. D., Waldmann, T. S., Goodman, D. S. and Gordon, R. R.: Protein-losing gastroenteropathy in congestive heart failure. Lancet, 1: 899, 1961.

Drinker, C. K. and Yoffey, J. M.: Lymphatics, Lymph and Lymphoid Tissue. Harvard University Press, Cambridge, 1941.

Emmett, A. J., Barron, J. N. and Veall, N.: The use of I-131 albumin tissue clearance measurements and other physiological tests for the clinical assessment of patients with lymphoedema. Br. J. Plast. Surg., 20: 1, 1967.

Escobar-Prieto, A., Gonzalez, G., Templeton, A. W., Cooper, B. R. and Palacios, E.: Lymphatic channel obstruction. Am. J. Roentgenol. Radium Ther. Nucl. Med., 113: 366, 1971.

Esterly, J. R.: Congenital hereditary lymphedema. J. Med. Genet., 2: 93, 1965.

Eustace, P. W. and Kinmonth, J. B.: The normal lymphatic vessels of the inguinal and iliac areas with special emphasis on the efferent inguinal vessels. Lymphology, 1976, in press.

Field, M. E. and Drinker, C. K.: Permeability of capillaries of dog to protein. Am. J. Physiol., 97: 40, 1931a.

Field, M. E. and Drinker, C. K.: Conditions governing the removal of protein deposited in the subcutaneous tissue of the dog. Am. J. Physiol., 98: 66, 1931b.

Firica, A., Ray, A., Murat, J. E. and Tompkins, R. K.: Alleviation of experimental lymphedema by lymphovenous anastomosis in 12 dogs. Am. Surg., 38: 409, 1972.

Foldi, M., Kepes, J., Papp, M., Rusznyak, I. and Szabo, G.: Significance of pulmonary lymph circulation in the fluid circulation of the lung. A contribution of the data concerning the pathogenesis of pulmonary oedema. MTA. Biol. Orvtud. Oszt., Kozi Hung., 5: 221, 1954.

Fonkalsrud, E. W.: Surgical management of congenital malformations of the lymphatic system. Am. J. Surg., 128: 152, 1974.

Fonkalsrud, E. W. and Coulson, W. F.: Management of congenital lymphedema in infants and children. Ann. Surg., 177: 280. 1973.

Fuchs, W. A., and Zuppinger, A.: Lymphographic and Tumor-diagnostic. Springer-Verlag, Berlin, 1965.

Goldsmith, H. S.: Long term evaluation of omental transposition for chronic lymphedema. Ann. Surg., 180: 847, 1974.

Gooneratne, B. W. M.: Lymphography of filarial infections. Lecture, St. Thomas' Hospital, 1969.

Handley, W. S.: Lymphangioplasty. Lancet, 1: 783, 1908.

Hirshowitz, B. and Goldan, S.: A bi-hinged chest-arm flap for lymphedema of the upper limb. Plast. Reconstr. Surg., 48: 52, 1971.

Homans, J.: Treatment of elephantiasis of legs. N. Engl. J. Med., 215: 1099, 1936.

Hughes, J. H. and Patel, A. R.: Swelling of the arm following radical mastectomy. Br. J. Surg., 53: 4, 1966.

Ivanov, G. F.: Pulmonaire de la circulation lymphatique. Bull. Histol. Appliquee Physiol. Pathol., 13: 401, 1936.

Jackson, B. T. and Kinmonth, J. B.: Pes cavus and lymphoedema. J. Bone Joint Surg. [Br.], 52B: 518, 1970.

Khamma, N. N.: Surgical treatment of elephantiasis of male genitalia. Plast. Reconstr. Surg., 46: 481, 1970.

Kinmonth, J. B.: Primary lymphedemas: classification and other studies based on oleolymphography and clinical features. J. Cardiovasc. Surg. (Torino), Special Supplement for XVII Congress of European Society of Cardiovascular Surgeons, 1969.

Kinmonth, J. B.: The Lymphatics: Diseases, Lymphography and Surgery. The Williams & Wilkins Co., Baltimore, 1972.

Kinmonth, J. B. and Taylor, G. W.: The lymphatic circulation in lymphedema. Ann. Surg., 139: 129, 1954.

Kinmonth, J. B., Taylor, G. W. and Jantet, G. M.: Chylous complications of primary lymphoedema. J. Cardiovasc. Surg. (Torino), 5: 327, 1964.

Kinmonth, J. B., Taylor, G. W., Tracy, G. D and Marsh, J. D.: Primary lymphoedema. Br. J. Surg., 45: 1, 1957.

Kittredge, R. D., Hashim. S., Roholt, H. B., Van Itallie, T. B. and Finby, M.: Demonstration of lymphatic abnormality in a patient with chyluria. Am. J. Roentgenol. Radium Ther. Nucl. Med., 90: 159, 1963.

Koehler, R. P., Chiang, T. C., Lin, C. T., Chen, K. C. and Chen, K. Y.: Lymphography in chyluria. Am. J. Roentgenol. Radium Ther. Nucl. Med., 102: 455, 1968.

Koehler, P. R. and Kyaw, M. M.: Lymphatic complications following renal transplantation. Radiology, 102: 539, 1972.

Kondoleon, E.: Die Chirurgische Behandlung der Elephantiastichen Oedeme. Munch. Med. Wochenschr., 59: 525, 1912.

Kreel, L. and George, P.: Post-mastectomy lymphangiography: detection of metastases and edema. Ann. Surg., 163: 470, 1966.

Kubik, I.: Die Hydrodynamischn und Mechanischen Faktoren in der Lymphzirkulation. Acta Morphol. Acad. Sci. Hung., 2: 95, 1952.

Kusick, H.: Technique of Lymphography and Principles of Interpretation, pp. 174–180. Warren H. Green, Inc., St. Louis, 1971.

Larson, D. L., Rodin, A. E., Roberts, D. K., O'Steen, W. K., Rappaport, A. S. and Lewis, S. R.: Perineural lymphatics: myth or fact. Am. J. Surg., 112: 488, 1966.

Larson, N. E., and Crampton, A. R.: A surgical procedure for postmastectomy edema. Arch. Surg., 106: 475, 1973.

Lee, F. C.: Establishment of collateral circulation following ligation of the thoracic duct. Bull. Johns Hopkins Hosp., 33: 21, 1922.

Lee, F. C.: Permeability of lymph vessels and lymph pressure. Arch. Surg., 48: 355, 1944.

Lewis, T. R.: On a hematazon inhabiting blood, its relation to chyluria and other diseases. Ind. Ann. Med. Sci., 16: 504, 1873.

Lloyd-Davies, R. W., Edwards, J. M. and Kinmonth, J. B.: Chyluria: a report of five cases with particular references to lymphography and direct surgery. Br. J. Urol., 39: 560, 1967.

Lorimer, W. S., Glassford, D. M., Sarles, H. E., Remmers, A. R. and Fish, J. C.: Lymphocele: a significant complication following renal transplantation. Lymphology, 8: 21, 1975.

Madura, J. A., Dunbar, J. D. and Cerilli, J. G.: Perirenal lymphocele as a complication of renal homotransplantation. Surgery, 68: 310, 1970.

Manson, P.: The Filaria Darginis-hominis. H. K. Lewis, London, 1883.

Mayerson, P.: Permeability characteristics of the lymph node. Senior thesis, presented at the 12th annual Senior Scientific Session of Tulane University School of Medicine, New Orleans, Louisiana, May 9, 1962.

Milroy, W. F.: An undescribed variety of hereditary oedema. N.Y. J. Med., 505, 1892.

Mistilis, S. P., Skyring, A. P. and Stephen, D. D.: Intestinal lymphangectasia: mechanism of enteric loss of plasma-protein and fat. Lancet, 1: 77, 1965.

Molen, H. R. and van der T'oth, L. M.: The conservative treatment of lymphedema of the extremities. Angiology, 25: 420, 1974.

Moreau, J. F., Leski, M., Beurton, D., Cukier, J., Michel, J. R., Kreis, J. and Lacombe, M.: Lymphoceles obstructives apres transplanation renale. Ann. Radiol. (Paris), 16: 471, 1973.

Negus, D., Edwards, J. M. and Kinmonth, J. B.: The iliac veins in relation to lymphedema. Br. J. Surg., 56: 481, 1969.

Nielubowicz, J. and Olszewski, W.: Surgical lymphaticovenous shunts in patients with secondary lymphedema. Br. J. Surg., 55: 440, 1968.

O'Connor, F. W.: The aetiology of the disease syndrome in Wuchereria bancrofti infection. Trans. R. Soc. Trop. Med. Hyg., 23: 13, 1932.

O'Donnell, T. F.: Congenital mixed vascular deformities of the lower limbs: the relevance of lymphatic abnormalities to their diagnosis and treatment. Ann. Surg., 185: 162, 1977.

O'Donnell, T. F., Edwards, J. M. and Kinmonth, J. B.: Lymphography in the mixed vascular deformities of the lower extremities. J. Cardiovasc. Surg. (Torino), 17: 1976a.

O'Donnell, T. F., Kalisher, L. Raines, J. K. and Darling, R. C.: Assessment of lymphedema by xeroradiography. Physiologist, 19: 3, 1976b.

Olszewski, W.: On the pathomechanism of development of postsurgical lymphedema. Lymphology, 6: 35, 1973.

Olszewski, W., Machowski, Z., Sawicki, A., and Wielubowicz, J.: Clinical studies in primary lymphedema. Pol. Med. J., 11: 1560, 1972a.

Olszewski, W., Machowski, Z., Sokolowski, J., Sawicki, Z., Zerbino, D. and Nielubowicz, J.: Primary lymphedema of lower extremities. I. Lymphangiographic and histologic studies of lymphatic vessels and lymph nodes in primary lymphedema. Pol. Med. J., 11: 1564, 1972b.

O'Reilly, K.: Treatment by nylon setons of lymphedema of the arm following radical mastectomy. Med. J. Aust., 1: 1269, 1972.

Peterson, V. P. and Hastrup, J.: Protein-losing enteropathy in constrictive pericarditis. Acta Med. Scand., 173: 401, 1963.

Peterson, V. P. and Ottosen, P.: Albumin turnover and thoracic-duct lymph in constrictive pericarditis. Acta Med. Scand., 176: 335, 1964.

Politowski, M., Bartkowski, S. and Dynowski, J.: Treatment of lymphedema of the limbs by lymphatic-venous fistula. Surgery, 66: 639, 1969.

Pomerantz, M. and Waldmann, T. A.: Systemic lymphatic abnormalities associated with gastrointestinal protein loss secondary to intestinal lymphangiectasia. Gastroenterology, 45: 703, 1963.

Pressman, J. J., Simon, M. B., Hand, K. and Miller, J.: Passage of fluids, cells and bacteria via direct communications between lymph nodes and veins. Surg. Gynecol Obstet., 115: 207, 1962.

Raines, J., O'Donnell, T. F., Kalisher, L. and Darling, R. C.: Selection of patients with lymphedema for compression therapy. Am. J. Surg., in press, 1977.

Rajaram, P. C.: Lymphatic dynamics in filarial chyluria and prechyluric state — lymphographic analysis of 52 cases. Lymphology, 3: 114, 1970.

Randolph, J. and Gross, R.: Congenital chylothorax. Arch. Surg., 74: 405, 1957.

Rashid, A., Posen, G., Couture, R., McKay, D. and Wellington, J.: Accumulation of lymph around the transplanted kidney (lymphocele) mimicking renal allograft rejection. J. Urol., 111: 145, 1974.

Reichert, F. L.: The regeneration of lymphatics. Arch. Surg., 13: 871, 1926.

Rigas, A., Vomoyannis, A., Gianoulis, K., Antipas, S. and Tsardakas, E.: Measurement of the femoral vein pressure in edema of the lower extremities. Report of 50 cases. J. Cardiovasc. Surg. (Torino), 12: 411, 1971.

Rusznyak, I., Foldi, M. and Szabo, G.: Lymphatics and Lymph Circulation. Pergamon Press, New York, 1960.

Saijo, M., Munro, I. R. and Mancer, K.: Lymphangioma, a long term follow-up study. Plast. Reconstr. Surg., 56: 642, 1975a.

Saijo, M., Munro, I. R., and Mancer, K.: Lymphedema: a clinical review and follow-up study. Plast. Reconstr. Surg., 56: 513, 1975b.

Sampson, D., Winterberger, A. R. and Murphy, G. P.: Lymphoceles complicating renal allotransplantation. NY State J. Med., 73: 2710, 1973.

Sawney, C. P.: Evaluation of Thompson's buried dermal flap operation for lymphedema of the limbs: a clinical and radioisotopic study. Br. J. Plast. Surg., 27: 278, 1974.

Selle, J. G., Synder, W. M. and Schreiber, J. T.: Chylothorax: indications for surgery. Ann. Surg., 177: 245, 1973.

Shanbrom, E. and Zheutlin, N.: Radiographic studies of lymphatic system. AMA Arch. Intern. Med., 104: 589, 1959.

Shimkin, P. M., Waldmann T. A. and Krugman, R. L.: Intestinal lymphangiectasia. Am. J. Roentgenol. Radium Ther. Nucl. Med., 110: 827, 1970.

Silver, D., and Puckett, J.: Lymphangioplasty: a ten year evaluation. Surgery, in press.

Silvester, C. F.: On the presence of permanent communications between the lymphatics and the venous system at the level of the renal vein in adult South American monkeys. Am. J. Anat., 12: 447, 1911–1912.

Sistrunk, W. E.: Modifications of the operation for elephantiasis. JAMA, 71: 800, 1918.

Stoelinga, G. B. A., van Munster, P. J. J. and Sloof, J. P.: Chylous effusions into the intestine in a patient with protein-losing gastroenteropathy. Pediatrics, 31: 1011, 1963.

Storen, E. J., Myhre, H. O. and Stiris, G.: Lymphangiographic findings in patients with leg edema after arterial reconstruction. Acta Chir. Scand., 140: 385, 1974.

Takahashi, M., Takeda, K., Ishibashi, T. and Kawanami, H.: Peritoneal extravasation of oily contrast medium following lymphography. Am. J. Roentgenol. Radium Ther. Nucl. Med., 104: 652, 1968.

Takashima, T., and Takekoshi, N.: Lymphographic evaluation of abnormal lymph flow in protein-losing gastroenteropathy secondary to chronic constricting pericarditis. Radiology, 90: 502, 1968.

Terrier, H., Ganascia-Goetschel, J., Lang, A. and Griton, P.: Therapy of lymphoid edema and of various edematic affections of the limbs by a new pneumatic compression instrument. Phlebologie, 26: 261, 1973.

Thompson, N.: Surgical treatment of chronic lymphedema of the lower limb. Br. Med. J., 2: 1566, 1962.

Thompson, N.: The surgical treatment of advanced postmastectomy lymphedema of the upper limb. With the later results of treatment by buried dermis flap operation. Scand. J. Plast. Reconstr. Surg., 3: 54, 1969.

Thompson, N.: Buried dermal flap operation for chronic lymphedema of the extremities. Ten year survey of results in 79 cases. Plast. Reconstr. Surg., *45:* 541, 1970.

Threefoot, S. A., Kent, W. T. and Hatchett, B. F.: Lymphaticovenous and lymphaticolymphatic communications demonstrated by plastic corrosion models of rats and by post mortem lymphangiography in man. J. Lab. Clin. Med., *61:* 9, 1963.

Vasko, J. S. and Tapper, R. I.: The surgical significance of chylous ascites. Arch. Surg., *95:* 355, 1967.

Vitek, J. and Kaspar, Z.: The radiology of the deep lymphatic system of the leg. Br. J. Radiol., *46:* 120, 1973.

Waldmann, T. A.: Protein-losing enteropathy. Prog. Gastroenterol., *50:* 422, 1966.

Wallace, S.: Dynamics of normal and abnormal lymphatic systems as studied with contrast media. Cancer Chemother. Rep., *52:* 31, 1968.

Wallace, S., Jackson, L., Dodd, G. D. et al.: Lymphatic dynamics in certain abnormal states. Am. J. Roentgenol. Radium Ther. Nucl. Med., *91:* 1187, 1964.

Wallace, S. and Jing, B.: Testicular malignancies and the lymphatic system. In *Testicular Tumors,* edited by D. Johnson. Medical Examination Publishing Co., Flushing, NY, 1972.

Weichert, R. F. and Jamieson, C. W.: Acute chylous peritonitis. A case report. Br. J. Surg., *57:* 230, 1970.

Wolfel, D. A.: Lymphatico-venous communications. Am. J. Roentgenol. Radium Ther. Nucl. Med., *95:* 766, 1965.

Wücherer, O.: Filaria. Gaz. Med. da Bohia, 1868.

Wutzer, C. W.: Einmundung des Duct Thoracicus in die Vena Azygos. Arch. Anat. Phys., 311, 1834.

Yoffey, J. M. and Courtice, F. C.: *Lymphatics, Lymph and Lymphoid Tissue.* Harvard University Press, Cambridge, 1956.

Young, A. E., Rutt, D. C. and Kinmonth, J. B.: The objective measurement of skin thickness in lymphedema. Eur. Surg. Res., *8:* 31, 1976.

Yune, H. Y. and Klatte, E. C.: Lymphography in lymphatic obstruction. Radiology, *92:* 824, 1969.

Zeissler, R. M., Rose, G. and Nelson, P. A.: Postmastectomy lymphedema: late results of treatment in 385 patients. Arch. Phys. Med. Rehabil., *53:* 159, 1972.

7

Benign Lymph Node Disease

MELVIN E. CLOUSE, M.D.

In the past, lymphography was seldom performed to demonstrate inflammatory disease in the lymph nodes. The most important reason for recognizing inflammatory disease was to distinguish it from lymphoma and metastatic carcinoma. More recently, the usefulness of lymphography in demonstrating sarcoid (Blaudow and Scharkoff, 1972) and tuberculosis (Suramo, 1974) has been reported, but specific indications for lymphography in inflammatory disease have still not been clearly defined.

Ruttner (1967) classified inflammatory diseases according to their morphologic appearance: follicular hyperplasia; reactive hyperplasia (hyperplasia of the histiocytes, reticular fibers, and lymphocytic cells); granulomatous inflammation; and abscess-forming or necrotizing inflammation. This is probably the best approach to a classification, but cellular reactions are not always specific even though they may be characteristic of certain inflammatory agents.

The lymphographic patterns of inflammatory reactions are even less specific because the lymph node (composed of lymphoid tissue, reticulum-supporting network, and endothelium-lined sinusoids) has a limited response to some inflammatory agents. The contrast material enters the afferent channels and is distributed throughout the sinusoids. If the inflammatory reaction is purely follicular, the node may appear more granular with a normal marginal sinus. If the response is hyperplastic, the sinusoids may become occluded and produce central filling defects. In both responses the node becomes more foamy and bubbly in appearance and is more difficult to differentiate from lymphoma. The granulomatous and abscess-forming inflammatory reactions interrupt the marginal sinus more frequently and produce filling defects similar to metastatic carcinoma.

ACUTE INFLAMMATION

Lymph nodes involved by acute inflammation are usually enlarged as a result of hyperplasia of lymph follicles and new follicle formation. The channels leading to and from the node as well as the sinusoids may be enlarged (Fig. 7.1). These changes are reflected in the lymphographic pattern. As the follicles enlarge, they compress the contrast-filled sinusoids. The normal ground-glass appearance gives way to discrete filling defects throughout the nodes, changing it to a more glandular or foamy pattern.

Tjernberg (1956) demonstrated the ability of lymphography to differentiate acute inflammation and metastatic carcinoma. When the sinusoids are dilated, more contrast material can be stored in the node giving it a more dense, homogeneous appearance. The contrast in the sinusoids may form droplets because it is not compressed by lymphoid follicles. This type of inflammation usually develops in the inguinal and axillary nodes because of infection in the extremities, but it may reflect systemic infection.

Viamonte et al. (1963) showed generalized enlargement of iliac and para-aortic nodes from infectious mononucleosis and enlarged nodes with preservation of nodal architecture in psoriatic arthropathy. Measles, poliomyelitis, and other viral infections (such as rheumatoid arthritis and ankylosing spondylitis) are also known to produce this response.

Wiljasalo et al. (1966) found normal lymph vessels and enlarged, coarsely granular lymph nodes with intact marginal sinuses in the early stages of rheumatoid arthritis and ankylosing

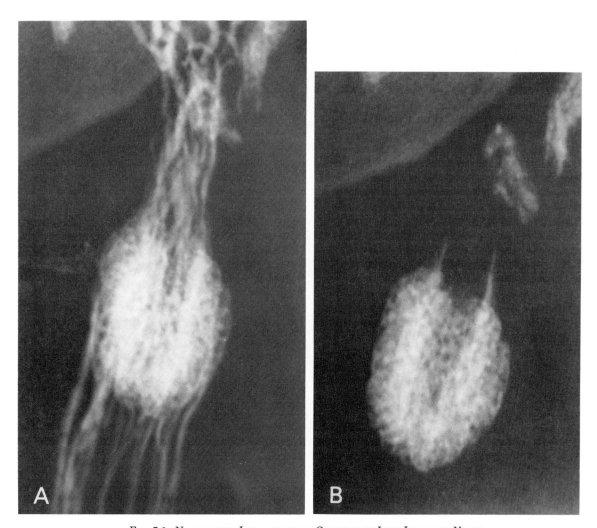

FIG. 7.1. NONSPECIFIC INFLAMMATORY CHANGES IN LEFT INGUINAL NODES
A: The afferent and efferent channels are enlarged. *B*: The follicles are enlarged. Droplets of contrast material are in enlarged sinusoids. *C*: Large right inguinal node in another patient with chronic dermatitis. There are marginal filling defects, enlarged follicles and large droplets of contrast material in large sinusoids. *D*: Another patient with generalized exfoliative dermatitis. The inguinal node is most involved because it is the first drainage node. The follicles are enlarged and a large number of sinusoids are obliterated. The external iliac nodes are involved to a lesser degree.

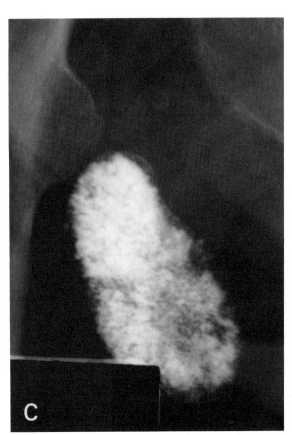

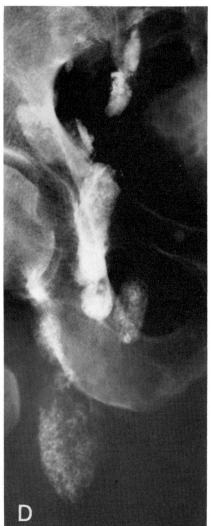

FIG. 7.1. *C–D*

spondylitis. The abnormal nodes were located in the iliac and para-aortic areas. The nodes gradually return to normal as inflammation subsides or after several years. Fornier et al. (1969)

found inflammatory changes in the lymph nodes to be proportional to the severity of spondyloarthritis. These nodal abnormalities preceded the bony changes.

REACTIVE HYPERPLASIA

Reactive hyperplasia is characterized histologically by proliferation of histiocytes, reticulum fibers, and lymphocytes. Hyalinization has also been seen (Castellino et al., 1974). It is regarded as inflammation induced by tumor cells and may imply a defense mechanism within the nodes (Fuchs, 1969). The lymphographic appearance of the lymph node does not differ significantly from nonspecific follicular hyperplastic inflammation. However, the site is

important: reactive hyperplasia is usually observed in areas other than inguinal drainage nodes unless the inguinal nodes are the primary drainage nodes. The regional lymph nodes are commonly involved in reactive hyperplasia (deRoo, 1973). This can be seen in Figure 7.2, a patient with carcinoma of the bladder. The iliac nodes showed reactive changes as did all the downstream drainage nodes including the common iliac and para-aortic nodes. The changes

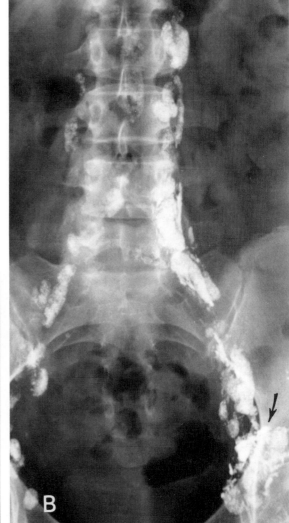

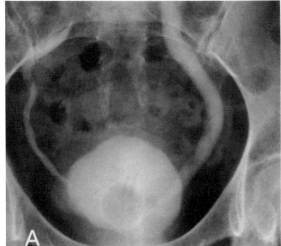

FIG. 7.2. REACTIVE HYPERPLASIA IN REGIONAL NODES DRAINING BLADDER CARCINOMA
Subject is a 60-year-old female with carcinoma invading the base of the bladder. *A*: Intravenous pyelogram. Coned view bladder shows dilated, partially obstructed left ureter with carcinoma involving the entire base of the bladder. *B*: Lymphangiogram. The left iliac and para-aortic nodes are enlarged with a foamy appearance. Biopsy (*arrow*) of common iliac node showed reactive hyperplasia. *C*: Left external iliac nodes.   ×2. *D*: Microscopy. Hematoxylin-eosin stain shows enlarged follicles and proliferation of histiocytic and endothelial lining cells.   ×40.

were more marked in the lower external iliac area. The same criteria hold for other solid tumors such as the seminoma in Figure 5.6. The primary drainage nodes of the testis showed reactive changes to the tumor that produced a histiocytic response progressing to complete caseation necrosis obliterating the sinusoids and producing the pseudolymphoma appearance. The lymphographic pattern was produced entirely by the inflammatory response and not by tumor cells. It is also interesting that the external iliac nodes show less striking inflammatory

changes not related to tumor cells but to the operation.

Lymphographically it is generally possible to distinguish reactive and follicular hyperplastic inflammatory reactions from metastatic carcinoma in lymph nodes, but inflammatory reactions are difficult to differentiate from lymphomas. Ruttner (1967) has suggested that the lymphographic appearance of follicular hyperplasia simulates follicular lymphoblastoma, and Butler (1969) has stated that reactive hyperplasia can simulate all patterns of lymphoma. Parker

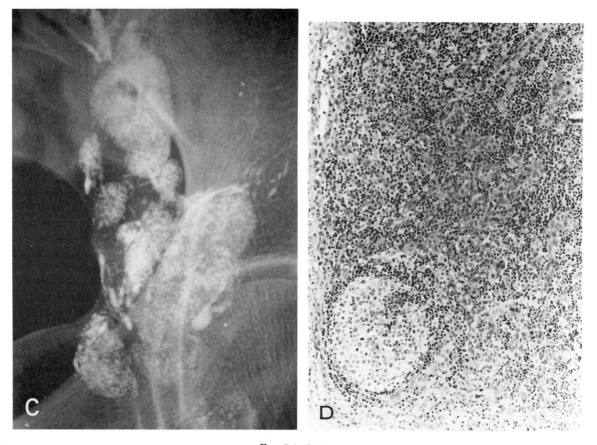

FIG. 7.2. *C–D*

et al. (1974) believe that reactive hyperplasia can be differentiated from lymphoma if all of the nodes are involved to the same degree and show a diffuse granular pattern (Fig. 7.3). In lymphoma all of the nodes are seldom involved to the same degree and the appearance is more bubbly. Although all the nodes in Figure 7.3 are involved more or less to the same degree, it is very difficult to be absolutely certain that the pattern is not that of follicular lymphoma or Hodgkin's disease other than nodular sclerosis cell type. The reason for the generalized inflammatory changes one sees in lymphoma is not understood. In a systemic inflammatory reaction one sees a generalized inflammatory response in the lymph nodes, whereas in a local inflammatory process one sees inflammatory changes only in the nodes draining the area.

HYPERPLASIA OF MEDIASTINAL LYMPH NODES

Enlarged mediastinal nodes containing hyperplastic germinal centers and focal areas of hyalinization in addition to scattered plasma cells have been seen in asymptomatic patients. Lymphographically the node appearance is coarsely granular with intact marginal sinuses. Such findings may represent a nonspecific inflammatory process (Castleman, 1954; Castleman and Iverson, 1956) or a developmental or growth disturbance of lymphoid tissue (Lattes and Pachter, 1962). These changes may also be seen in lymphoma (Nishimine et al., 1974).

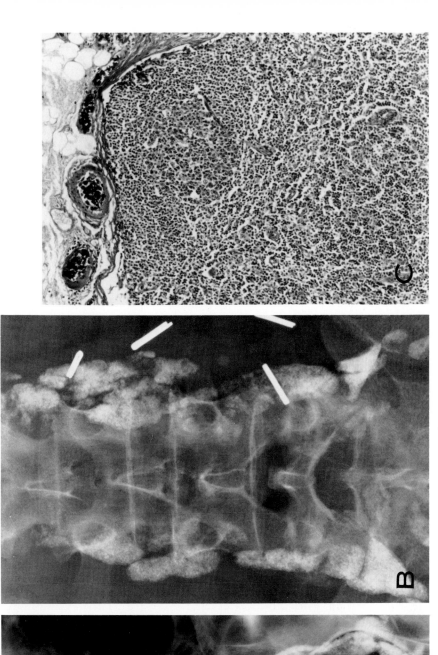

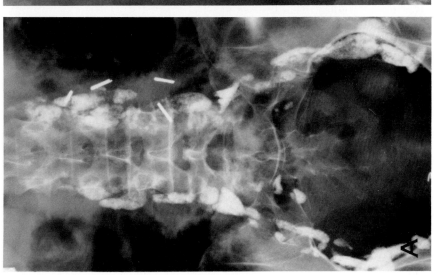

FIG. 7.3. REACTIVE HYPERPLASIA IN 42-YEAR-OLD FEMALE WITH LOCALIZED LYMPHOSARCOMA OF STOMACH

A: Lymphogram shows enlarged foamy nodes in the iliac and para-aortic area. All nodes are involved to the same degree. Biopsy taken in area of clips. B: Para-aortic nodes. ×2. C: Microscopy. Reactive hyperplasia. ×100.

RETROPERITONEAL FIBROSIS

Retroperitoneal fibrosis, first described by Ormond in 1948, is a relatively uncommon clinical entity. The etiology of the disease is unknown but is considered to be related to hypersensitivity or an autoimmune reaction. The disease most frequently occurs in the retroperitoneum. It has also been reported in the mediastinum obstructing the superior vena cava (Kunkel et al., 1954; Barrett, 1958; Hache et al., 1962) as well as involving the inferior vena cava, bile ducts and duodenum (Schneider, 1964), aorta (Furlong and Connerty, 1958), and mesenteric vessels (Baum, 1972). The colon and bile ducts have also been affected and an associated vasculitis reported (Arger et al., 1973).

The clinical symptoms are nonspecific, and irreversible renal damage may result before a diagnosis is made. Abdominal pain, anorexia, renal dysfunction, hypertension, anemia, and dysproteinemia are suggestive symptoms.

The process may be localized (involving a segment of one ureter) or extensive (involving the entire retroperitoneum from the renal pedicles to the sacrum and encasing all of the retroperitoneal structures). Conventional roentgenograms may reveal loss of the normal contour of the psoas shadows (Holmes and Robbins, 1955).

Urography may reveal delayed excretion of contrast material, dilatation of the collecting system, and a smooth tapered obstruction of one or both ureters. The ureters may taper gradually at the point of obstruction and deviate medially. Medial displacement of the ureters has been considered a significant finding in the diagnosis of idiopathic retroperitoneal fibrosis. Arger et al. (1973) have recently shown that the ureters are encased in the fibrotic process, but there is no medial displacement. The position of the ureters in patients with idiopathic retroperitoneal fibrosis is not statistically different from the position of the ureters in normal patients. The fibrotic process may also obstruct the lymphatics.

The pertinent lymphographic findings in retroperitoneal fibrosis are secondary to obstruction with collateral filling and reflux into lymphatic channels not visualized in normal patients (Fig. 7.4). There is a marked delay in passage of contrast material through the iliac and para-aortic channels. There is frequent, irregular nodal filling defects in delayed films. Lymphatic obstruction predisposes to lymphaticovenous communications, and it is imperative to routinely fluoroscope and film especially in the pelvis during the procedure (Fig. 7.5). Pa-

tients presenting these lymphographic findings have been reported (Clouse et al., 1964; Lemmon and Kiser, 1966; Hahn, 1966; Suby et al., 1965; Bookstein, 1966; Gregl et al., 1967). The lymphatics above L4 are usually not visualized.

Aortography and cavography also have diagnostic importance in retroperitoneal fibrosis. The fibrotic process also compresses and obstructs the major vessels resulting in complete obstruction of the inferior vena cava. Collateral

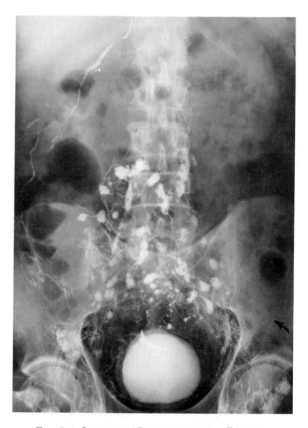

FIG. 7.4. IDIOPATHIC RETROPERITONEAL FIBROSIS
Lymphangiogram shows no filling of lymphatics above L4 with marked reflux and filling of presacral, bladder wall lymphatic, superficial epigastric (*arrow*), and a large lymphatic in retroperitoneal area on the right eventually emptying into the thoracic duct.

circulation develops in the venous system similar to the lymphatic collateral circulation. It is most frequently seen in the second to fourth lumbar area (Fig. 7.5C).

Microscopic examination reveals fibrous tissue and granulomatous fibroelastic areas, containing histiocytes, lymphocytes, and plasma cells. There may be secondary fatty degeneration with areas of necrosis.

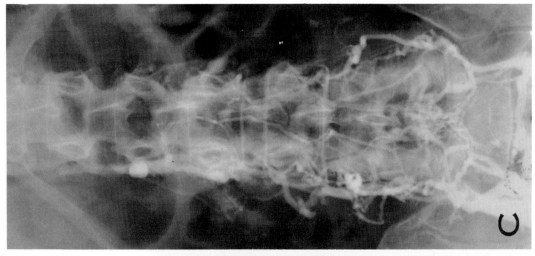

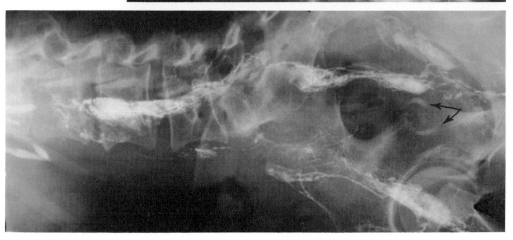

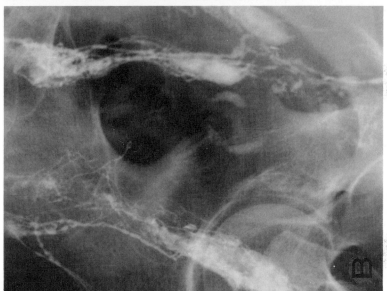

FIG. 7.5. ANOTHER PATIENT WITH IDIOPATHIC RETROPERITONEAL FIBROSIS

A: The right common iliac lymphatics are obstructed. Contrast material outlines a pelvic vein (*arrows*). B: Coned view of lymphaticovenous communication. C: Bilateral femoral venogram shows obstruction of the inferior vena cava with extensive filling of lumbar veins. D: Retrograde urogram shows obstruction and encasement of the ureter at the exact site of obstruction of the right common iliac lymphatics (*arrow*). E: Lymphogram 24 hr after injection shows no nodal filling on the right above L4.

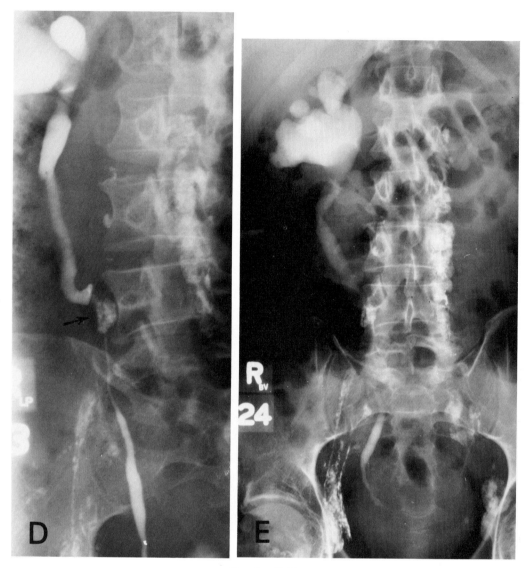

FIG. 7.5. *D–E*

RETROPERITONEAL PANNICULITIS

Retroperitoneal panniculitis is presumed to be related to mesenteric panniculitis and may represent an early stage of retroperitoneal fibrosis (Harbrecht, 1967; Rogers et al., 1961). It is characterized by fat necrosis (Clemett and Tracht, 1969) and inflammation of adipose tissue containing lymphocytes, plasma cells, and fibrocytes. The lymphographic findings include central and peripheral filling defects in the nodes similar to the inflammatory changes of retroperitoneal fibrosis, granulomatous processes, and metastatic disease (Giustra et al., 1973). The lymphatic channels are not disturbed (Fig. 7.6).

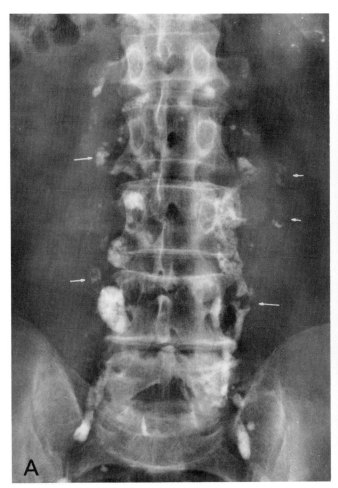 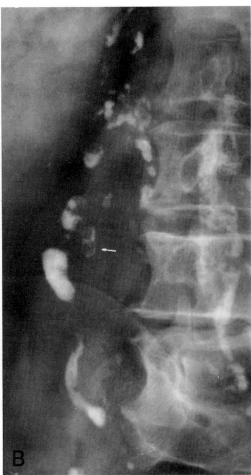

FIG. 7.6. RETROPERITONEAL PANNICULITIS
Common iliac and para-aortic lymph nodes after 24 hr are abnormal with areas of peripheral and central "replacement" (*arrows*). The filling defects resulted from an inflammatory process with loss of normal architecture. *A:* Frontal view. *B:* Right posterior oblique view. (Courtesy of Peter E. Giustra, M.D., Rockland, Maine.)

FIBROLIPOMATOSIS

Infiltration of the lymph node by fat and fibrous tissue is a degenerative change related to the process of aging and is seen in patients of middle and older age groups. The center of lymph node is replaced by fat and fibrous tissue leaving an incomplete rim of lymphatic tissue at the periphery (Fuchs et al., 1960; Fischer et al., 1962; Ditchek et al., 1973). The appearance on the lymphogram is that of a large central filling defect with contrast material in the peripheral lymphatic tissue (Fig. 7.7).

The findings must be differentiated from metastatic carcinoma. Fibrolipomatosis is most commonly seen in the inguinal and axillary nodes because they are the first order drainage nodes of the extremities. It may also be seen in the common iliac nodes following pelvic inflammatory disease.

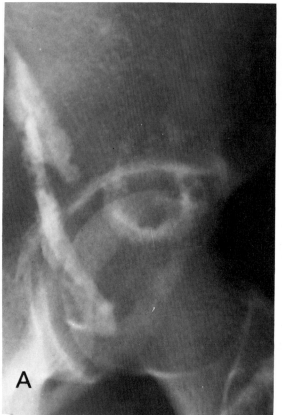

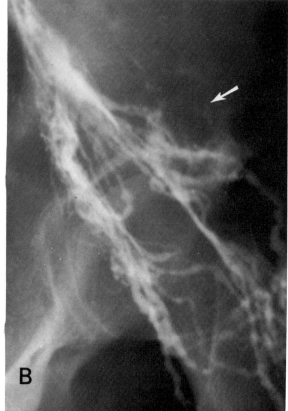

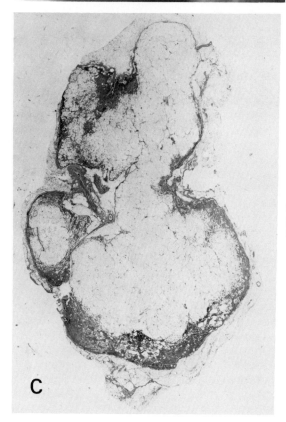

FIG. 7.7. FIBROLIPOMATOUS LYMPH NODE CHANGES IN
34-YEAR-OLD MALE WITH HODGKIN'S DISEASE IN
SUBMANDIBULAR LYMPH NODE
A: Coned view of lymphogram. Early channel filling shows
paucity of efferent vessels in external iliac node. *B*: Nodal
phase shows large filling defect (*arrow*). *C*: Microscopy, whole
node mount, shows fatty replacement. ×4.

LIPOPLASTIC LYMPHADENOPATHY

This process is associated with aging, is more common in women, and is characterized by mature adipose cells in the hilum of the lymph node. Morehead and McClure (1953) and Morehead (1965) have described the excessive accumulation of fat within axillary nodes. The nodes are usually normal in size, but they may become large enough to bother the patient. Wolfel and Smalley (1971) and Platzbekder et al. (1973) have reported marked enlargement due to lipoplastic changes in the external iliac and para-aortic nodes. The etiology is obscure.

GRANULOMATOUS EPITHELIOID INFLAMMATION

Granulomatous reactions are produced by a large variety of organisms including:
1. Sarcoidosis
2. Bacterial infections: tuberculosis, leprosy, tularemia, *Treponema pallidum*, brucellosis
3. Fungi: histoplasmosis, coccidioidomycosis
4. Protozoan: toxoplasmosis, leishmaniasis
5. Parasites: filariasis
6. Regional enteritis

Sarcoidosis

Sarcoidosis is a systemic disease of unknown etiology. The patients have an altered immunologic response with hypergammaglobulinemia (Goldstein et al., 1971) and nonspecific hypercomplementemia (H50, C4, C2) (Sheffer et al., 1971). Viamonte et al. (1963) described the lymphographic changes in sarcoid and reported 6 cases (Fig. 7.8). Albrecht et al. (1967) reported abnormal pelvic and retroperitoneal nodes in 55% of 20 patients in whom there was no other clinical evidence of node enlargement. Bacsa and Mandi (1966) in lymphography of 12 patients and Rauste (1974) in 136 patients observed a correlation of hilar node enlargement with abnormal pelvic and retroperitoneal nodes.

Blaudow and Scharkoff (1972) in 96 cases of sarcoid also found concomitant retroperitoneal involvement in 33% of patients with stage 1 disease. In stage 2, 45% had retroperitoneal node involvement when the disease was less than 1 year, and 75% when the disease had been present for more than 1 year. In contrast, Akisada et al. (1969) and Zalar (1973) found no consistent relationship between abnormal paratracheal and mediastinal nodes and severity of lung changes with abnormal retroperitoneal nodes.

LaMarque et al. (1971a, b) described the lymphographic changes in sarcoid as occurring in three stages. The first stage of adenitis produces a granular appearance to the nodes with droplets of contrast material in slightly dilated sinusoids. An intermediate stage produces a foamy appearance. In the late stage the node undergoes fibrosis with obstruction of sinusoids and lymph channels between the nodes, resulting in nodes which may be only partially filled.

Blaudow and Scharkoff (1972) consider the occurrence of a granular pattern with sharply defined filling defects to favor spontaneous remissions. They recommend lymphography only in therapy-resistant and reactivated cases as well as the suspicion of intra-abdominal sarcoidosis. The lymphographic pattern is not specific for sarcoid in any stage of the disease. It mimics acute and reactive hyperplastic inflammatory reactions or lymphomas. In contrast, Strickstrock and Weissleder (1968) do not recommend routine lymphography in patients with histologically verified pulmonary sarcoidosis because demonstration of retroperitoneal nodes has no therapeutic importance. The response to therapy in this disease is best followed by chest roentgenograms.

Tuberculosis

Infections with the tubercle bacillus produce central and marginal filling defects of varying sizes on the lymphograms. The nodes may be normal to enlarged. The bacillis enter via the afferent channels, lodge in the marginal sinus or sinusoids, and produce a caseous area of necrosis with obstruction of the sinusoids. The node appearance more closely resembles metastatic carcinoma, but it may also be indistinguishable from lymphoma (Schaffer et al., 1963; Viamonte et al., 1963; Ruttiman, 1964; Babeau and Fourier, 1965; Betoulieres et al., 1968).

Albrecht et al. (1967) studied 15 patients with tuberculosis and only cervical adenopathy; 6 were found to have abnormal retroperitoneal nodes. They suggest that tuberculosis infection should not be considered a regional disease. In support of this concept Gregl and Kienle (1969) reported a case of carcinoma of the breast with ipsilateral old tuberculous node involvement

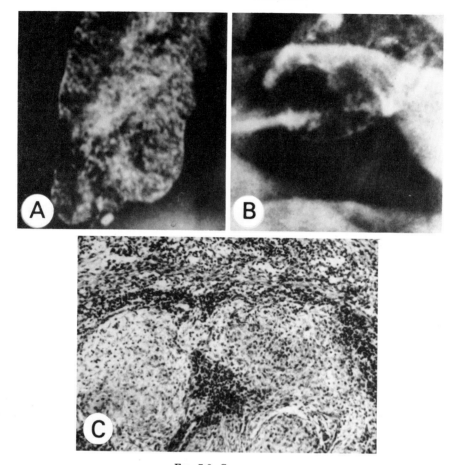

FIG. 7.8. SARCOIDOSIS

A: Right inguinal node changes indistinguishable from lymphoma. *B*: Left supraclavicular node. *C*: Magnification shows discrete noncaseating granulomas.   ×100. (Courtesy of Manuel Viamonte, Jr., M.D., Miami, Florida.)

that was indistinguishable from metastatic carcinoma.

In 100 patients with tuberculosis Suramo (1974) found diseased lumbar nodes in 71 and iliac nodes in 11. In 61 patients the nodes were normal in size. Abnormal iliac and lumbar nodes were present in 41 of 52 patients with cervical or axillary lymph node tuberculosis, and in 17 of 18 patients with urogenital tuberculosis. The diagnosis of tuberculosis was considered reasonably certain when the nodes were enlarged, showed marginal filling defects produced by caseation necrosis, and when the central architecture of the node was destroyed. When the central architecture of the node is disrupted, the appearance more closely resembles lymphoma. The diagnosis of tuberculosis is less certain when the sinusoids are mildly dilated and not disrupted. The caseating areas produce filling defects slightly larger than normal follicles. These changes result in a lymph node that is more granular or foamy without marginal filling defects (Fig. 7.9).

Other Granulomatous Diseases

The lymphographic pattern in brucellosis, syphilis, and histoplasmosis also simulates lymphoma. LaMarque et al. (1971a, b) described the lymphographic changes in 11 patients with brucellosis. The study showed generalized lymph node involvement associated with nonspecific adenitis and lymph node fibrosis. During the acute stage of brucellosis, the lymph nodes are moderately enlarged in a coarse granular lymphographic pattern. In the chronic stage the nodes increase in size; as irregular filling defects increase, the pattern becomes more foamy.

In syphilis capsular fibrosis, vascular endothelial proliferation, granuloma, and follicular hyperplasia with sheets of plasma cells produce a generalized pattern throughout the nodes that is indistinguishable from lymphoma (Kerk and

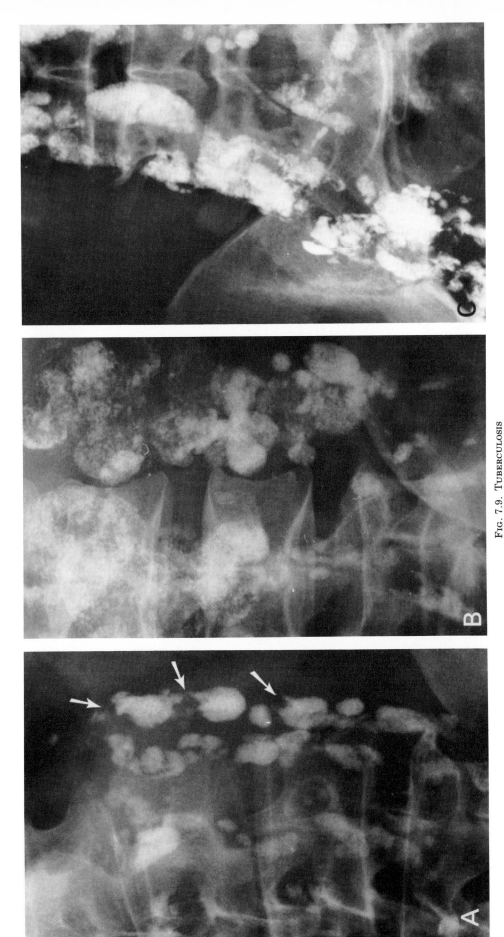

FIG. 7.9. TUBERCULOSIS

A: There are marginal filling defects in para-aortic nodes (*arrows*). *B*: The para-aortic nodes are more foamy with destruction of central nodal architecture. *C*: Common iliac nodes show uneven granular nodes, coarser than normal with large globules of contrast material in large sinusoids. (Courtesy of Ilkka Suramo, M.D., Oulu, Finland.)

Schilling, 1969; Bergstrom and Navin, 1973). Histoplasmosis also produces changes in the lymph node indistinguishable from the malignant lymphoma. Viamonte et al. (1963) observed a nonspecific inflammatory reaction with preservation of the internal architecture of the lymph nodes. Bottcher (1974) reported toxoplasmosis lymphadenitis superimposed on Hodgkin's disease. The nodes were slightly enlarged with small follicular filling defects characteristic of inflammatory disease.

RADIATION CHANGES

The sensitivity of lymphocytes to irradiation was described by Heineke (1905). Excellent papers have described the rapid death of lymphocytes in lymphoid tissue and decrease in circulation. Cytoplasmic disintegration follows nuclear disruption (Trowell, 1952; Schrek, 1961). Histiocytes containing cellular debris can be seen 3 hr after 300 R and are more numerous after 8 hr

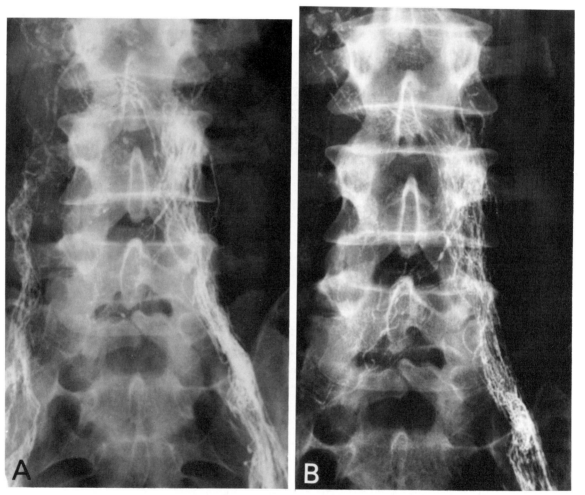

FIG. 7.10. RADIATION CHANGES IN LYMPHATICS
A: Normal para-aortic lymphatics. *B*: Lymphatics 3 years after 3500 R.

lating lymphocytes after irradiation. Trowell (1952), using the light microscope, described the changes of chromatin clumping followed by nuclear vacuolization, pyknosis, and fragmentation and disappear after 24–48 hr (DeBruyn, 1948).

Smith et al. (1967), using the electron microscope, demonstrated prominent histiocytic pseudopodia near damaged lymphocytes within 30 min after 500 R whole body irradiation. Damaged lymphocytes showed aggregation of chromatin near the nuclear membrane, electrondense mitochondria, and widening of the perinuclear space with separation of the nucleus and cytoplasm. Three hours later the chromatin had condensed near the nuclear membrane and the center of the nucleus became electronlucent. Nuclear disintegration was complete within 6 hr, and remnants of nuclei and other cytoplasmic organelles were noted within histiocytes. Similar findings have been reported by Holsten (1970).

Irradiation of the lymph nodes causes destruction of lymphocytes even in low doses of 50–800 R (Cottier, 1966). Engeset (1964) irradiated the lymph nodes of rats with a single dose of 3000 R. Lymphocyte destruction was complete within 24 hr, and after 9 months the node was replaced by fibrous tissue with no follicles or sinuses. The ability of the lymph node to regenerate appears to be variable, however. Hall and Morris (1964) have reported re-establishment of node lymphocyte population by circulating lymphocytes.

There has been considerable controversy as to the ability of irradiated nodes to filter particulate matter and tumor cells. Virchow (1863) suggested that lymph nodes are effective barriers to particulate matter. Many investigators con-

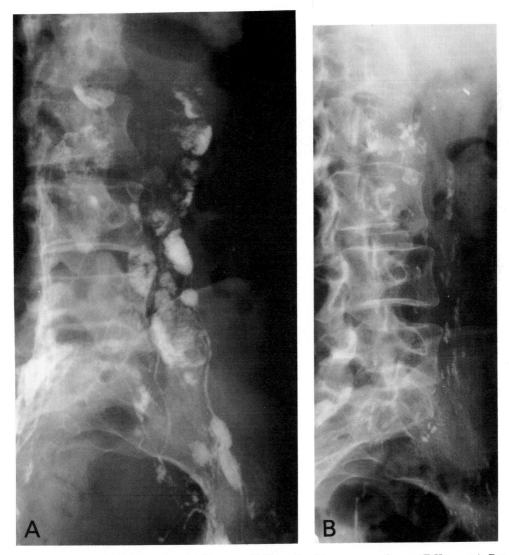

FIG. 7.11. RADIATION CHANGES IN LYMPH NODES IN 26-YEAR-OLD FEMALE WITH STAGE 4E HODGKIN'S DISEASE

A: Lymphogram (1969) showing extensive involvement of the para-aortic nodes. *B*: Lymphogram 6 years later (1975) showing small atrophic lymph nodes without recurrent Hodgkin's disease.

firmed his observation (Drinker et al., 1934; Engeset, 1962; Ludwig and Titus, 1967) while others (Yoffey and Sullivan, 1939; Herman et al., 1968; Dettman et al., 1966) have seen no effective barrier by the nodes. The same type of experiments using live tumor cells have resulted in additional conflicting data (Engeset, 1964; Fisher and Fisher, 1967). Ujiki et al. (1970), using V2 rabbit carcinoma, found that the irradiated lymph node acted as an effective barrier for 2–3 weeks. Three weeks after tumor infusion, distant tumor growth was increased in rabbits receiving 1–3000 R, but after 6 weeks both groups had a similar incidence of distant tumor growth. They concluded that the earlier presence of distant metastases in the irradiated rabbit was the result of a decrease in barrier function allowing immediate passage of tumor cells during the process of infusion and that irradiated nodes are unable to retain growing cancer cells for the same length of time as the normal nodes.

The effect of irradiation on lymphatic vessels has been studied extensively. Van Den Brenk (1957), using the Sandison-Clark type of ear chamber on rabbits, observed lymphatic vessel regeneration with doses of 1000 R but not doses of 2000 R. Preformed lymphatics survived after doses of 4000 R, and irradiation failed to produce swelling of the lymphatic endothelium and obstruction. Lenzi and Bassani (1963), studying pelvic organs after irradiation, found tortuous vessels but no obstruction after doses of 15,000 R. Obstruction was only found in areas receiving 25,000–30,000 R with tissue necrosis.

Other authors reviewing clinical material (Wiljasalo and Perttala, 1966; Ariel et al., 1967) also report no obstruction in normal lymphatics after therapeutic doses of radiation. Reduction in size of lymph nodes secondary to fibrosis and fine delicate lymphatic vessels are seen on second-look lymphography (Fig. 7.10). The lymph nodes do not retain large amounts of contrast material (Fig. 7.11). Irradiation of lymph nodes and vessels infiltrated by tumors may produce obstruction by tumor and tissue necrosis, fibrosis, or recurrent tumor. In these patients constant monitoring is necessary in order to observe collateral lymphatic circulation and to discontinue the procedure when lymphovenous communications are present.

REFERENCES

Akisada, M., Tasaka, A. and Mikami, R.: Lymphography in sarcoidosis: comparison with roentgen findings in the chest. Radiology, 93: 1273, 1969.

Albrecht, A., Taenzer, V. and Nickling, H.: Lymphographische befunde sei Sarkoidose und Lymphkrotentuberkulose. Fortschr. Roentgenstr., 106: 178, 1967.

Arger, P. H., Stolz, J. L. and Miller, W. R.: Retroperitoneal fibrosis. An analysis of the clinical spectrum and roentgenographic signs. Am. J. Roentgenol., 119: 812, 1973.

Ariel, I. M., Resnick, M. I. and Oropeza, R.: The effect of irradiation (external and internal) on lymphatic dynamics. Radiology, 99: 404, 1967.

Babeau, P. and Fourier, A.: Rapport clinique de la lymphographie lipiodolee dans certaines formes de lymphadenite tuberculereuse. J. Belge. Radiol., 48: 332, 1965.

Bacsa, S. and Mandi, L.: Abdominal lymphography in thoracic sarcoidosis. Scand. J. Respir. Dis., 47: 244, 1966.

Barrett, N. P.: Idiopathic mediastinal fibrosis. Br. J. Surg., 46: 207, 1958.

Baum, S.: Case records, Massachusetts General Hospital. N. Engl. J. Med., 287: 33, 1972.

Bergstrom, J. F. and Navin, J. J.: Luetic lymphadenitis: lymphographic manifestations simulating lymphoma. Radiology, 106: 287, 1973.

Betoulieres, P., LaMarque, J. L., Ginestie, J. F. and Caubes, C.: Etude des aspects lymphographiques de la tuberculose ganglionnaire. J. Radiol. Electrol. Med. Nucl., 49: 1, 1968.

Blaudow, K. and Scharkoff, T.: Lymphographie des retroperitonealen Lymphsystems bei Sarkoidose. Z. Erkr. Atmungsorgane, 136: 311, 1972.

Bookstein, J. J., Schroeder, K. F. and Batsakis, J. G.: Lymphangiography in the diagnosis of retroperitoneal fibrosis: case report. J. Urol., 95: 99, 1966.

Bottcher, J.: Lymphographie bei dem Zusammentreffen von Lymphknoten-Toxoplasmose und Stationarer Lymphogranulomatose. Roentgenblaetter, 27: 257, 1974.

Butler, J. J.: Non-neoplastic lesions of lymph nodes in man to be differentiated from lymphomas. Natl. Cancer Inst. Monogr., 32: 233, 1969.

Castellino, R. A., Billingham, M. and Dorfman, R. F.: Lymphographic accuracy in Hodgkin's disease and malignant lymphoma with a note on the "reactive" lymph node as a cause of most false-positive lymphograms. Invest. Radiol., 9: 155, 1974.

Castleman, B.: Case records of the Massachusetts General Hospital: hyperplasia of mediastinal lymph nodes. N. Engl. J. Med., 250: 26, 1954.

Castleman, B. and Iverson, L.: Localized mediastinal lymph node hyperplasia resembling thymoma. Cancer, 9: 822, 1956.

Clemett, A. R. and Tracht, D. G.: The roentgen diagnosis of retractile mesenteritis. Am. J. Roentgenol., 107: 787, 1969.

Clouse, M. E., Fraley, E. E. and Lituim, S. B.: Lymphographic criteria for diagnosis of retroperitoneal fibrosis. Radiology, 83: 1, 1964.

Cottier, H.: Histopathologie der Wirkung ionisierender Strahlen auf hohere Organismen (Tier und Mensch). In Encyclopedia of Medical Radiology II/2, p. 100, New York, Springer-Verlag, 1966.

DeBruyn, P. P. H.: Lymph node and intestinal lymphatic tissue. In Histopathology of Irradiation from External *and Internal Sources,* edited by W. Bloom, pp. 348-445. New York, McGraw-Hill Co., 1948.

deRoo, T.: *Atlas of Lymphography,* p. 34. Sandoz, 1973.

Dettman, P. M., King, E. R. and Zinberg, Y. H.: Evaluation of lymph node function following irradiation or surgery. Am. J. Roentgenol., *96:* 711, 1966.

Ditchek, T., Blahut, J. and Kittelson, A. C.: Lymphadenography in normal subjects. Radiology, *80:* 175, 1973.

Drinker, C. K., Field, M. E. and Ward, H. K.: The filtering capacity of lymph nodes. J. Exp. Med., *59:* 393, 1934.

Engeset, A.: Barrier function of lymph glands. Lancet, *1:* 324, 1962.

Engeset, A.: Irradiation of lymph nodes and vessels. Acta Radiol. Suppl., 229, 1964.

Fischer, H. W., Lawrence, M. S. and Thornbury, J. R.: Lymphography of the normal adult male. Radiology, *78:* 399, 1962.

Fisher, B. and Fisher, E.: Barrier function of lymph node to tumor cells and erythrocytes. II. Effect of x-ray, inflammation, sensitization and tumor growth. Cancer, *20:* 1914, 1967.

Fornier, A. M., Denizet, D. and Delagrange, A.: La lymphographie dans la spondylarthrite ankylosante. J. Radiol. Electrol. Med. Nucl., *50:* 773, 1969.

Fuchs, W. A.: In *Lymphography in Cancer,* edited by P. Rentchnick, p. 94. New York, Springer-Verlag, 1969.

Fuchs, W. A., Ruttiman, A. and DelBuono, M. S.: Zur Lymphographie bei Chronischen sekundaren Lymphodemen. Fortschr. Geb. Roentgenstr. Nuklearmed., *92:* 608, 1960.

Furlong, J. H., Jr. and Connerty, H. V.: Compression of the aorta and ureters by a retroperitoneal inflammatory mass; case report. Del. Med. J., *30:* 63, 1958.

Giustra, P. E., Killoran, P. J., Opper, L. and Root, J. A.: Abnormal excretory urogram and lymphangiogram in retroperitoneal panniculitis. Radiology, *106:* 545, 1973.

Goldstein, R. A., Israel, H. L. and Rawnsley, H. M.: Effect of race and stage of disease on the serum immunoglobulins in sarcoidosis. In *5th International Conference on Sarcoidosis, Prague Karolinum June 16-21, 1969,* edited by L. Levinsky and F. Macholda, p. 178. Universita Karlova Praha, Prague, 1971.

Gregl, A. and Kienle, J.: Axillary lymph node tuberculosis presenting lymphological signs of metastasis from ipsilateral breast cancer. Radiology, *93:* 1107, 1969.

Gregl, A., Truss, F., Grabner, F. and Kienle, U. J.: Lymphographie und Cavographie bei der idiopathischen retroperitonealen Fibrose. Fortschr. Roentgenstr., *107:* 329, 1967.

Hache, L., Woolner, L. B. and Bernatz, P. B.: Idiopathic fibrous mediastinitis. J. Dis. Chest, *41:* 9, 1962.

Hahn, B. D.: The use of lymphangiography for the diagnosis of idiopathic retroperitoneal fibrosis. Am. J. Obstet. Gynecol., *14:* 539, 1966.

Hall, J. G. and Morris, B.: Effect of x-radiation of the popliteal lymph node on its output of lymphocytes in immunological responsiveness. Lancet, *1:* 1077, 1964.

Harbrecht, P. J.: Variants of retroperitoneal fibrosis. Ann. Surg., *165:* 388, 1967.

Heineke, H.: Experimentelle Untersuchungen uber die Einwirkung der Roentgenstrahlen auf inner Organe. Mitt. Grenzgeb. Med. Chir., *14:* 21, 1905.

Herman, P. G., Benninghoff, D. L. and Mellins, H. Z.: Radiation effect on the barrier function of the lymph node. Radiology, *91:* 698, 1968.

Holmes, G. W. and Robbins, L. L.: *Roentgen Interpretation,* 8th ed., p. 372. Philadelphia, Lea & Febiger, 1955.

Holsten, D. R.: Die Strahleneinwirkung auf den lymphnoten, eine elektronenmikroskopische Untersuchung. Strahlentherapie (Munchen), *139:* 41, 1970.

Kerk, E. and Schilling, L.: Lymphographische Befunde bei Uenerischen Erkrankungen. Fortschr. Geb. Roentgenstr. Nuklearmed., *111:* 22, 1969.

Kunkel, W. M., Clagett, O. T. and MacDonald, J. R.: Mediastinal granulomas. J. Thorac. Cardiovasc. Surg., *27:* 565, 1954.

LaMarque, J. L., Ginestie, J. F., Senac, J. P. and Harson, B.: Etude lymphographique de la brucellose. Ann. Radiol. (Paris), *14:* 79, 1971a.

LaMarque, J. L., Ginestie, J. F., Senac, J. P. and Mathieu, F.: Apport de la lymphographie dans la maladie de Besnier-Boech-Schaumann. Ann. Radiol. (Paris), *14:* 437, 1971b.

Lattes, R. and Pachter, M. R.: Benign lymphoid masses of probable hamartomatous nature. Cancer, *15:* 197, 1962.

Lemmon, W. T. and Kiser, W. S.: Idiopathic retroperitoneal fibrosis. Diagnostic enigma: report of a case simulating diabetes insipidus and a review of the literature. J. Urol., *96:* 658, 1966.

Lenzi, M. and Bassani, G.: The effect of radiation on the lymph and on lymph vessels. Radiology, *80:* 814, 1963.

Ludwig, J. and Titus, J. L.: Experimental tumor cell emboli in lymph nodes. Arch. Pathol., *84:* 304, 1967.

Morehead, R.: *Human Pathology,* p. 1307. New York, McGraw-Hill Co., 1965.

Morehead, R. and McClure, S.: Lipoplastic lymphadenopathy (abstr.). Am. J. Pathol., *26:* 615, 1953.

Nishimine, M., Sako, M., Kubota, A. and Okada, S.: Lymphography in mediastinal lymph node hyperplasia: report of two cases. Lymphology, *7:* 22, 1974.

Ormond, J. K.: Bilateral ureteral obstruction due to involvement and compression by inflammatory retroperitoneal process. J. Urol., *59:* 1072, 1948.

Parker, B. R., Blank, N. and Castellino, R. A.: Lymphographic appearance of benign conditions simulating lymphoma. Radiology, *111:* 267, 1974.

Platzbekder, H., Kohler, K., Hanefeld, M. and Kunze, D.: Zur sogenannten, Lipomatose der Lymphknoten im Lymphogramm. Radiol. Diagn. (Berl.), *6:* 677, 1973.

Rauste, J.: Lymphography in granulomatous inflammations. Scand. J. Respir. Dis. [Suppl.], *89:* 186, 1974.

Rogers, C. E., Demetrakopoulos, N. J. and Hyamns, V.: Isolated lipodystrophy affecting the mesentery, the retroperitoneal area and the small intestines. Ann. Surg., *153:* 277, 1961.

Ruttiman, A.: Die Lymphographie. In *Ergebnisse der medizinischen Strahlenforschung,* Neue Folge, Band I, Hrsg. Schinz-Glauner-Ruttimann. Stuttgart, G. Thieme, 1964.

Ruttner, J. R.: Pathological anatomy of "benign" lymph node disease. In *Progress in Lymphology,* p. 98. Stuttgart, G. Thieme, 1967.

Schaffer, B., Koehler, R. P., Daniel, C. R., Wohl, G. T., Rivera, E., Meyers, W. A. and Skelley, J. F.: A critical evaluation of lymphography. Radiology, *80:* 917, 1963.

Schneider, C. F.: Idiopathic retroperitoneal fibrosis producing vena caval, biliary, ureteral and duodenal obstruction. Ann. Surg., *159:* 316, 1964.

Schrek, R.: Qualitative and quantitative reactions of lymphocytes to x-rays. Ann. N.Y. Acad. Sci., *95:* 839, 1961.

Sheffer, A. L., Ruddy, S., and Israel, H. L.: Serum complement levels in sarcoidosis, In *5th International Conference on Sarcoidosis, Prague Karolinum, June 16-21, 1969,* edited by L. Levinsky and F. Macholda, ch. 5, p.

195. Universita Karlova Praha, Prague, 1971.

Smith, E. B., White, D. C., Hartsock, R. J. and Dixon, A. C.: Acute ultrastructural effects of 500 roentgens on the lymph node of mouse. Am. J. Pathol., *50:* 159, 1967.

Strickstrock, K. H. and Weissleder, H.: Lymphographische Diagnose und Differentialdiagnose bei der Sarkoidose. Fortschr. Roentgenstr., *108:* 576, 1968.

Suby, H. J., Kerr, W. S., Grahm, J. R. and Fraley, E. G.: Retroperitoneal fibrosis: a missing link in the chain. J. Urol., *93:* 144, 1965.

Suramo, I.: Lymphography in tuberculosis. Acta Radiol. Suppl., *339:* 1, 1974.

Tjernberg, B.: Lymphography as an aid to examination of lymph nodes. Acta Soc. Med. Upsalien., *61:* 207, 1956.

Trowell, O. A.: The sensitivity of lymphocytes to ionising radiation. J. Pathol. Bact., *64:* 687, 1952.

Ujiki, G. T., O'Brien, P. H., Moss, W. T., Putong, P., and Towne, W.: The lymph node barriers to viable tumor cells before and after irradiation. J. Surg. Oncol., *2:* 193, 1970.

Van Den Brenk, H. A. S.: The effect of ionizing radiations on the regeneration and behavior of mammalian lymphatics. Radiology, *78:* 837, 1957.

Viamonte, M., Altman, D., Parks, R., Blum, E., Bevilacqua, M. and Recher, L.: Radiographic-pathologic correlation in the interpretation of lymphangioadenograms. Radiology, *80:* 903, 1963.

Virchow, R.: *Cellular Pathology*. London, John Churchill, 1863.

Wiljasalo, M., Julkunen, H. and Saluen, I.: Lymphography in rheumatic diseases. Ann. Med. Intern. Fenn., *55:* 125, 1966.

Wiljasalo, M. and Perttala, Y.: Lymphographic changes caused by radiotherapy. Ann. Med. Intern. Fenn, *55:* 57, 1966.

Wolfel, D. A. and Smalley, R. H.: Lipoplastic lymphadenopathy. Am. J. Roentgenol. *112:* 610, 1971.

Yoffey, J. M. and Sullivan, E. R.: The lymphatic pathways from the nose and pharynx. J. Exp. Med., *69:* 133, 1939.

Zalar, J.: Limfografija u Dijagnostici Retroperitonealne Sarkoidoze. Plucne Bolesti Tuberk., *25:* 183, 1973.

8

Lymphoma

THE FUNCTIONAL APPROACH TO THE PATHOLOGY OF MALIGNANT LYMPHOMA

ROBERT J. LUKES, M.D.*

In the decade since the Rye Conference on Hodgkin's disease, there has been remarkable progress in the understanding of the pathology of the disease and the effectiveness of therapy; however, in the non-Hodgkin's lymphomas there has been little progress until recently.

The non-Hodgkin's lymphomas through the decades have been involved in disputes over terminology and classification, apparently as a result of a lack of fundamental understanding of lymphopoiesis and the associated imprecision in cytologic characterization and identification. The traditional terms lymphosarcoma and reticulum cell sarcoma, have been applied in an extraordinarily variable fashion. Each included a number of cytologic types and presently has achieved a meaningless status in communication (Gall, 1958; Lukes, 1968). In addition, follicular lymphoma was regarded as a lymphoma of the follicular structure in the traditional cytologic classification, but apparently accounted for only 50% of the nodular proliferations (Jones et al., 1973). The approach of Rappaport et al., proposed in 1956 long before the modern developments in immunology, provided important emphasis on cytologic features and the significance of nodularity. Its clinical and prognostic value only recently became appreciated. Unfortunately, the classification of Rappaport does not appear conceptually relevant since it lacks a relationship to our modern understanding lymphocytes and immunology.

* The reporting of this investigation has been supported in part by National Institute of Health training grants PO1 CA-19449-01 and CA-09025-01A1. There was partial support by the Beaumont Foundation.

Lukes and Collins initially outlined the basis for a new functional approach for the malignant lymphomas relating these neoplasms to the recent remarkable developments in immunology, the T and B cell systems, and alterations in lymphocyte transformation (Collins and Lukes, 1971; Lukes and Collins, 1973). A functional approach was outlined subsequently for the redefinition of the lymphomas applying a variety of immunologic and cytochemical techniques to characterize these processes according to the T and B cell systems (Lukes and Collins, 1974a). In these initial publications it was proposed that (1) malignant lymphomas principally involve the T and B lymphocytic systems; (2) lymphomas of "true" histiocytes are rare, and reticulum cell sarcoma and histiocytic lymphoma of the past with rare exceptions are lymphomas of transformed lymphocytes of either the T or B cell systems; and (3) lymphomas commonly develop as a block for a "switch on" (derepression) in lymphocyte transformation. A functional classification initially was presented at the Congress of Radiologists Meeting in 1972 in Freiburg, West Germany, and subsequently defined in detail (Lukes and Collins, 1974a). On the basis of this conceptual approach the lymphomas are regarded as aggregates of immune-deficient cells that migrate, target, and function to varying degrees similar to their normal counterparts. It was suggested also that the study of lymphomas from an immunologic approach might lead to a better understanding of the basic mechanism of these disorders and eventually permit the design of a more ideal biologic approach for therapy.

Following the presentation of our new functional approach and classification at a series of international meetings in 1973 (Lukes and Collins, 1974b and 1975), a number of other classifications were proposed (Bennett et al., 1974; Dorfman, 1974; Gerard-Marchant et al., 1974; and Lennert et al., 1975), but all the authors were reluctant to relate the lymphomas to the T and B cell systems. With the exception of the Kiel Classification (Gerard-Marchant et al., 1974), these new classifications are modifications of the Rappaport approach. The results of a number of studies using immunologic surface markers on non-Hodgkin's disease and related leukemias support the T and B cell nature of lymphomas (Aisenberg and Long, 1975; Berard et al., 1976; Braylan et al., 1975; Brouet et al., 1975; Davey et al., 1976; Gajl-Peczalska et al.,

1975; Green et al., 1975; and Leech et al., 1975). Our combined study of 384 cases of non-Hodgkin's disease and related leukemias evaluated by my associate, Dr. Robert Collins' group at the Vanderbilt University, and the author's at the University of Southern California School of Medicine, demonstrate that lymphomas with few exceptions mark as T and B cells and rarely as histiocytes (Lukes and Collins, 1977). The lymphomas of large cells for the most part mark as transformed lymphocytes.

In this presentation, I will review briefly (1) the immunologic and morphologic basis of our proposal; (2) the functional classification and cytologic types of both Hodgkin's and non-Hodgkin's lymphomas; (3) the functional approach and the results of our multiparameter studies; and (4) clinical-pathologic correlations.

IMMUNOLOGIC AND MORPHOLOGIC BASIS

Malignant lymphomas now appear established as neoplasms of the immune system. From our studies lymphoma cells can be related to their normal counterparts according to their morphologic features, distributional characteristics, and immunologic surface markers (Lukes and Collins, 1977). The dramatic progress in immunology in the past 15 years, particularly the establishment of the T and B lymphocytic systems in man with their distinctive functions and the remarkable phenomenon of lymphocyte transformation, are fundamental phenomena essential for our understanding of malignant lymphomas. The terminology and classification of the past, including that of Rappaport et al. (1956), lack any relationship to modern immunology, since they were all proposed long before these phenomena were demonstrated.

Lymphocytic Systems

The recent progress in immunology has been a subject of numerous reviews and its relationship to malignant lymphomas has recently been emphasized by Hansen and Good (1974). The T and B lymphocytic systems, originally discovered through ablation experiments in animals, were confirmed in man through studies of immune deficiency states. A third lymphocytic system, the precursor cell for T and B lymphocytes, possibly the marrow stem cell, also appears to exist. We have proposed the term, U cell (undefined or unmarked), since it lacks both T or B cell markers. The U cell includes, therefore, the theoretical null cell and those cells presently without specific demonstrable surface

markers or definable characteristics or functions. In all three systems the remarkable lymphocyte transformation phenomenon apparently occurs and each has small, intermediate and transformed cells. Recognition of these three systems with their individual variants, accounts for the remarkable diversity of the morphologic and functional expressions of both normal lymphocytes and their lymphomatous counterparts.

The proposed development of the T and B cell systems is well documented in experimental animals. The T cell acquires its membrane characteristics when the precursor cell or U cell migrates to the thymus during a limited period in immunologic development, and comes in contact with thymic epithelium at which time the cell membrane is modified in an unknown fashion. In a similar manner in the avian species the precursor cell, after migrating to the bursa of Fabricius, acquires its B cell characteristics. The precise location of the bursal equivalent in man has never been identified in spite of extensive search, although it apparently exists in some form, possibly in Peyer's patches. The precursor cell seems to possess the membrane characteristics of both T and B cells that apparently are uncovered selectively in the thymus and the bursa of Fabricius.

The T cell or thymic dependent system is involved in cellular immunity and is measured clinically by delayed hypersensitivity responsiveness and in vitro lymphocyte transformation response to certain mitogens. T cell function is associated with the formation of a variety of soluble substances known as lymphokines and the functional cells producing the substances are designated as suppressor, helper, and killer T cells. The diversity and complexity of the functioning T cells only now are becoming appreciated, although their morphologic expressions are unknown. Undoubtedly malignant lymphomas of T cells at times may possess some of these functions, as recently suggested by Broder's proposal of the helper T cell nature of the cells in Sézary's syndrome (Broder et al., 1976). The B cell or thymic independent system, also known as the bursal equivalent system, is involved in immunoglobulin and antibody production.

The topographical distribution of the T and B lymphocytic system is now well established and is important morphologically in the understanding of normal immune reactions in various tissues and the morphologic interpretation of malignant lymphomas. From the ablation experiments in animals and parallel findings in congenital immune defects in man, the B cell system has been related to follicular centers and the distribution of plasma cells, while the T cell system is distributed in the paracortical areas of lymph nodes, perivascular regions of the spleen, and in small foci in the gastrointestinal tract. B cells are found in primary and secondary follicles wherever they exist and in the Malpighian bodies of the spleen, the lamina propria of the gastrointestinal tract, and interspersed in the bone marrow. The lymphocytic systems are not static. The T lymphocytes circulate four to six times a day and account for approximately 70% of normal peripheral blood lymphocytes. It is estimated that 20–25% of peripheral blood lymphocytes are B cells, although recent studies suggest that the proportion of B cells may be considerably lower. Thus, there is an extremely complex daily circulating traffic of lymphocytes through blood and tissue with a highly selective "homing" phenomenon of the T and B cell systems to preferential anatomic sites throughout the body. From our morphologic studies the lymphomas essentially are distributed in a highly predictable fashion parallel to the migration and distributional characteristics of their normal counterparts.

Lymphocyte Transformation

This remarkable phenomenon has been studied extensively in vitro, but its morphologic expressions and implications, both in normal immunologic reactions and the malignant lymphomas, have been unappreciated by pathologists until our recent proposals (Lukes and Collins, 1973; 1974a,b; 1975). Lymphocytes under the influence of certain plant mitogens, such as phytohemagglutinin, pokeweed, concanavalin A, and antigens to which an individual has been immunized, change from a small lymphocyte to a large hyperbasophilic blast cell or transformed lymphocyte. The exact mechanism of initiating transformation is not precisely established (O'Brien et al., 1977). Phytohemagglutinin and concanavalin A are thought to be highly selective transformers of T cells, while pokeweed is believed to transform both T and B cells. The only selective mitogen for human B cells appears to be Nocardia apaca, although the EB virus is a B cell transformer in human lymphoblastoid cell lines. From our morphologic studies, both the small lymphocyte and the fully transformed cell are regarded as expressions of lymphocytes. The small lymphocyte represents the dormant form and the transformed lymphocyte, the metabolically active dividing state. Lymphocytes in vivo seem to modulate between the dormant and the dividing form. The morphologic expression encountered is contingent upon the immunologic requirements. If our proposal is correct, the concept of differentiation in lymphocytes is inappropriate with the exception of the change to functional expressions, such as the plasma cell in the B cell system. In this situation the use of a term for differentiation does not appear as meaningful as the use of a functional designation.

The transformed lymphocyte is four to six times the size of a small lymphocyte and has primitive finely distributed chromatin, one or more prominent nucleoli, and abundant deeply basophilic cytoplasm in Romanowski's stained preparations. The cytoplasm is intensively pyroninophilic. The in vitro transformed lymphocytes grow in cohesive clusters. In sections of concentrated specimens these cells present wide variations in cell size and resemble a primitive appearing neoplastic process with numerous mitotic figures. Upon comparison study we were impressed by the remarkable resemblance of in vitro transformed lymphocytes and the large cells in both normal reactive lymphoid tissue and malignant lymphomas with the exception of obvious macrophages. Large transformed lymphocytes (immunoblasts) were identified in small numbers in the interfollicular tissue in benign reactions and in severe degrees in infectious mononucleosis, and in the regional lymph nodes of smallpox vaccination. Binucleated transformed immunoblasts, indistinguishable from diagnostic Reed-Sternberg cells of Hodgkin's disease, were found in every case of infectious mononucleosis on which morphologic material was available for study (Lukes et al., 1969; Tindle et al., 1972). There are also transformed lymphocytes in reactive follicular centers, varying in size and number, apparently as a reflection of the state of reactivity. The morphologic features of transformed lymphocytes most effectively are demonstrated in methyl green pyronine and Giemsa-stained sections. The follicular center is established as a B cell region, and therefore we regard the large transformed lymphocyte of the follicular center as a transformed B cell. Transformed lymphocytes (immunoblasts) of both T and B cell types apparently occur in the interfollicular tissue and are presently difficult to differentiate in histologic sections, although it seems likely that the B immunoblast is larger and possesses more densely staining amphophilic cytoplasm which at times may have plasmacytoid features.

B Cells

In lymph nodes normal B cells principally are found in primary and secondary follicles, in the peripheral blood in small numbers, and in the medulla of lymph nodes in functional expression as plasma cells. Transformed B cells are located in follicular centers, in interfollicular tissue with transformed T cells, and in widespread sites of reaction often with plasma cells. Following the recognition of transformed B cells in follicular centers, we proposed the follicular

center cell (FCC) concept (Lukes and Collins, 1973; 1974a,b; 1975). Camera lucida studies of normal follicular centers revealed four cell types: (1) cleaved FCC, (2) noncleaved FCC, (3) tingible body macrophages, and (4) dendritic reticulum cells. The wide range in size of both the cleaved and noncleaved cell revealed by the camera lucida drawings (Fig. 8.1) of normal FCC were attributed to stages in B cell transformation. Identification of nuclear cleavage planes depends upon the technical quality of the fixation, processing, and histologic sections. In the average formalin-fixed, thick lymph node section, the cytologic features, particularly nuclear cleavage planes, are not readily discernible. Methyl green pyronine-stained, well fixed tissue most ideally demonstrates the character of the noncleaved (transformed) FCC.

In the FCC concept we proposed the sequence in B cell transformation from the small B lymphocyte of the lymphocytic mantle to the large noncleaved FCC as illustrated in Figure 8.2. In this concept, the small lymphocyte, under the influence of antigen trapped in the follicular center primarily on the surface of dendritic reticulum cells illustrated schematically as a perifollicular center, is induced to undergo transformation as shown by Nossal et al. (1968). In the first stage the small lymphocyte changes to the small cleaved FCC. By gradual enlargement and acquisition of a small amount of pyroninophilic cytoplasm, it reaches the second stage, the large cleaved FCC.

NORMAL FOLLICULAR CENTER CELLS

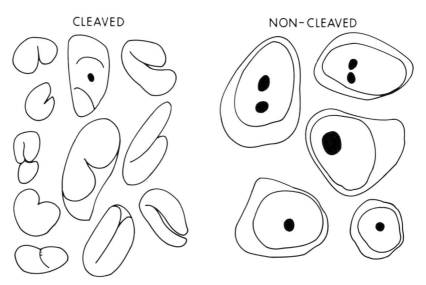

FIG. 8.1

SCHEMATIC REPRESENTATION OF DEVELOPMENT OF MALIGNANT LYMPHOMAS
OF FOLLICULAR CENTER CELLS

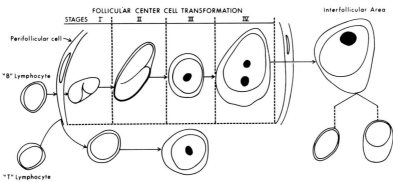

FIG. 8.2

In the third designated stage, the small non-cleaved FCC, the nucleus becomes round, the nuclear chromatin finely dispersed in association with a small nucleolus, and the cytoplasm prominently pyroninophilic. In the fourth stage, the large noncleaved FCC is similar, but larger; has more abundant pale acidophilic cytoplasm; and one to three more prominent nucleoli are often situated on the nuclear membrane. The cleaved cells of the follicular center are essentially nondividing cells, while the noncleaved cells are dividing cells. From the studies of Dr. Clive Taylor, of our group, cytoplasmic immunoglobulin initially can be demonstrated in the large cleaved FCC in small amounts and with increasing prominence in the small and large noncleaved FCC stages (Taylor, 1976; Taylor and Mason, 1974). The large noncleaved FCC appears in histologic sections to migrate out of the follicular center into the interfollicular tissue where we have designated it an immunoblast of B cell type. This apparent migration is supported by the recent ultrastructural studies of follicular centers of tonsils by Kojima and Tsunoda (1976), also using the immunoperoxidase technique. The demonstration of cytoplasm immunoglobulin in FCC and some immunoblasts of the interfollicular tissue provides strong supportive evidence of their relationship and B cell nature. The proposed direction of in vivo transformation of B cells in the follicular center is in contradiction to the generally held view. Our proposal is based on our in vitro lymphocyte transformation experience. The in vitro phenomenon occurs from the small lymphocyte to the transformed lymphocyte in both T and B cell systems. The proposed sequence in the FCC concept also parallels the evolution observed in FCC lymphomas in which the process is observed initially as the small cleaved FCC type with limited aggressiveness and later there is change to the highly aggressive noncleaved FCC type. The FCC concept provides the basis for relating the cytologic types of FCC neoplasms to their normal counterparts, and permits an understanding of the evolution of the process in the B cell system.

T Cells

The morphologic differentiation between T and B cells remains a subject of debate even though functional studies are beginning to provide strong support for the distinctiveness of some cytologic types in both systems. The transformed lymphocytes (immunoblasts) of the T and B cell systems are generally similar, but the B immunoblast at times may be larger, have more abundant, denser, amphophilic cytoplasm, and even have plasmacytoid features. The demonstration of cytoplasmic immunoglobulin by the immunoperoxidase technique developed by Taylor and Mason (1974) is a helpful method for distinguishing transformed T and B cell types of the interfollicular tissue because of the cytoplasmic content of immunoglobulin in B cells. Transformation in T cells occurs in a somewhat parallel fashion to B cells, but outside of the follicular center in the paracortical region without the formation of cleaved nucleated cells or plasma cells. The intermediate stage of transformation consists of medium size cells with round nuclei, finely dispersed chromatin, small nucleoli, and a moderate amount of pyroninophilic cytoplasm. The T cell lymphomas observed thus far possibly may represent extreme expansions of defective counterparts of normal cells that ordinarily occur in small numbers and as yet have not been described. The convoluted T cell we described in children and young adults possibly is a development abnormality of the pre-T cell (Barcos and Lukes, 1975; Stein et al., 1976). The cerebriform cell of Sézary's syndrome has been proposed as lym-phoma of helper cells by Broder et al. (1976). Both cells will be described in some detail with the cytologic types of lymphoma.

A FUNCTIONAL CLASSIFICATION OF MALIGNANT LYMPHOMAS

The immunologic basis of the functional classification of malignant lymphomas outlined briefly in the previous section can be summarized in the following points: (1) malignant lymphomas are neoplasms of the immune system; (2) they involved primarily T and B cell and U cell (undefined) systems and rarely histiocytes and monocytes; (3) malignant lymphomas possibly develop as a block or a "switch on" (derepression) of lymphocyte transformation in the various lymphocytic systems; and (4) the cytologic types of lymphoma are counterparts to normal immunologic cells and are similar in varying degrees morphologically and functionally. The cytologic types of lymphoma are related to positions in B and T cell transformation illustrated in Figure 8.2, with the exception of the true histiocytic lymphoma, the convoluted lymphocyte that possibly represents a pre-T cell (Barcos and Lukes, 1975; Stein et al., 1976), and the cerebriform cell of Sézary's syndrome and mycosis fungoides, the precise nature of which remains uncertain. The involved cell in Hodgkin's disease is unknown.

Our functional classification initially was proposed before the application of multiparameter studies. The results of our recent study of 384 cases of lymphomas and related leukemias using these techniques have confirmed the immunologic approach and the cytologic types (Lukes and Collins, 1977). Only the lymphoma of small T lymphocytes has been added to the original cytologic types. It is acknowledged that the final acceptance of any classification is dependent upon the soundness of the conceptual basis as well as the clinical relevance and effectiveness of its application. Acceptance may require a number of years of trial by numerous centers.

The classification of malignant lymphoma is listed in Table 8.1 according to the following major groups: (1) U cell (undefined), (2) T cell, (3) B cell, (4) histiocytic, (5) cell type of uncertain origin—Hodgkin's disease; and (6) unclassifiable. The U cell (undefined) type is hypothetical and was developed for the proliferations of cells that lack discriminating primitive morphologic features or have undetectable immunologic or cytochemical markers according to presently available techniques. It includes the theoretical null cell and the primitive lymphocytes or true stem cells, such as those found in acute

lymphocytic leukemia (ALL) in childhood without specific markers. The unclassifiable type is designed for those lymphomatous appearing proliferations on which the histologic and cytologic findings are indistinct or obscured for technical reasons, and the process cannot be classified precisely.

In both the T and B cell group there is a small lymphocytic type and a large transformed lymphocytic type or immunoblastic sarcoma. The T cell group also includes cytologic types with the extraordinary nuclear configuration, the primitive appearing convoluted T cell and the cerebriform cell of Sézary's syndrome and mycosis fungoides. The B cell group contains the FCC variants which are regarded as plasma cell precursors and the plasmacytoid lymphocytic type which is frequently associated with dysglobulinemias, such as Waldenström's syndrome. The histiocytic type refers to those disorders that lack the immunologic surface markers and features of T or B cells and exhibit the cytochemical expression of histiocytes for which we have used the alpha naphthyl butyrate cytochemical

TABLE 8.1
FUNCTIONAL CLASSIFICATION

U CELL (undefined)
T CELL
  Small lymphocyte
  Convoluted lymphocyte
  Sézary – mycosis fungoides
  Immunoblastic sarcoma of T cells
B CELL
  Small lymphocyte
  Plasmacytoid lymphocyte
  Follicular center cell (FCC)
    Follicular, diffuse, follicular and diffuse, and with or without sclerosis
    Small cleaved
    Large cleaved
    Small noncleaved
    Large noncleaved
  Immunoblastic sarcoma of B cells
  Hairy cell leukemia
HISTIOCYTIC
CELL OF UNCERTAIN ORIGIN
  Hodgkin's disease
    Lymphocyte predominance
    Mixed cellularity
    Lymphocyte depletion
    Nodular sclerosis
UNCLASSIFIABLE

method (Yam et al., 1971b) and the cytoplasmic immunoperoxidase technique for muramidase. Hodgkin's disease is subclassified according to the well established and accepted types of the Rye Classification (Lukes et al., 1966b) which is a modification of the original Lukes-Butler classification (Lukes et al., 1966a). The classification and cytologic types have been described in detail in a number of publications (Lukes et al., 1966a; Lukes, 1971). Only the essential features will be considered in the following presentations.

T Cell Types

Small Lymphocyte (T Cell)

The existence of a lymphoma-leukemia of small T cells has been documented by multiparameter studies in a small number of cases, but the distinctiveness of the morphologic features has not been established. The cytologic features we have observed in a small group of cases are those of a small lymphocyte that resemble the normal small lymphocyte. The nucleus has compact nuclear chromatin, and there is a small amount of pale staining cytoplasm. The nucleus at times has a somewhat irregular nuclear configuration. The distinctiveness of this configurational change is uncertain at the present time.

Convoluted Lymphocyte (Fig. 8.3)

This process is a diffuse proliferation of primitive appearing noncohesive cells occurring in widely infiltrated masses or in partially or totally involved lymph nodes. The lymphoma cells vary in size ranging from that of a small

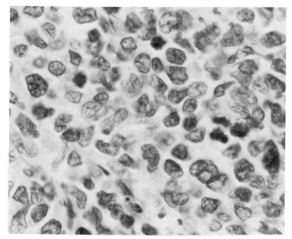

FIG. 8.3. CONVOLUTED LYMPHOCYTIC TYPE
The nuclei vary widely in size and configuration, have finely dispersed chromatin, numerous fine linear subdivisions, and no apparent nucleoli. The cytoplasm is scant.

lymphocyte to four to five lymphocyte nuclear diameters. The nuclei have distinctive, fine distributed chromatin and inconspicuous or small nucleoli. The nuclei of the smaller cells are round in configuration, while the larger cells commonly have deep subdivisions of varying prominence. At times these subdivisions present an image of a "chicken footprint." Usually the linear subdivisions resemble a convolutional phenomenon in a round nucleus, but the nucleus may be irregular and almost lobated from the deep convolutions. The small and large cells vary in frequency. The frequency of mitoses typically ranges from five to seven per high power field and is proportional to the number of large cells. The cytoplasm is indistinct or scanty and relates to the noncohesive character of the cells. Occasionally reactive "starry-sky" phagocytes are interspersed, and for this reason the proliferation may be mistaken for a Burkitt lymphoma in overly thick sections.

Cerebriform Cell of Sézary's Syndrome and Mycosis Fungoides

The lymphoma cells in these closely related conditions are medium size and approximately two to three normal lymphocytes in diameter. They have barely discernible linear subdivisions in cells found in the peripheral blood and tissue, but in the later aggressive stage the cells may be large, the chromatin finely dispersed, and the configurational outline remarkably abnormal. There is only a narrow rim of cytoplasm that usually contains numerous periodic acid-Schiff (PAS)-positive globules at times in a "necklace" distribution. Ultrastructural studies dramatically demonstrate the deep cerebriform subdivisions (Lutzner et al., 1975; Rosas-Uribe et al., 1974).

Immunoblastic Sarcoma of T Cells

We are just becoming acquainted with this proliferation. It exhibits a lymphocytic spectrum ranging from a small irregular peculiar lymphocyte to the fully transformed lymphocyte. The median and large cells closely resemble in vitro transformed lymphocytes and in histologic sections have pale staining to almost water-clear cytoplasm with well defined cohesive interlocking cytoplasmic membranes. The nucleus is round to oval with finely distributed chromatin and usually one central prominent nucleolus. The process generally extends throughout the lymph node and is unassociated with follicle or nodule formation. The small peculiar lymphocyte appears to be a definite component of an apparently evolving process.

B Cell Types

Small Lymphocyte of B Cells

This is a diffuse proliferation of noncohesive small lymphocytes closely resembling normal lymphocytes. They have uniform round nuclei with compact basophilic chromatin, inapparent nucleoli, and a small rim of pale staining cytoplasm. Large transformed lymphocytes and mitoses usually are infrequent and plasma cells essentially are absent. Lymphomatous follicles or nodules are absent.

Plasmacytoid Lymphocytic Type (Fig. 8.4)

This lymphomatous proliferation is generally similar to the small lymphocyte of B cells with the exception of an abnormal plasma cell component with a nucleus that resembles a lymphocyte. There is also a component of cells intermediate between the small lymphocyte and the abnormal plasma cell. A large pale acidophilic staining globule which is PAS-positive occasionally overlies the nucleus (Dutcher body) in Waldenström's macroglobulinemia (Dutcher and Fahey, 1959). A similar cellular proliferation is found with other types of dysglobulinemias, but often no dysglobulinemia is detected.

Follicular Center Cell (FCC) Types

The four FCC types may occur with follicular, follicular and diffuse, or diffuse histologic patterns, with or without sclerosis. The small cleaved FCC type usually is associated with some degree of follicle (nodular) formation, the large cleaved FCC, in approximately one-half of the cases, and the noncleaved FCC occasionally (10%).

Small Cleaved FCC. The range in size and configuration of normal cleaved FCC is illustrated schematically in Figure 8.1. The small cleaved FCC varies in size from a small lymphocyte to that of a reactive histiocyte nucleus (Fig. 8.5). The nuclei are basically of irregular configuration and a variable portion of the cells exhibit typical nuclear cleavage planes similar to normal cells. The degree of irregularity and cleavage increases in prominence with nuclear size. The nuclear chromatin is compact and basophilic and nucleoli are inconspicuous. Mitotic figures are rare. The cytoplasm is scanty or indistinct. A small proportion of noncleaved (transformed) FCC are intermixed usually in small numbers, but on occasion reach 10–20%. The small cleaved cells usually extend throughout the lymphomatous follicles into the interfollicular tissue and commonly infiltrate the capsule.

Large Cleaved FCC. The nucleus of the large cleaved cell is larger than a reactive histiocyte nucleus and consistently irregular in configuration. Often the nuclear cleavage planes result in exaggerated nuclear forms. The cytoplasm is moderate in amount and pyroninophilic, and frequently this proliferation is associated with a deposit of pale staining intercellular material and early sclerosis. Small and large cleaved FCC commonly occur together in different parts of a lymphomatous proliferation when the large cleaved FCC is prominent, particularly with sclerosis.

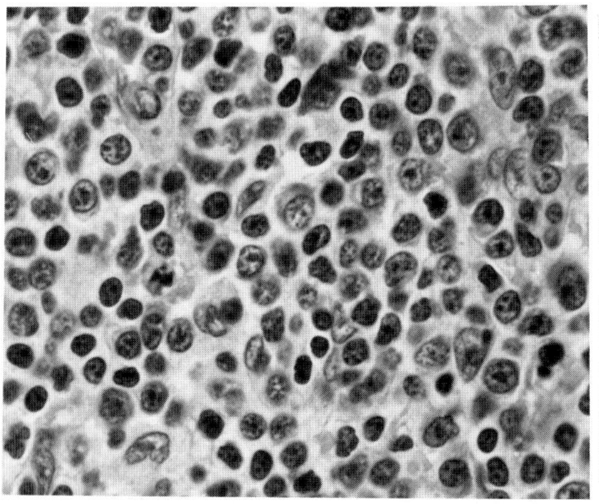

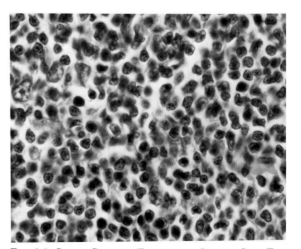

FIG. 8.4. PLASMACYTOID LYMPHOCYTIC TYPE
The proliferation appears predominantly lymphocytic but a proportion of the cells have plasmacytoid cytoplasm in varying amounts.

FIG. 8.5. SMALL CLEAVED FOLLICULAR CENTER CELL TYPE
These cells are small and have irregular nuclei often with a single linear subdivision. Mitoses are rare. The cytoplasm is scanty.

Small Noncleaved (Transformed) FCC. This lymphoma is composed of medium size cells with features of small transformed lymphocytes. The nuclei are round and regular in configuration, and the nuclei predominantly do not exceed the size of the phagocyte nucleus. The nuclear chromatin is finely dispersed, and there are several small nucleoli. There is a narrow rim of pyroninophilic cytoplasm and the cellular borders are cohesive in well fixed tissue. Reactive phagocytes of "starry-sky" type commonly are regularly interspersed throughout the tumor. This lymphoma fulfills the criteria of the Burkitt lymphoma of Africa when the cells are uniform in size and configuration (Berard et al., 1969). In the United States the small noncleaved FCC usually exhibits considerably more variation in cytologic features, and is designated commonly as the non-Burkitt type. In a few reported cases of the Burkitt lymphoma, a follicular (nodular) pattern has been observed in a small portion of the proliferation (Mann et al., 1976). This observation provides support for our proposal that the Burkitt lymphoma is of FCC type (Lukes and Collins, 1973; 1974a,b; 1975).

Large Noncleaved (Transformed) FCC. This lymphoma in general possesses similar cytologic features to the small noncleaved FCC type with the exception that the cells are larger and have more abundant cytoplasm, the nuclei are larger, and the nucleoli are more prominent. Often two prominent nucleoli are found situated on the nuclear membrane in a characteristic pattern on the short axis of an oval nucleus. Mitoses are numerous. Both individual cell necrosis and areas of necrosis are common.

Immunoblastic Sarcoma of B Cells (Fig. 8.6)

This lymphoma of transformed B cells resembles the large noncleaved FCC, but in general it is a larger cell with more dense amphophilic cytoplasm and often exhibits plasmacytoid features. It lacks the typical features of the FCC types, specifically the cleaved FCC component and follicular pattern. The process often initially is observed partially involving an abnormal immune process of various types and presents as monomorphous areas (clones) of large abnormal immunoblasts. Later in the process the proliferation may totally involve and replace the lymph node or present as a tumor mass. The immunoblasts of B cell types are differentiated from T immunoblasts on the basis of the density of the amphophilic cytoplasm and their frequent plasmacytoid character. The demonstration of the cytoplasmic immunoglobulin by the immunoperoxidase technique (Taylor, 1976; Taylor and Mason, 1974) offers supportive evidence, particularly if monoclonal in character.

Histiocytic

A true histiocytic type appears to exist as an interrelated histiocyte-monocyte proliferation. The number of proven cases with functional studies is too small at the present time to establish an accurate description of its morphologic expressions. To be acceptable as a true histiocytic type, the lymphoma cells in our view require cytochemical demonstration of their macrophage-monocyte enzyme with the alpha naphthyl butyrate esterase (Yam et al., 1971a). Ideally, the lack of immunologic surface markers for T and B cells also is shown. The small number of proven cases Dr. Collins and I have had the opportunity to study have been variable in their histologic appearance, but have had both an identifiable histiocyte component such as a macrophage and also a monocyte component. Several of these cases have terminated with a leukemic process resembling a monocytic leukemia.

Uncertain Cell Type — Hodgkin's Disease

The precise nature of the Reed-Sternberg cell remains controversial, although the histologic types of the Rye Classification (Lukes et al.,

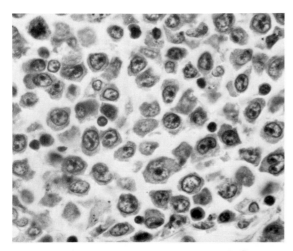

FIG. 8.6. IMMUNOBLASTIC SARCOMA OF B CELLS
The cells are large and resemble the in vitro transformed lymphocytes. The nuclei are round to oval and occasionally irregular in configuration. The chromatin is finely dispersed and the nucleoli are prominent. The cytoplasm is abundant and deeply staining.

1966b) adapted from the original Lukes and Butler types (Lukes et al., 1966a) have long been accepted. The histologic types of both classifications are designed to characterize the host response and are based on our concept that the basic process in Hodgkin's disease is a struggle between host and the factors involved in the induction of Reed-Sternberg cells. The lymphocyte predominance, histologic type is regarded as an expression of an extremely effective host response, characterized morphologically by a predominance of lymphocytes and a rarity of diagnostic Reed-Sternberg cells, and clinically by disease of limited extent.

The lymphocyte depletion type, by contrast, is associated with an ineffective host response reflected morphologically by decreased numbers of lymphocytes associated with either a distinctive type of diffuse fibrosis or numerous diagnostic Reed-Sternberg cells and clinically by stage III or IV disease. The mixed cellularity type occupies an intermediate position between lymphocyte predominance and lymphocyte depletion, and indicates a failing host response expressed clinically by changing disease. Nodular sclerosis is regarded separately as a result of its dominant association with the anterior superior mediastinum and adjacent cervical, hilar, and axillary lymph nodes and is regarded as a regional expression of Hodgkin's disease. It includes cases with both quiescent and aggressive disease. The spread of nodular sclerosis appears to be contiguous and predictable, while in the remaining types it usually skips the mediastinum and is noncontiguous in its spread.

In the following, each histologic type of the Rye Classification will be briefly defined.

Lymphocyte Predominance. This type includes both the lymphocytic and histiocytic, nodular and diffuse types of our original classification (Lukes et al., 1966a). The proliferation may be composed dominantly of lymphocytes or histiocytes or in varying proportions, although a predominance of lymphocytes is most commonly encountered. In approximately half of the cases the proliferation is aggregated into large vague nodules and is associated usually with stage I disease. The lymphocytic and histiocytic components are regarded as reactive host responses. The lymphocytes are small and have round to irregular nuclei, and scanty cytoplasm. The histiocytes occur singly or in small clusters and at times resemble small sarcoid-like aggregations. Scattered throughout the lymphocytic and histiocytic proliferation is a

prominent component of large polyploid appearing cells with pale cytoplasm, folded and overlapping large nuclei, and small or inconspicuous nucleoli. We have designated these cells the L & H variants of the Reed-Sternberg cell, since they have proved extremely reliable in recognizing this histologic type (Lukes, 1971). By contrast the diagnostic Reed-Sternberg cell with huge nucleoli typically is extremely rare in this type.

Mixed Cellularity. This type, as the name implies, contains a variety of components in variable degrees. Diagnostic Reed-Sternberg cells with large nucleoli are conspicuous; histiocytes, eosinophils, and disorderly fibrosis are also commonly prominent. The mixed type also provides a category for those cases in which the histologic findings do not fulfill the criteria for any of the other histologic types.

Lymphocyte Depletion. This type includes the diffuse fibrosis and reticular types of our original classification (Lukes et al., 1966a). In the former there is typically marked reduction in cellularity associated with a distinctive type of disorderly fibrosis characterized by loose amorphous, poorly formed connective tissue that extends throughout the majority of the lymph node. Diagnostic Reed-Sternberg cells are often difficult to find. Lymphocytes may be infrequent or limited to a portion of the node. In the reticular variant, diagnostic Reed-Sternberg cells are extremely numerous and, on rare occasions, appear sarcomatous. Features of both the reticular and diffuse fibrosis types at times may be found together.

Nodular Sclerosis. This histologic type exhibits numerous variations in expression both in the degree of sclerosis and in its cellular composition. The sclerosis varies from a single broad collagen band extending from a thickened lymph node capsule to almost total sclerosis of a mass. The cellularity varies from predominantly lymphocytic to a dominance of lacunar cell variants of the Reed-Sternberg cell. There are two essential criteria for the diagnosis of the nodular sclerosing type: (a) thick birefringent collagen bands and (b) typical lacunar cells with well demarcated cellular borders, abundant water-clear cytoplasm, and a tendency to multiple lobation with small nucleoli. Often the lacunar cells occur in distinctive cohesive clusters in the center of lymphocytic nodules that are often surrounded by a collagen band. Central necrosis of these lacunar cell clusters associated with mature granulocyte infiltration is common.

RESULTS OF FUNCTIONAL STUDIES

The functional approach employs a variety of techniques in the study of lymphomas and related leukemias including special morphology, cytochemistry, electron microscopy, and immunologic surface marker techniques to characterize the type of proliferation. When possible, other techniques such as immunoglobulin synthesis and cell kinetics are used to evaluate their functional capacity. The immunologic surface marker techniques have been helpful in the study of immune abnormalities and defects for a number of years, and more recently they have been applied to the study of malignant lymphomas and their leukemic expressions. The results of these studies in general support our initial proposal that these disorders, with the exception of a portion of acute lymphocytic leukemia (ALL), mark as T or B cells and rarely as histiocytes. The morphologic features of our cytologic types of lymphoma are predictive of the T and B cell type in a high proportion of cases (Lukes and Collins, 1977).

The most commonly employed and effective techniques in the study of malignant lymphomas are listed in Table 8.2. These techniques have been the subject of numerous reviews (Braylan et al., 1975; Green et al., 1975; Kunkel, 1975); therefore they will be briefly summarized. The collection of fresh biopsies of lymph nodes or masses, or specimens of peripheral blood is an essential requirement for all except the immunoperoxidase technique. Suspensions of live cells are required for the immunologic surface marker techniques and freshly prepared imprints and unfixed frozen tissue for most of the cytochemical techniques. These include a battery of stains that are distinctive for granulocytes, histiocytes, monocytes, and special cells such as those of hairy cell leukemia and ALL. Ideal fixation for histopathology is achieved with the collection of fresh biopsy material by the preparation of thin (2–3 mm) tissue blocks which permit rapid and thorough penetration by the fixative. We have found a modified Zenker's solution to be the best fixative for hematopoietic tissues.

Sheep erythrocytes attach to lymphocytes in suspension and form rosettes under a variety of controlled conditions and help in the discrimination between T and B cells and histiocytes (Jondal et al., 1972). Spontaneous rosettes of sheep erythrocytes (E) form consistently about T cells. Similar rosette formation of complement-dependent type (EAC) occurs with both B cells and histiocytes if the sheep erythrocytes are previously exposed to antibody IGM and complement, whereas rosette formation (EA) occurs with histiocytes and monocytes, if the erythrocytes are pretreated with antibody (IgG) only. Application of the EAC and EA techniques to frozen unfixed tissue sections effectively identifies the B cell nature of reactive follicles and lymphomatous nodules, and the distributional character of histiocytes and monocytes in lymph nodes and spleen (Jaffe et al., 1974). The detection of surface immunoglobulins is generally regarded as the most effective method of identifying B cells (Kunkel, 1975). Immunoglobulin is identified on live cells using fluorescent-labeled monospecific antibodies for heavy and light immunoglobulin chains. The population of B cells found in the peripheral blood of normal individuals and in reactive lymphoid tissue exhibits a variety of immunoglobulins (polyclonal immunoglobulin) on their surface. Typically the lymphomas and leukemias of B cell type display monoclonal surface immunoglobulin, i.e., a single heavy and a single light chain on their surface. Monoclonicity is interpreted as evidence of a neoplastic clonal proliferation similar to the immunoglobulin production observed typically in myeloma.

Demonstration of immunoglobulin synthesis is acknowledged as the most precise method for

TABLE 8.2

TECHNIQUES FOR IDENTIFICATION OF T AND B CELLS AND HISTIOCYTES

	T Cells	B Cells	Histiocytes-Monocytes
Sheep RBC rosettes			
E	+	−	−
EAC (IgM)*	−	+	+
EA (IgG)	−	−	+
Surface Ig†	−	+	−
Cytoplasmic immuno-peroxidase			
Immunoglobulin	−	+	−
Muramidase	−	−	+
Antiserum			
HTLA‡	+	−	−
HBLA‡	−	+	−
Alpha naphthyl butyrate	−	−	+

* The convoluted T cell has been observed with complement receptors.

† T cells have a small amount of surface Ig.

‡ HTLA, human T lymphocyte antibody; HBLA, human B lymphocyte antibody.

characterizing a B cell proliferation. In paraffin sections of fixed tissue it is possible to demonstrate cytoplasmic immunoglobulin and characterize the immunoglobulin monospecifically according to heavy and light immunoglobulin chains using the immunoperoxidase technique as described by Taylor and Mason (1974, 1976). The basis of the technique is similar to the fluorescent method with horseradish peroxidase substituted for the fluorescent label on the specific antibody. The stained peroxidase serves as the marker for the site of the immunoglobulin. The immunoperoxidase technique may also be used on fixed paraffin sections for the demonstration of cytoplasmic muramidase, an enzyme found normally in histiocytes, monocytes, granulocytes, and a variety of tissues other than T and B cells. The alpha naphthyl butyrate cytochemical technique detects an enzyme found in histiocytes and monocytes, and identifies a somewhat wider range of histiocytes and monocytes than the immunoperoxidase for muramidase, but this cytochemical technique is limited to relatively fresh tissue imprints, peripheral blood, and bone marrow smears and unfixed frozen tissue sections (Yam et al., 1971a). Prior exposure of the specimen to sodium fluoride blocks the staining of monocytes and permits the distinction between histiocytes and monocytes. The tartrate-resistant acid phosphatase technique of Yam et al. (1971b) is a useful method of precisely identifying cases of hairy cell leukemia through its demonstration of a single isoenzyme. Effective antiserum for human T lymphocytes (HTLA) and B lymphocytes (HBLA) has been claimed, but specific membrane antigens for these cells in humans have not been identified. The value of such antiserums for this reason has always been questioned. Nevertheless, if relatively specific antiserums for T and B cells can be reliably produced, this approach has great potential value in both diagnosis and therapy.

The results of a number of studies on malignant lymphomas and leukemias of lymphocytes evaluated by the various surface marker techniques have now appeared in the literature (Aisenberg and Long, 1975; Berard et al., 1976; Braylan et al., 1975; Brouet et al., 1975; Davey et al., 1976; Gajl-Peczalska et al., 1975; Green et al., 1975; and Leech et al., 1975).

In general the results of these studies support our original proposal that (a) malignant lymphomas are neoplasms of the immune system, (b) for the most part these proliferations mark as T and B cell types, and (c) lymphomas of

histiocytes as macrophages are rare (Lukes and Collins, 1977). It is clear from these reports and our experience that the techniques are complex procedures vulnerable to erroneous and at times confusing results. Unquestionably refinement of these techniques and the development of more precise methods will ultimately add greater precision and reproducibility to the functional approach. The results of our combined study of 384 cases of malignant lymphoma and related leukemia collected and evaluated both at Vanderbilt University under my colleague, Dr. Robert Collins, and my group at University of Southern California School of Medicine using essentially similar techniques have provided verification of the cytologic types of our functional classification and the value of the immunologic approach outlined in this presentation (Lukes and Collins, 1977). The results of this study will be briefly summarized and related to the other recent reports.

The non-Hodgkin's lymphomas and the closely related leukemias of past classifications appear to be groups of disorders rather than homogeneous entities. Acute lymphocytic leukemia (ALL) of childhood has been demonstrated to be heterogeneous (Haegert et al., 1975; Kersey et al., 1973; Williams et al., 1977); 20–25% are of T cell type, a small portion are of B cell type resembling small immunoblasts, and the remainder that fail to mark are included in our U cell group. Using special B antiserums, the recent studies of Winchester et al. (1975) and Schlossman et al. (1976) have suggested that the unmarked cells of ALL may represent a special B cell type, possibly involving the bone marrow B cell. Chronic lymphocytic leukemia (CLL) and its tissue counterpart, the lymphoma of small lymphocytes, also are heterogeneous, although only 1–2% are of T cell type and the remainder mark as B cells.

We regard CLL of both T and B cell types as lymphomas of small lymphocytes that have a propensity for peripheral blood and bone marrow involvement. The cerebriform cell of Sézary's syndrome (Brouet et al., 1973) and mycosis fungoides is accepted as a T cell (Lutzner et al., 1975), although the precise nature of the process and origin of the cell is uncertain. Recently, Broder et al. (1976) have shown evidence of the possible helper T cell character of Sézary cells. Similarly the T cell nature of the convoluted lymphocyte appears to be confirmed from our study of 26 cases (Lukes and Collins, 1977) and Stein et al. (1976) who also demonstrated strong focal acid phosphatase positivity. Similar strong acid phosphatase positivity also was found by Catovsky et al. (1974) in a small group of proven T cell ALL cases. It is acknowledged that the degree of convolutional nuclear change varies widely from case to case in both lymphomatous and leukemic expressions. Recognition of nuclear convolutions also may be difficult in less than optimal histologic sections. The combination of variable frequency and technical factors may account for the difference in the findings reported by Nathwani et al. (1976). Thus far, all 16 cases interpreted morphologically as the convoluted lymphocytic type with surface marker studies have formed E rosettes in varying numbers (Lukes and Collins, 1977). Nuclear convolutions are more difficult to discern in smear preparations. This proliferation is interrelated with the T cell type of ALL of childhood mentioned above (Kersey et al., 1973; Williams et al., 1977).

The study of lymphomas previously included in the histiocytic type of Rappaport have presented a problem in investigation apparently because of the fragile nature of these high turnover rate types of cellular proliferations and the difficulty of cell separation. Nevertheless, in our study these cells have marked almost always as T or B cells when a sufficient number of viable cells were obtained for evaluation (Lukes and Collins, 1977). Morphologically these cells usually presented the features of transformed lymphocytes either as immunoblastic sarcoma of T or B cell types, or large noncleaved (transformed) FCC. Only 4 cases in our study marked as the histiocytic types, and these were distinguishable morphologically from the lymphomas of transformed lymphocytes. However, Epstein and Kaplan (1974) believe that the large cells essentially are of histiocytic type as a result of their studies of transplantable lymphomas in nude mice. These lymphomas, however, were not evaluated prior to transplantation by the multiparameter techniques.

Lymphomas with a follicular (nodular) histologic pattern have been shown by Jaffe et al. (1974), using the frozen section EAC and EA rosette techniques, to be of B cell type. In our study of 130 cases of FCC lymphomas with follicular or diffuse histologic patterns, monoclonal type surface immunoglobulin was demonstrated in the majority of cases (Lukes and Collins, 1977). The follicular nature of lymphomatous follicles was demonstrated in the comparative ultrastructural studies of normal and lymphomatous follicles by Glick et al. (1975). In the same study the morphologic identity of FCC lymphomas whether nodular or diffuse was also observed (Leech et al., 1975). The ultrastructural similarity of normal follicular centers and nodular lymphomas also was reported by Levine and Dorfman (1975). These studies confirm the views of Lennert (1973) and the original ultrastructural findings of Kojima et al. (1973) that nodular lymphomas consisted of lymphomatous follicles.

The controversial nature of hairy cell leukemia seems to have been clarified by demonstrations of monoclonal surface immunoglobulin in the majority of cases we reported (Lukes and Collins, 1977), and the observation of immunoglobulin synthesis following trypsinization by Dr. Collins' group.

In Hodgkin's disease the results of surface marker studies have provided further evidence in support of a possible T cell abnormality. A reduction in the number of T cells has been reported by a number of observers, but evidence recently has been reported by Fuks et al. (1976) of a serum factor that interferes with E rosette formation. The possibility of interference with T cell function by this serum factor has considerable potential significance.

CLINICAL AND MORPHOLOGIC CORRELATIONS

In the past the morphologic types of malignant lymphomas and related leukemias included a number of cytologic types as a result of the lack of precision in methodology. Homogeneous cell proliferations have now been recognized using the multiparameter approach and a number of new clinical, morphologic, immunologic entities are emerging, such as the convoluted T cell type, the FCC types, and the immunoblastic sarcomas of both T and B cell types (Lukes and Collins, 1977). It is possible that there are as many as 9 or 10 entities presently included in malignant lymphomas. Unquestionably the identification and investigation of homogeneous cell proliferations will permit an improved understanding of their biologic character, and also an appreciation of their clinical expressions and therapeutic responsiveness that previously have been obscured in the heterogeneous groups.

The degree of aggressiveness of the T and B cell types can be related to their morphologic features and presumed proliferative rates. The cytologic types are arranged according to their aggressiveness in Table 8.3, together with their potential evolutionary changes. In general the small cells of both T and B cells are of limited aggressiveness while the larger cells, the transformed lymphocytic types, are highly aggressive.

The change in the small cell types from the low aggressive to the highly aggressive expressions occurs in varying frequency with the cytologic types. This change, we believe, represents a "switch on" (derepression) of the lymphocyte transformation mechanism. In the seven types included in the B cell groups, four are of limited aggressiveness (low turnover rate proliferations): the small B lymphocyte, the plasmacytoid lymphocyte, and the small and large cleaved FCC types. There are three highly aggressive (high turnover rate) proliferations: the small and large noncleaved (transformed) FCC type and immunoblastic sarcoma of B cells. Both the small and large cleaved FCC types commonly evolve into the highly aggressive proliferations of the noncleaved FCC type in the later phases of the disease after variable periods of time up to many years. The plasmacytoid lymphocytic type occasionally terminates as immunoblastic sarcoma of B cells, while the small

B lymphocyte including CLL rarely evolves to immunoblastic sarcoma of B cells. The latter in the past has been designated as the Richter syndrome. The degree of aggressiveness of the T cell types has not been established. In Sézary's syndrome and mycosis fungoides, the limited aggressiveness of the prolonged earlier phases is well known and is associated predominantly with small cells. The later highly aggressive tumor phase is accompanied by either large cerebriform cells, or at times by large cells of possibly transformed T cell type. The convoluted T cell is a high turnover rate proliferation throughout its course. The full range of T cell expressions and the evolution of T cell immunoblastic sarcoma have yet to be elucidated. Successful therapy of the low aggressive types in our view depends to a large extent on the prevention of the evolution to the highly aggressive types or the prevention of the "switch on" (derepression) of the transformation mechanism.

Clinically in our experience the low aggressive types of T and B cell types both have an insidious onset; are generally widespread when initially evaluated apparently because of their noncohesive, mobile character; and have prolonged median survivals. The lymphoma of the small B lymphocyte, the prototype of the lym-

TABLE 8.3
EVOLUTION OF CYTOLOGIC TYPES OF MALIGNANT LYMPHOMA IN RELATIONSHIP TO
AGGRESSIVENESS*

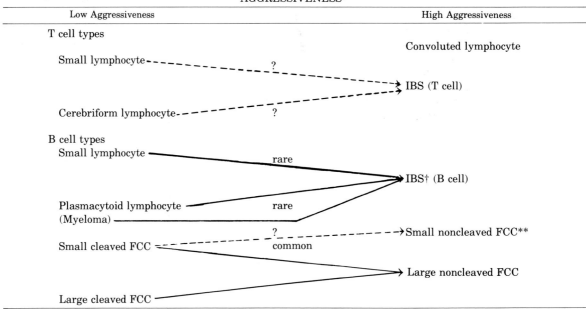

* The position of histiocytic lymphoma is unknown.

** FCC (follicular center cell).

† Most cases of IBS (immunoblastic sarcoma) of B cell type evolve from previous non-neoplastic abnormal immune states.

phomas of low aggressiveness, predominantly is expressed as chronic lymphocytic leukemia (CLL). The plasmacytoid lymphocytic lymphoma at times is associated with IgM gammopathy and Waldenström syndrome, but occasionally it is associated with IgG gammopathy, commonly without any serum globulin abnormality. The small cleaved FCC type usually has a follicular pattern, and presents with asymptomatic lymphadenopathy. On detailed clinical staging, over 70% of the cases have widespread disease involving bone marrow, spleen, and retroperitoneal nodes. The large cleaved FCC type has a follicular pattern of limited degree in approximately 50% of the cases, is often associated with a sclerosing component, and has a lower frequency of widespread disease. The large cleaved FCC lymphoma with sclerosis most commonly presents in the retroperitoneum, mesentery, and inguinal region and is widespread in less than half of the cases. The sclerosing lymphomas were initially described by Bennett and Millett in the retroperitoneum under the term nodular sclerosing lymphosarcoma as a slowly progressive process (Bennett, 1975; Bennett and Millet, 1969). The highly aggressive Burkitt lymphoma of Africa and the American counterparts appear to be included in the small noncleaved FCC type, and on rare occasions have a follicular pattern (Mann et al., 1976).

In American children from our recent study, the proliferation is more variable, but of the small noncleaved FCC type, and usually diffuse (Schneider et al., 1977). Clinically over 70% of the cases have an abdominal presentation often in the terminal ileum or cecum, or as a mesenteric or retroperitoneal mass. It is in dramatic contrast to the convoluted T cell type, the most common cytologic type in this childhood case series, that presented primarily with either a mediastinal mass, peripheral lymphadenopathy, or a bone lesion (Barcos and Lukes, 1975; Schneider et al., 1977). The large noncleaved FCC and the immunoblastic sarcoma of B cells are somewhat similar morphologically, but usually present clinically in different situations. The large noncleaved FCC represents the later aggressive phase of the small cleaved FCC type, and at times may be the initially observed presentation in lymph nodes, tonsils, or gastrointestinal tract. It may represent the initial site or a primary lymphoma in the tonsil or gastrointestinal tract and offers the opportunity for effective therapy, if observed sufficiently early. We have observed immunoblastic sarcoma of B cells, on the other hand, usually developing in a variety of abnormal immune states, including immunoblastic lymphadenopathy (Lukes and Tindle, 1975), systemic lupus erythematosus, immunosuppressed states for graft rejection, malabsorption disease, both alpha chain disease and sprue, in the thyroid in Hashimoto's disease, and Sjögren's syndrome (Lukes and Collins, 1974a, b; 1975). Senescence also appears to represent a failing or defective immune state. Immunoblastic sarcoma also is found at times with the plasmacytoid lymphocyte in Waldenström's macroglobulinemia, and rarely with the small B lymphocytes associated with CLL, and on a few occasions in younger individuals without an apparent underlying immunologic abnormality. Thus far, immunoblastic sarcoma of T cells has not been preceded by an abnormal state in our experience. The distinctiveness of immunoblastic sarcoma as a clinical morphologic entity has been supported by Mathé and associates (1975).

Of the T cell types Sézary's syndrome and mycosis fungoides are well known clinically and generally accepted as T cell types. On the other hand, there are an insufficient number of cases of lymphoma of small T lymphocytes and immunoblastic sarcoma of T cells to define their clinical expressions with certainty, although there are suggestive features of their distinctiveness. The convoluted T cell lymphoma is the prototype of the new emerging entities and was previously included in ALL or one of several types of the lymphomas depending upon the initial clinical manifestations and the available material for diagnosis. The process principally is observed in children and, more commonly, in teenagers. It presents with a prominent mediastinal mass in over half the cases, but at times with lymphadenopathy and bone lesions, or a diffusely leukemic marrow (Barcos and Lukes, 1975; Schneider et al., 1977; and Stein et al., 1976). The initial presentation often is outside of the marrow, such as a mediastinal mass or lymphadenopathy, and involves the marrow in a leukemic fashion during relapse. In our original study both lymphoid masses and leukemic marrows were observed at times in individual cases and demonstrated the potential for both lymphoma and leukemic expressions (Barcos and Lukes, 1975). For this reason, we regard the convoluted T cell as a lymphoma-leukemic process. In our experience the convoluted T cell process dramatically responds to ALL therapy, but relapses generally within 6 months. The central nervous system commonly is involved either initially or at relapse. The L-asparagine dependence of T cell ALL reported by Ohnuma et al. (1976) demonstrates the distinctive biologic characteristic of this T cell neoplasm that in our view interrelates closely with the convoluted T cell type.

The clinical expressions of the new histiocytic lymphoma defined as a macrophage by enzymatic studies is uncertain, since only a small number of cases have been identified as of this date.

Comparison of our cytologic types of the functional classification with those of the classification of Rappaport in terms of clinical pathologic correlations demonstrates that most of the emerging entities were lost in the heterogeneous cytologic types of Rappaport. The classification of Rappaport et al. (1956) is based essentially on cell size and the potential of each cytologic type to occur in either nodular or diffuse histologic forms. The nodular proliferations have been demonstrated to be lymphomatous follicles (Jaffe et al., 1974), FCC types (Glick et al., 1975; Leech et al., 1975; Lukes and Collins, 1977), and heterogeneous cytologic types (Lukes and Collins, 1977). The prognostic significance in our view relates to the behavior of the FCC types. For example, the small T and B lymphocytes and the plasmacytoid lymphocytic type were included in the well differentiated lymphocytic type. The histiocytic type of Rappaport included the large cleaved FCC, the large non-cleaved FCC type, the immunoblastic sarcomas of both B and T cell types, as well as the new histiocytic lymphoma. The convoluted lymphocytic lymphoma apparently was classified variably as either the undifferentiated type and the poorly differentiated lymphocytic diffuse types. When nodular, the poorly differentiated lymphocytic type appears to be essentially similar to the small cleaved FCC type, as do many of the mixed nodular type. The diffuse poorly differentiated lymphocytic and mixed types, however, are of variable composition.

In Hodgkin's disease the correlation of clinical features and the histologic types are generally well known. There are three distinctive entities—lymphocyte predominance, lymphocyte depletion, and nodular sclerosis. Lymphocyte predominance is observed principally in young asymptomatic males in clinical stage I with disease presenting most commonly in the upper cervical region. The median survival is prolonged and there is an excellent chance of cure. Lymphocyte depletion presents a contrasting type, occurring in older males with symptomatic febrile disease, often with pancytopenia and lymphocytopenia and disease principally in abdominal lymph nodes, spleen, liver, and bone marrow. The median survival is 4 months and response to therapy generally is poor (Neiman et al., 1973). Nodular sclerosis predominantly occurs in younger individuals, and there is a definite sex association since the majority of women exhibit the nodular sclerosing type. It also has a regional association with the mediastinum, even though it may be observed initially in any stage. Those patients with disease of limited extent have a prolonged median survival and an excellent opportunity for cure.

SUMMARY

1. The non-Hodgkin's lymphomas of past decades have been involved in terminologic and conceptual disputes with lack of progress. Advances in pathology and therapy of Hodgkin's disease by comparison have been dramatic.

2. Recently we outlined a functional approach for the malignant lymphomas with the goal of relating these disorders to the T and B cell systems and alterations in lymphocyte transformation. Five general groups were proposed: (1) U cell (undefined); (2) T cell; (3) B cell, including the follicular center cell (FCC) types; (4) histiocytic; and (5) cell of uncertain origin—Hodgkin's disease.

3. A multiparameter investigative approach—including special morphology, cytochemistry, electron microscopy, immunologic surface marker, in vitro, and immunoperoxidase techniques—has been employed in the redefinition of these disorders according to the T and B cell systems. The results of a number of studies including our own on 384 cases of non-Hodgkin's disorders and related leukemias reveal that the majority mark as T or B cells with the exception of a portion of acute lymphocytic leukemia (ALL) and the rare true histiocytic type. Our studies indicate that the majority of lymphomas previously regarded as reticulum cell sarcoma or histiocytic lymphoma involve transformed lymphocytes with the exception of the true histiocytic type. Of major importance is the predictive nature of the morphologic types, but it is dependent upon excellent histologic material and an experienced observer.

4. The results of the functional studies demonstrate the heterogeneity of the histologic types of the past, including the histiocytic type and the diffuse types of Rappaport and ALL of

childhood. A number of homogeneous cytologic types have been identified and are emerging as clinical, morphologic, immunologic entities, such as the convoluted T cell lymphoma-leukemia that interrelates with T cell ALL, the plasmacytoid lymphocyte type often associated with dysglobulinemias of various types, the cerebriform type associated with Sézary's syndrome and mycosis fungoides, the FCC types and immunoblastic sarcoma of B cells that commonly develop in abnormal immune disorders. In Hodgkin's disease the long suspected immunologic abnormality has been related to decreased numbers of T cells in the peripheral blood and to a recently identified serum factor that interferes with E rosette formation.

5. The implications of the functional approach both immediate and future are important and far reaching. Use of the new approach by pathologists will require a change in the collection and processing of biopsy material to achieve the excellent cytologic detail required for evaluation. Acquisition of considerable experience with proven cases of new cytologic types will be necessary for effective application. The only new techniques necessary for general use in pathology may be the immunoperoxidase stain on paraffin sections of fixed tissue for cytoplasmic immunoglobulin in B cells and for muramidase in histiocytes and monocytes. The most ideal method for identifying histiocytes and monocytes is the nonspecific esterase method (i.e., the alpha naphthyl butyrate) which requires tissue imprints or frozen unfixed tissue. Use of this procedure may be essential for reliably establishing the diagnosis of histiocytic lymphoma. Establishment of the T cell type of ALL at the present time requires the use of the E rosette procedure, but the acid phosphatase stain may prove to be helpful. In the future, use of specific antiserums for T and B cells may prove to be the most effective approach, if relatively specific and reliable antiserums are developed.

6. Relating the malignant lymphomas to modern immunology and the resultant establishment of homogeneous cytologic types will permit the reliable investigation of the basic biologic mechanism of these disorders and ultimately the design of fundamental biologic approaches to their therapy.

REFERENCES

Aisenberg, A. C. and Long, J. C.: Lymphocyte surface characteristics in malignant lymphoma. Am. J. Med., 58: 300–306, 1975.

Barcos, M. P. and Lukes, R. J.: Malignant lymphoma of convoluted lymphocytes: a new entity of possible T-cell type. In Conflicts in Childhood Cancer, pp. 147–178. New York, Alan R. Liss, Inc., 1975.

Bennett, M. H.: Sclerosis in non-Hodgkin's lymphomata. Br. J. Cancer, 31: 44–52, Suppl. II, 1975.

Bennett, M. H., Farrer-Brown, G., Henry, K. and Jelliffe, A. M.: Classification of non-Hodgkin's lymphomas. Lancet, ii: 405, 1974 (Letters).

Bennett, M. H. and Millett, Y. L.: Nodular sclerotic lymphosarcoma: a possible new clinico-pathological entity. Clin. Radiol., 20: 339–343, 1969.

Berard, C. W., Gallo, R. C., Jaffe, E., Green, I. and DeVita, V. T.: Current concepts of leukemia and lymphoma: etiology, pathogenesis and therapy. Ann. Intern Med., 85: 351–366, 1976.

Berard, C., O'Conor, G. T., Thomas, L. B. and Torloni, H.: Histopathologic definition of Burkitt's tumor. Bull. WHO, 40: 601–607, 1969.

Braylan, R. C., Jaffe, E. S. and Berard, C. W.: Malignant lymphomas: current classification and new observations. In Hematologic and Lymphoid Pathology Decennial 1966–1975, edited by S. C. Sommers. New York, Appleton-Century-Crofts, 1975.

Broder, S., Edelson, R. L., Lutzner, M. A., Nelson, D. L., MacDermott, R. P., Durm, M. E., Goldman, C. K., Meade, B. D. and Waldmann, T. A.: The Sézary syndrome – a malignant proliferation of helper T cells. J. Clin. Invest., 58: 1297–1306, 1976.

Brouet, J., Flandrin, G. and Seligmann, M.: Thymus-derived nature of the proliferating cells in Sézary's syndrome. N. Engl. J. Med., 289: 341–344, 1973.

Brouet, J., LaBaume, S. and Seligmann, M.: Evaluation of T and B lymphocyte membrane markers in human non-Hodgkin's malignant lymphomas. Br. J. Cancer, 31: 121–127, Suppl. II, 1975.

Catovsky, D., Galetto, J., Okos, A., Milliani, E. and Galton, D. A. G.: Cytochemical profile of B and T leukaemic lymphocytes with special reference to acute lymphoblastic leukaemia. J. Clin. Path., 27: 767–771, 1974.

Collins, R. D. and Lukes, R. J.: Studies on possible derivation of some malignant lymphomas from follicular center cells. Am. J. Path., 62: 63a, 1971.

Davey, F. R., Goldberg, J., Stockman, J. and Gottlieb, A. J.: Immunologic and cytochemical cell markers in non-Hodgkin's lymphomas. Lab. Invest., 35: 430–438, 1976.

Dorfman, R. F.: Classification of non-Hodgkin's lymphomas. Lancet, i: 1295, 1974 (Letter).

Dutcher, T. F. and Fahey, J. L.: The histopathology of the macroglobulinemia of Waldenström. J. Natl. Cancer Inst., 22: 887–916, 1959.

Epstein, A. L. and Kaplan, H. S.: Biology of the human malignant lymphomas. I. Establishment in continuous cell culture and heterotransplantation of diffuse histiocytic lymphomas. Cancer, 34: 1851–1872, 1974.

Fuks, Z., Strober, S. and Kaplan, H. S.: Interaction between serum factors and T lymphocytes in Hodgkin's disease. Use as a diagnostic test. N. Engl. J. Med., 295: 1273–1278, 1976.

Gajl-Peczalska, K. J., Bloomfield, C. D., Coccia, P. F.,

Sosin, H., Brunning, R. D. and Kersey, J. H.: B and T cell lymphomas. Am. J. Med., *59:* 674-685, 1975.

Gall, E. A.: The reticulum cell, the cytological identity and interrelation of mesenchymal cells of lymphoid tissue. Ann. N. Y. Acad. Sci., *73:* 120, 1958.

Gerard-Marchant, R., Hamlin, I., Lennert, K., Rilke, F., Stansfeld, A. G. and Van Unnik, J. A. M.: Classification of non-Hodgkin's lymphomas. Lancet, *ii:* 406, 1974 (Letter).

Glick, A. D., Leech, J. H., Waldron, J. A., Flexnder, J. M., Horn, R. G. and Collins, R. D.: Malignant lymphomas of follicular center cell origin in man. II. Ultrastructural and cytochemical studies. J. Natl. Cancer Inst., *54:* 23-36, 1975.

Green, I., Jaffe, E., Shevach, E. M., Edelson, R. L., Frank, M. M. and Berard, C. W.: Determination of the origin of malignant reticular cells by the use of surface membrane markers. In *The Reticuloendothelial System,* edited by Rebuck, Berard, and Abell, pp. 282-300. Baltimore, Williams & Wilkins, 1975.

Haegert, D. G., Stuart, J. and Smith, J. L.: Acute lymphoblastic leukaemia: a heterogeneous disease. Br. Med. J., *1:* 312-315, 1975.

Hansen, J. A. and Good, R. A.: Malignant disease of the lymphoid system in immunologic perspective. Hum. Pathol., *5:* 567-599, 1974.

Jaffe, E. S., Shevach, E. M., Frank, M. M., Berard, C. W. and Green, I.: Nodular lymphoma – evidence for origin from follicular B lymphocytes. N. Engl. J. Med., *290:* 813-819, 1974.

Jondal, M., Holm, G. and Wigzell, H.: Surface markers on human T and B lymphocytes. J. Exp. Med., *136:* 207-215, 1972.

Jones, S. E., Fuks, Z., Bull, M., Kadin, M., Dorfman, R. F., Kaplan, H. S., Rosenberg, S. A. and Kim, H.: Non-Hodgkin's lymphomas. IV. Clinicopathologic correlation in 405 cases. Cancer, *32:* 682-691, 1973.

Kersey, J. H., Sabad, A., Gajl-Peczalska, K. et al.: Acute lymphoblastic leukemic cells with T (thymus derived) lymphocyte markers. Science, *182:* 1355-1356, 1973.

Kojima, M., Imai, Y. and Mori, N.: A concept of follicular lymphoma. A proposal for the existence of a neoplasm originating from the germinal center. In *GANN Monograph on Cancer Research 15, Malignant Diseases of the Hematopoietic System,* edited by K. Akazaki et al., p. 195. Baltimore, University Park Press, 1973.

Kojima, M. and Tsunoda, R.: Localization of immunoglobulins in germinal centers of human tonsils. In *The Reticuloendothelial System in Health and Disease: Immunologic and Pathologic Aspects,* edited by H. Friedman et al., pp. 77-86. New York, Plenum Publishing Corp., 1976.

Kunkel, H. G.: Surface markers of human lymphocytes. Johns Hopkins Med. J., *137:* 216-223, 1975.

Leech, J., Glick, A., Horn, R. and Collins, R.: Immunologic histochemical and ultrastructural studies of malignant lymphomas presumed to be of follicular center cell origin. J. Natl. Cancer Inst., *54:* 11-21, 1975.

Lennert, K.: Follicular lymphoma. A tumor of the germinal centers. In *GANN Monograph on Cancer Research 15, Malignant Diseases of the Hematopoietic System,* edited by K. Akazaki et al., p. 217. Baltimore, University Park Press, 1973.

Lennert, K., Mohri, N., Stein, H. and Kaiserling, E.: Histopathology of malignant lymphomas. Br. J. Haematol., *31:* 193-203, 1975.

Levine, G. D. and Dorfman, R. F.: Nodular lymphoma: an ultrastructural study of its relationship to germinal centers and a correlation of light and electron micro-

scopic findings. Cancer, *35:* 148-164, 1975.

Lukes, R. J.: The pathological picture of the malignant lymphomas. In *Proceedings of the International Conference on Leukemia-Lymphoma,* edited by Zarafonetis, pp. 333-356, Philadelphia, Lea & Febiger, 1968.

Lukes, R. J.: Criteria for involvement of lymph node, bone marrow, spleen and liver in Hodgkin's disease. Cancer Res., *31:* 1755-1767, 1971.

Lukes, R. J., Butler, J. J. and Hicks, E. B.: Natural history of Hodgkin's disease as related to its pathologic picture. Cancer, *19:* 317-344, 1966a.

Lukes, R. J. and Collins, R. D.: New observations on follicular lymphoma. In *GANN Monograph on Cancer Research 15, Malignant Diseases of the Hematopoietic System,* edited by K. Akazaki, et al., pp. 209-215. Baltimore, University Park Press, 1973.

Lukes, R. J. and Collins, R. D.: A functional approach to the classification of malignant lymphoma. Recent Results Cancer Res., *46:* 18-30, 1974a.

Lukes, R. J. and Collins, R. D.: Immunologic characterization of human malignant lymphomas. Cancer, *34:* 1488-1503, 1974b.

Lukes, R. J. and Collins, R. D.: New approaches to the classification of the lymphomata. Br. J. Cancer, *31:* 1-28, Suppl. II, 1975.

Lukes, R. J. and Collins, R. D.: The Lukes-Collins classification and its significance. Conference on the Non-Hodgkin's Lymphomas, San Francisco, September 30-October 2, 1976. Cancer Treatment Reports, *61:* June, 1977.

Lukes, R. J., Craver, L. L., Hall, T. C., Rappaport, H. and Ruben, P.: Hodgkin's disease, report of Nomenclature Committee, Cancer Res., *26:* 1311, 1966b.

Lukes, R. J. and Tindle, B. H.: Immunoblastic lymphadenopathy. A hyperimmune entity resembling Hodgkin's disease. N Engl. J. Med., *292:* 1-8, 1975.

Lukes, R. J., Tindle, B. H. and Parker, J. W.: Reed-Sternberg-like cells in infectious mononucleosis. Lancet, *ii:* 1003-1004, 1969.

Lutzner, M., Edelson, R., Schein, P., Green, I., Kirkpatrick, C. and Ahmed, A.: Cutaneous T cell lymphoma: the Sézary syndrome, mycosis fungoides and related disorders. Ann. Intern. Med., *85:* 534-552, 1975.

Mann, R. B., Jaffe, E. S., Braylan, R. C., Nanba, K., Frank, M. M., Ziegler, J. L. and Berard, C. W.: Non-endemic Burkitt's lymphoma. A B-cell tumor related to germinal centers. N. Engl. J. Med., *295:* 685-691, 1976.

Mathé, G., Belpomme, D., Dantchev, D., Khalil, A., Afifi, A. M., Taleb, N., Pouillart, P., Schwarzenberg, L., Hayat, M., De Vassal, F., Jasmin, C., Misset, J. L. and Musset, M.: Immunoblastic lymphosarcoma, a cytological and clinical entity? Biomedicine, *22:* 473-488, 1975.

Nathwani, B. N., Kim, H. and Rappaport, H.: Malignant lymphoma, lymphoblastic. Cancer, *38:* 964-983, 1976.

Neiman, R. S., Rosen, P. J. and Lukes, R. J.: Lymphocyte-depletion Hodgkin's disease. N. Engl. J. Med., *288:* 751-755, 1973.

Nossal, G. J. V., Abbot, A., Mitchell, J. and Lummus, Z.: Antigens in immunity. XV. Ultrastructural features of antigen capture in primary and secondary lymphoid follicles. J. Exp. Med., *127:* 277-289, 1968.

O'Brien, R. O., Parker, J. W. and Dixon, J. F. P.: Mechanisms of lymphocyte transformation. In *Progress in Molecular and Subcellular Biology,* Vol. 6, edited by F. Hahn. New York, Springer-Verlag, 1977.

Ohnuma, T., Orlowski, M., Minowada, J. and Holland, J. F.: Differences in amino acid metabolism of human T-

and B-cells in culture. Presented at the Proceedings of the 16th International Congress of Hematology, Kyoto, Japan, September 5–11, 1976.

Rappaport, H., Winter, W. J. and Hicks, E. B.: Follicular lymphoma; re-evaluation of its position in the scheme of malignant lymphoma, based on survey of 253 cases. Cancer, *9:* 792–821, 1956.

Rosas-Uribe, A., Variakojis, D., Molnar, Z. and Rappaport, H.: Mycosis fungoides: an ultrastructural study. Cancer, *34:* 634–645, 1974.

Schlossman, S. F., Chess, L., Humphreys, R. E. and Strominger, J. L.: Distribution of Ia-like molecules on the surface of normal and leukemic human cells. Proc. Natl. Acad. Sci. USA, *73:* 1288–1292, 1976.

Schneider, B. K., Higgins, G. R., Swanson, V., Isaacs, H., Tindle, B. H. and Lukes, R. J.: Malignant lymphomas of childhood. Submitted for publication.

Stein, H., Peterson, N., Gaedicke, G., Lennert, K. and Landberg, C.: Lymphoblastic lymphoma of convoluted or acid phosphatase type-a tumor of T precursor cells. Int. J. Cancer, *17:* 292–295, 1976.

Taylor, C. R.: An immunohistological study of follicular lymphoma, reticulum cell sarcoma and Hodgkin's disease. Eur. J. Cancer, *12:* 61–75, 1976.

Taylor, C. R. and Mason, D. Y.: The immunohistological detection of intracellular immunoglobulin in formalin-paraffin sections from multiple myeloma and related conditions using the immunoperoxidase technique. Clin. Exp. Immunol., *18:* 417–429, 1974.

Tindle, B. H., Parker, J. W. and Lukes, R. J.: "Reed-Sternberg cells" in infectious mononucleosis? Am. J. Clin. Path., *58:* 607–617, 1972.

Williams, A. H., Taylor, C. R., Higgins, G. R., Quinn, J. J., Schneider, B. K., Swanson, V., Parker, J. W., Pattengale, P. K., Chandor, S. B., Powars, D., Lincoln, T. L., Tindle, B. H. and Lukes, R. J.: Childhood leukemia and lymphoma. I. Correlation of morphology and functional studies. Submitted for publication.

Winchester, R. J., Fu, S. M., Wernet, P., Kunkel, H. G., Dupont, B. and Jersild, C.: Recognition by pregnancy serums of non-HL-A alloantigens selectively expressed on B lymphocytes. J. Exp. Med., *141:* 924–929, 1975.

Yam, L. T., Li, C. Y. and Crosby, W. H.: Cytochemical identification of monocytes and granulocytes. Am. J. Clin. Path., *55:* 283–290, 1971a.

Yam, L. T., Li, C. Y. and Lam, K. W.: Tartrate resistant acid phosphatase isoenzyme in the reticulum cells of leukemic reticuloendotheliosis. N. Engl. J. Med., *284:* 357–360, 1971b.

LYMPHOGRAPHY IN LYMPHOMA*

SAMUEL J. HESSEL,† M.D., DOUGLASS F. ADAMS, M.D., AND HERBERT L. ABRAMS, M.D.

The development over the past two to three decades of effective radiotherapeutic approaches to lymphoma, particularly Hodgkin's disease, has been based upon the recognition of the stepwise progression of disease from one lymph node region to the other. Therapeutic radiation is directed to the involved and contiguous node-bearing regions (Peters, 1966; Kaplan, 1966). With the availability of such therapy, it became critical to define as precisely as possible the extent of nodal disease. The axillary, cervical, and mediastinal nodes were amenable to evaluation by easily employed clinical and radiologic examinations. There were no such effective approaches for evaluating the iliac and para-aortic nodes. The development of pedal lymphography has permitted us to evaluate these areas in order to improve diagnosis, patient care, and ultimate prognosis in lymphomatous disease.

Indications

Pedal lymphography has three primary applications in patients with lymphoma: (1) staging of disease believed to be localized for radiation treatment planning; (2) evaluating the response to radiation or chemotherapy; and (3) detecting the recurrence or progression of disease.

The Initial Examination: Staging Disease

Since radiation therapy in asymptomatic patients with truly localized Hodgkin's disease can lead to long term survival and cure, pedal lymphography is indicated. Similarly, lymphosarcoma and reticulum cell sarcoma isolated to the para-aortic nodes can be eradicated by irradiation, although the localized forms of these lymphomas are less common than that of Hodgkin's disease. Thus, lymphography is indicated in all patients with clinically localized lymphoma (e.g., Hodgkin's disease, primarily stages IA and IIA) (Table 8.4).

Lymphography is valuable because of its sensitivity in detecting retroperitoneal disease. Farrell (1967) reported lymphography to be

* Supported by USPHS GM18674, HL11668, and HL05832.

† James Picker Foundation Fellow in Academic Radiology.

twice as sensitive as inferior vena cavography (Fig. 8.7) and more than three times as sensitive as intravenous urography (Fig. 8.8) in detecting retroperitoneal lymphoma. Schwarz et al. (1965) pointed out that while 37 of 45 patients with stage I or stage II Hodgkin's disease showed nodal involvement, only 12 of the 45 had positive cavograms. However, cavography can evaluate the lower thoracic through upper lumbar

TABLE 8.4
HODGKIN'S DISEASE: ANN ARBOR MODIFICATION OF RYE STAGING SYSTEM (1971)*

Stage I	Involvement of a single lymph node region (1) or of a single extralymphatic organ or site (1$_E$).
Stage II	Involvement of two or more lymph node regions on the same side of the diaphragm (II) or localized involvement of an extralymphatic organ or site and of one or more lymph node regions on the same side of the diaphragm (II$_E$).
Stage III	Involvement of lymph node regions on both sides of the diaphragm (III), which may also be accompanied by localized involvement of an extralymphatic organ or site (III$_E$) or by involvement of the spleen (III$_S$) or both (III$_{SE}$).
Stage IV	Diffuse or disseminated involvement of one or more extralymphatic organs or tissues with or without associated lymph node enlargement. Reasons for classifying the patient as stage IV should be identified.

* Note: In Hodgkin's disease, all patients are subclassified A or B to indicate the absence or presence, respectively, of (1) unexplained weight loss of more than 10% body weight; (2) unexplained fever with temperatures above 38° C; and (3) night sweats.

region (T10 through L1) where lymphography is of little value. In Schwarz's series, 2 of 56 patients showed retroperitoneal disease only on cavography which would have been missed without this examination. Davidson et al. (1967) reported 50 patients believed to have stage I or II Hodgkin's disease, 18 of whom (36%) had unsuspected retroperitoneal disease detected by lymphography. The staging of these patients' disease was altered with a concomitant change

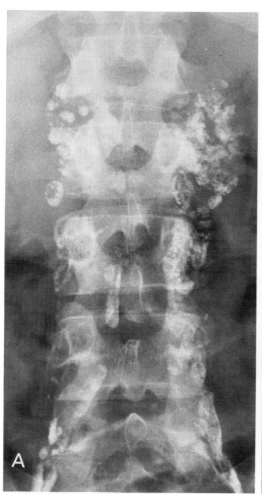

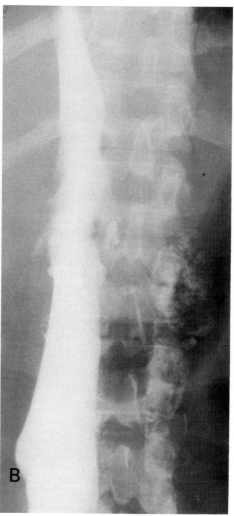

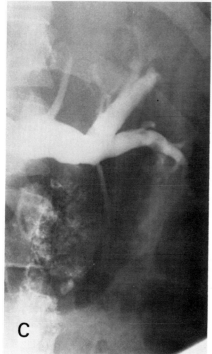

FIG. 8.7. HODGKIN'S DISEASE IN 20-YEAR-OLD PATIENT
A: Lymphangiogram shows gross filling defects and lateral displacement of nodes at the left L2 level. Laparotomy documented Hodgkin's involvement of the nodes. *B:* Inferior vena cavogram is normal. *C:* Left renal venogram is also normal.

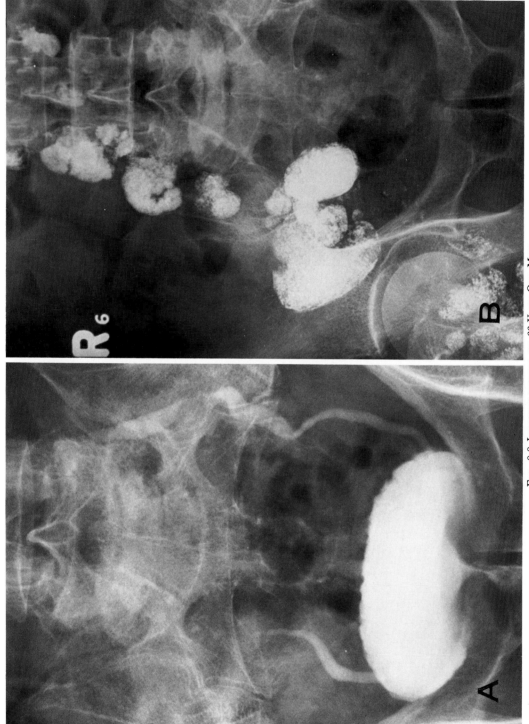

FIG. 8.8 LYMPHOSARCOMA IN 66-YEAR-OLD MAN

A: Medial deviation of right ureter was initially interpreted as normal. *B*: Lymphangiogram shows enormously enlarged bulky lymphomatous nodes in this same area. The relative subtlety of the ureteral deviation is in sharp contrast to the obvious nature of the nodal disease.

in therapy. Juttner et al. (1973) reported occult retroperitoneal disease in 21% of patients with stage I and II lesions. These data are similar to our own in which 32% of patients have the staging of their disease changed by lymphography (Table 8.5). Thus, short of laparotomy, lymphography provides a direct and sensitive means for evaluating the retroperitoneum in patients with presumed localized lymphoma. When staging laparotomy is planned, lymphography can direct the surgeon to abnormal or

TABLE 8.5
RELATIONSHIP BETWEEN PRE- AND POSTLYMPHOGRAM STAGING IN HODGKIN'S DISEASE

Stage before Lymphography	Stage after Lymphogram			
	I	II	III	IV
I	29	1	12	1
II		39	28	0
III			5	0
IV				16

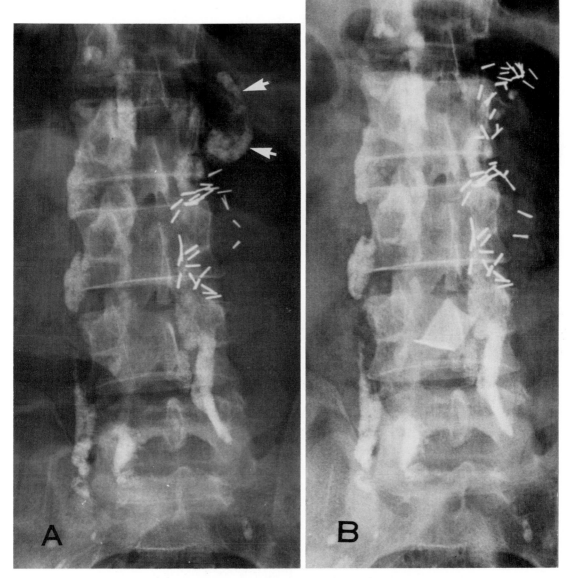

FIG. 8.9. HODGKIN'S DISEASE IN 35-YEAR-OLD MAN

A: Initial intraoperative film shows surgical clips and an obviously enlarged node with a gross filling defect at the L1 level (*arrows*). *B:* Second intraoperative film shows that the node has been removed. Sequential intraoperative films are valuable in assuring that the appropriate nodes are biopsied.

suspicious lymph nodes in order to maximize the value of his nodal biopsies. Our standard procedure is to identify the most suspicious nodes for the surgeon. He makes every effort to find and remove them. He marks the region with metallic clips and obtains an intraoperative film to assure that the proper nodes have been excised (Fig. 8.9).

The role of lymphography in patients with widespread disease is much less clear since (a) lymphograms reveal retroperitoneal nodal disease at least 90% of the time; (b) there is a greater incidence of pulmonary complications reported in stage III and stage IV patients undergoing lymphography; and (c) lymphographic findings will only rarely affect or help to determine the choice of therapy in generalized disease.

Follow-Up Films: Evaluating the Response to Therapy and Detecting Recurrences or Progression of Disease

Since the oily, iodinated contrast material remains in lymph nodes for a considerable pe-

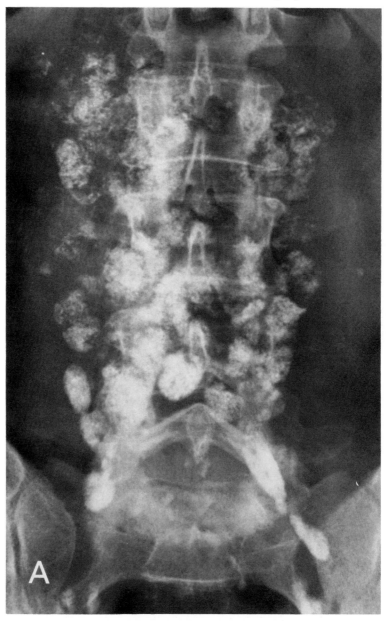

FIG. 8.10. MALIGNANT LYMPHOMA IN 47-YEAR-OLD MAN

A: Grossly abnormal lymphangiogram with lateral displacement, nodal foaminess, and filling defect. *B:* Follow-up abdominal film 4 months after radiation therapy shows dramatic reduction in nodal size.

riod, many patients may have sufficient contrast at 15 months to permit re-evaluation of lymph nodes on a follow-up plain abdominal film (Fabian et al., 1966). Other workers feel there is insufficient filling beyond 6 months to permit precise diagnoses (Gregl et al., 1970). Nevertheless, the response to treatment, both radiotherapy (Fig. 8.10) and chemotherapy (Fig. 8.11) can be evaluated at varying intervals after the lymphangiogram without resorting to a repeat study (Figs. 8.12, 8.13).

Diagnostic Criteria

Lymphographically visualized lymphomatous nodes have been variously described as "foamy," "lacy," "reticular," "granular," "blotchy," and "salt and pepper" in appearance (De Jesus, 1970). These appearances result from infiltration of tumor cells throughout the nodal reticulum. Irregular radiolucent filling defects occur when relatively large tumor deposits are found within a node. With diffuse nodal involvement,

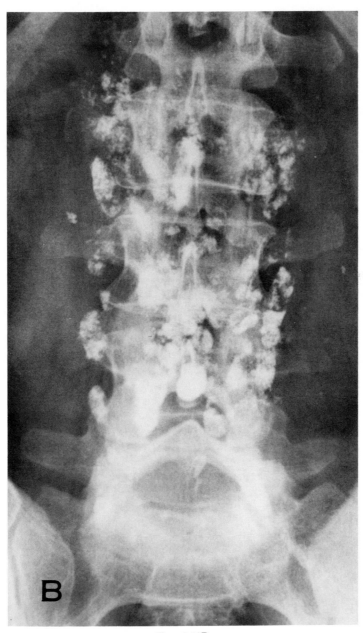

Fig. 8.10B

small foci of neoplasm appear as radiolucent dots outlined by contrast material surrounding dilated sinuses. These produce ring-
like margins, also known as the "rim" sign
(Dhawan et al., 1974). Nodes are typically enlarged (Kiely et al., 1970), although the degree
of enlargement for nodes to be considered abnormal has been disputed (De Jesus, 1970). Replacement of lymph nodes by tumor is noted by
unopacified areas representing malignant de-

posits (Fig. 8.14). Takahashi and Abrams (1967)
quantified the radiologic findings which separated normal from abnormal lymph nodes. The
criteria they formulated included (1) foaminess
of nodes greater than grade I (Fig. 8.15); (2)
filling defects occupying 33% or more of the node
(Fig. 8.16); (3) para-aortic nodes greater than
2.6 cm in size (Fig. 8.17); (4) anterior extension
of nodes greater than 3 cm from a line drawn
along the concavity on the anterior aspect of the

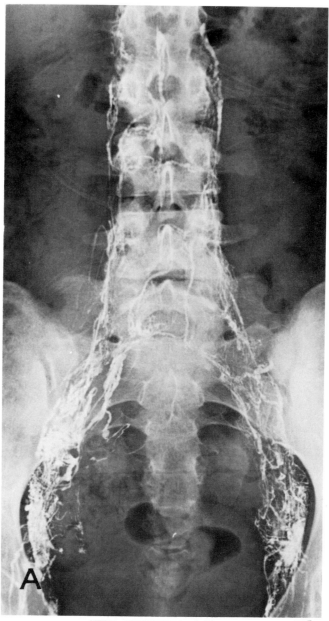

FIG. 8.11. HODGKIN'S DISEASE IN 15-YEAR-OLD FEMALE AFTER 6 CYCLES OF CHEMOTHERAPY
A: Filling phase shows para-aortic lymph channels without evident nodes. *B:* Nodal phase shows a few tiny nodes in the
para-aortic chains. This pattern can be seen after chemotherapy.

vertebral bodies (Fig. 8.18A); (5) lateral displacement of nodes greater than 2 cm from the concave border of the adjacent vertebral body (Fig. 8.18B). Since the para-aortic nodes lie in close approximation to the abdominal aorta (Fig. 8.19), the displacement criteria must be evaluated carefully in patients with tortuous or dilated aortae. Overall, these criteria were instrumental in their achieving an 81% accuracy in interpreting 206 lymphograms for lymphoma (Takahashi and Abrams, 1967). These criteria have been valuable particularly when there are questionable findings.

In addition to nodal findings, the effects of lymphatic obstruction may be manifested by the filling of collateral channels (Fig. 8.20), ectasia, backflow, and occasionally lymphaticovenous communications (Kiely et al., 1970). The latter finding has been associated with a poor prognosis due to rapid hematogenous spread of disease (Roxin and Bujar, 1970).

Accuracy of Lymphographic Interpretation

Although bipedal lymphography is a sensitive method of detecting lymphomatous involvement of the abdomen, it has significant limita-

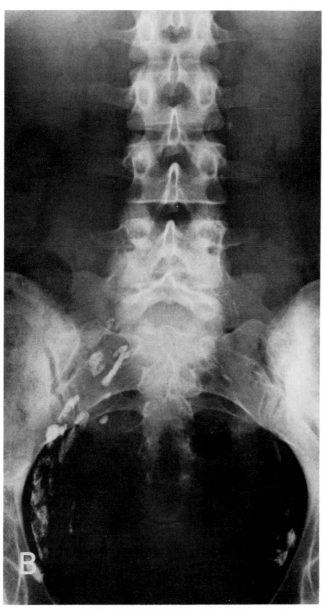

FIG. 8.11B

tions. Small, early microscopic lesions cannot be detected. This accounts for many of the false negative studies (Greening and Wallace, 1963). Various nonspecific benign or "reactive patterns may simulate lymphoma rendering diagnosis difficult" (Figs. 8.21, 8.22) (Parker et al., 1974). The radiologist's experience in interpreting lymphograms is another factor (Takahashi and Abrams, 1967). In addition, certain abdominal lymph nodes (i.e., skeletal, porta hepatic, splenic hilar, and mesenteric) cannot be visual-

ized by this technique. Thus, the extent of involvement in these areas cannot be determined by lymphography but must await staging laparotomy.

The reported accuracy of lymphography in lymphoma has ranged from approximately 75% (Schwarz et al., 1965) to over 90% (Castellino et al., 1974a, b). In the study of 166 Hodgkin's patients by Castellino et al. (1974a), there were no false negatives and only 14 false positives for an overall accuracy of 92%. In a similar study of

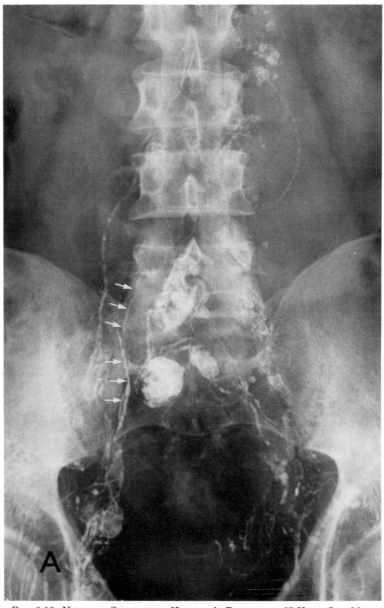

FIG. 8.12. NODULAR SCLEROSING HODGKIN'S DISEASE IN 37-YEAR-OLD MAN

A: Lymphatic channels (*arrows*) bypassing enlarged, spherical nodes involved with Hodgkin's disease. *B:* Follow-up abdominal film 10 months later shows decreased nodal size after chemotherapy.

a group of non-Hodgkin's lymphoma patients (Castellino et al., 1974b), 36 of 39 lymphograms called negative were confirmed on histologic examination, and 31 of 35 called positive were similarly confirmed. In 125 pathologically proven cases of Hodgkin's disease from the Peter Bent Brigham and the New England Deaconess Hospitals, there were 16 false positive and 3 false negative interpretations of disease in para-aortic nodes. This corresponded to a true positive ratio of 95% and a false positive ratio of 23%. The overall accuracy was 85%. In part, the relative incidence of false positive and false negative diagnoses will depend on how strictly one applies criteria of abnormality. This in turn will reflect one's own a priori judgment of the likelihood of a positive examination in any given population and the consequences of undercalling or overcalling disease.

Lymphographic-Histologic Correlation

There have been varying opinions regarding the degree of lymphographic-histologic correlation possible from lymphography. The current

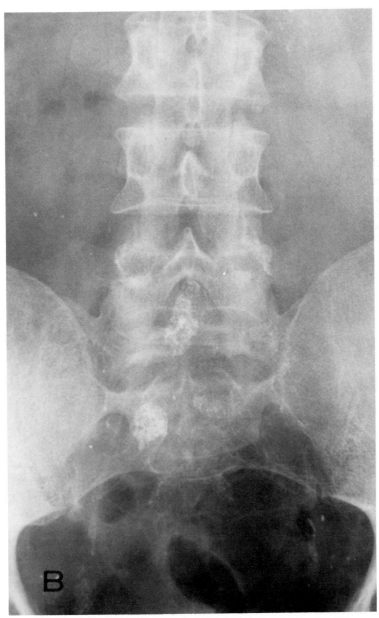

FIG. 8.12B

consensus is that while certain tumors may be more likely to manifest particular forms of nodal changes (Figs. 8.23–8.25), precise lymphographic-histologic correlation is usually unreliable (Takahashi and Abrams, 1967). Viamonte et al. (1963) noted that just as different pathologic processes may show similar lymphographic patterns, the same pathologic process may reveal varying abnormalities in nodal architecture. The lymph nodes can respond in only a limited way to a wide variety of external stimuli including inflammation and infection, systemic diseases, and immunologic disorders as well as neoplastic disease. Therefore, although a lymphogram is highly accurate in detecting gross structural changes regardless of their specific etiology, it is rarely pathognomonic of a specific disease process.

Data from the Peter Bent Brigham and New England Deaconess Hospitals (Table 8.6) show a 58-67% incidence of positive lymphograms in all Hodgkin's patients except those with the nodular sclerosing type. Similar results have been reported by Glatstein et al (1970).

Benign Changes Mimicking Lymphoma

The lymphographic appearance of certain nonspecific "reactive" changes mimics the typical lymphographic changes encountered in malignant lymphoma and accounts for the majority of false-positive exams (Parker et al., 1974). In the study by Castellino et al. (1974a), 16 of 18 false positive lymphangiograms showed pronounced nonspecific changes. Such changes, including fibrosis, sinus histiocytosis, reactive follicular hyperplasia (Figs. 8.21, 8.22), amorphous hyaline deposition, granuloma formation (Fig. 8.26), and vascular transformation (Koehler and Salmon, 1966) distort the internal nodal architecture.

Lymphography and Laparotomy

The role of laparotomy in staging lymphoma has evolved over several years. Laparotomy is

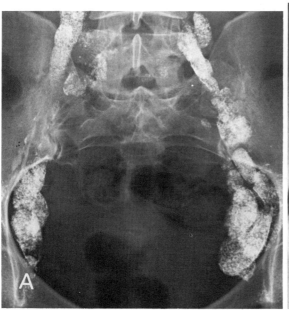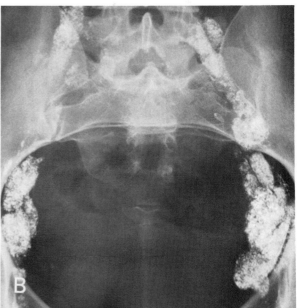

FIG. 8.13. LYMPHOSARCOMA IN 42-YEAR-OLD WOMAN

A: Initial films show enlargement and foaminess of iliac node. *B:* Follow-up film 2 months later after total nodal irradiation demonstrates a minimal response to therapy. Subsequent abdominal films may be used for follow-up, taking advantage of the previously injected contrast material.

TABLE 8.6
RELATIONSHIP OF LYMPHOGRAM RESULTS TO CELL TYPE

Cell Type	Positive Lymphography	Negative Lymphography	% Positive
Nodular sclerosing	12	34	26%
Lymphocyte predominant	6	3	67%
Lymphocyte depleted	9	6	60%
Mixed cellularity	22	16	58%

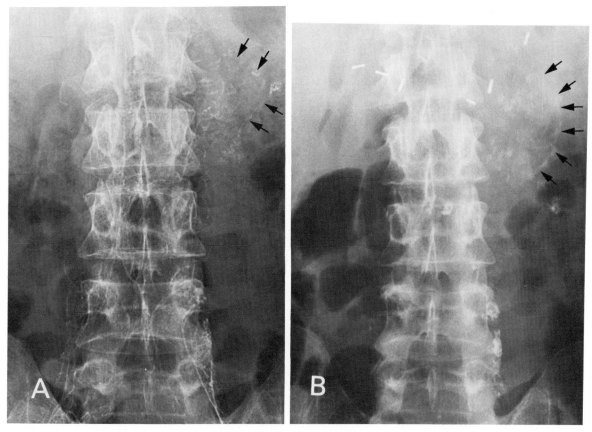

FIG. 8.14. MIXED CELLULARITY HODGKIN'S DISEASE IN 40-YEAR-OLD MAN

A: Filling phase showed para-aortic lymph channels with poorly defined masses (*arrows*) opposite the L1-L2 vertebral bodies. *B:* Nodal phase film immediately after exploratory laparotomy shows only minimal filling of para-aortic nodes with large, laterally deviated, poorly filling masses at the L2 and L3 vertebral levels (*arrows*). These are enlarged and virtually completely replaced lymph nodes. This degree of replacement is relatively unusual for Hodgkin's disease.

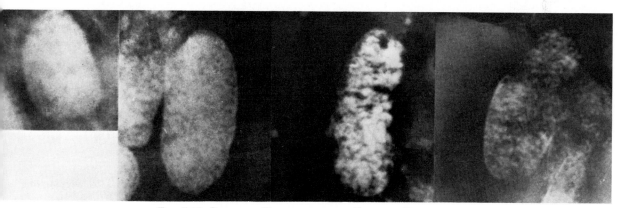

FIG. 8.15. STANDARD ROENTGENOGRAMS SHOWING FOAMINESS
From left to right: grade 0, grade 1, grade 2, and grade 3.

necessary in Hodgkin's disease for biopsy of suspicious nodes on lymphography and for evaluation of the spleen and liver (Glatstein et al., 1970; Hass et al., 1971). The latter purpose is particularly important since splenic involve-

ment in the face of a negative lymphogram occurs in a significant number of cases (Table 8.7). The liver, however, is only occasionally involved when the periaortic nodes are free of disease (Table 8.8). Furthermore, the liver is

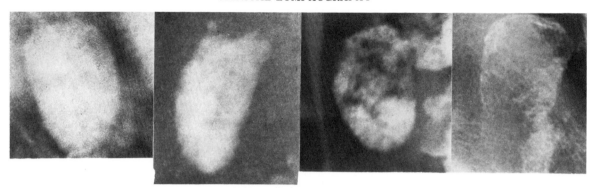

FIG. 8.16. STANDARD ROENTGENOGRAMS WITH FILLING DEFECTS

From left to right: grade 0 (no filling defects), grade 1 (less than one-third of node), grade 2 (one- to two-thirds of node), and grade 3 (more than two-thirds of node).

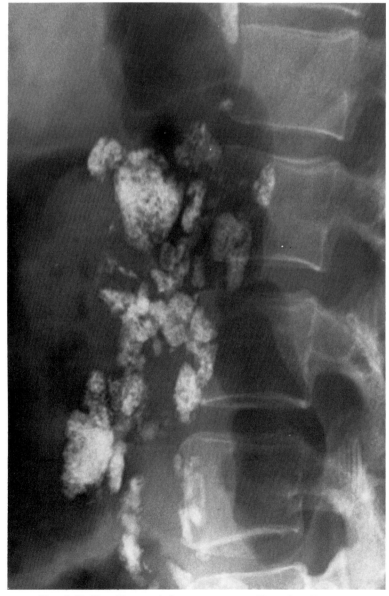

FIG. 8.17. NON-HODGKIN'S LYMPHOMA IN 50-YEAR-OLD WOMAN

Lymphangiogram shows markedly enlarged para-aortic nodes with anterior displacement at the L2-L3 level.

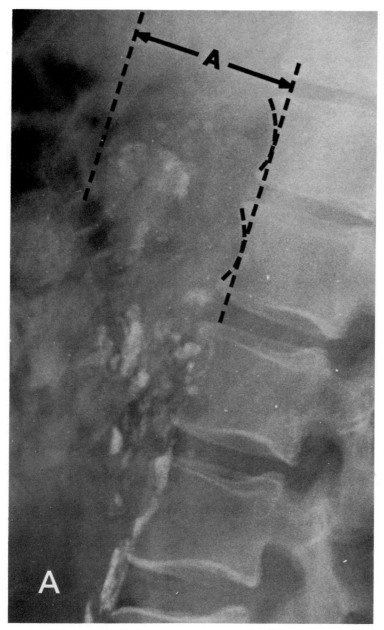

FIG. 8.18. MEASUREMENT OF LATERAL SPINE TO NODE DISTANCE

A: Measurement *A* in this case of Hodgkin's disease is 5.5 cm. The upper limit of normal is 3 cm. If the lateral film had been omitted, correct evaluation of this proven case would have been difficult. *B:* Spine to node distances. The right lateral spine to node distance (measurement *B*) is from the right lateral border of a lumbar vetebral body in its midportion to the most lateral border of the right paracaval node group. In this case, it measures 2.5 cm and is beyond the normal limits of 2 cm. The left lateral spine to node distance (measurement *C*) is the same measurement on the left side. In this case it is within the normal range, measuring 1.8 cm.

only rarely positive when the spleen is free of disease (Table 8.9).

Second Look Lymphography

While repeat abdominal films may provide information on the progress of disease for sev-

eral months, the status of a significant number of patients requiring re-evaluation will not be obtainable from repeat abdominal films.

Gregl et al. (1970) reported 38 patients who underwent second look lymphography. Of these, 16 had progression of disease, 7 had

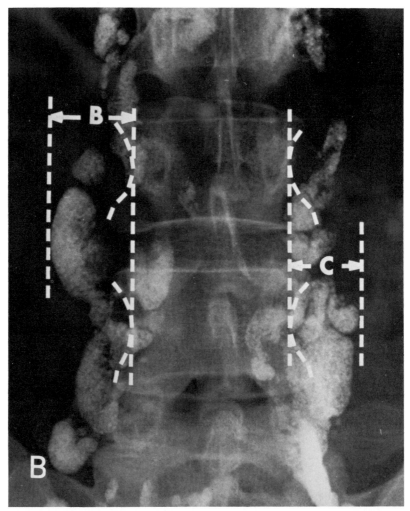

FIG. 8.18B

TABLE 8.7
RELATIONSHIP BETWEEN LYMPHOGRAM
RESULTS AND SPLENIC INVOLVEMENT

Lymphogram	Spleen	Number	% of Total
Positive	Positive	27	28%
Positive	Negative	12	13%
Negative	Positive	12	13%
Negative	Negative	44	46%

TABLE 8.8
RELATIONSHIP BETWEEN LYMPHOGRAM
RESULTS AND LIVER INVOLVEMENT

Lymphogram	Liver	Number	% of Total
Positive	Positive	3	3%
Positive	Negative	32	35%
Negative	Positive	2	2%
Negative	Negative	54	59%

TABLE 8.9
RELATIONSHIP BETWEEN SPLENIC AND HEPATIC
INVOLVEMENT

Spleen	Liver	Number	% of Total
Positive	Positive	5	5%
Positive	Negative	34	35%
Negative	Positive	1	1%
Negative	Negative	56	58%

regression, and 15 had no signs of tumor (Fig. 8.27). The author indicated that while a second look lymphogram may be technically more difficult, it can provide vital data not otherwise easily obtainable. When second look lymphography is performed, changes secondary to therapy (see Fig. 8.10, 8.11) and the effects of intervening surgery or infection must be considered when searching for tumor containing lymph nodes.

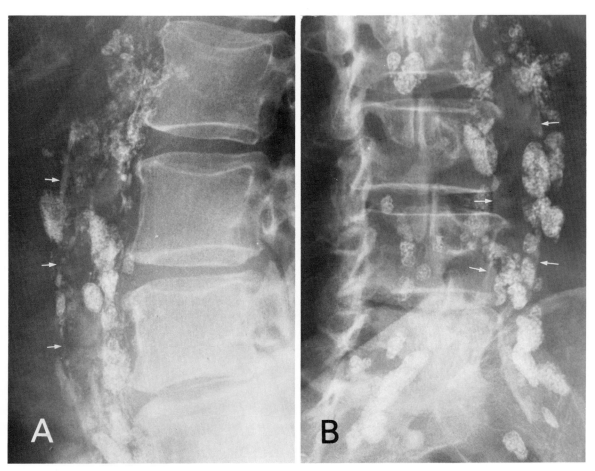

FIG. 8.19. HISTORY OF HODGKIN'S DISEASE AND AORTIC CALCIFICATION IN 68-YEAR-OLD PATIENT
The relationship of the para-aortic lymph nodes to the calcified abdominal aorta (*arrows*) is seen in the lateral (*A*) and oblique (*B*) views. There are grade 2 foamy nodes at the L1 level.

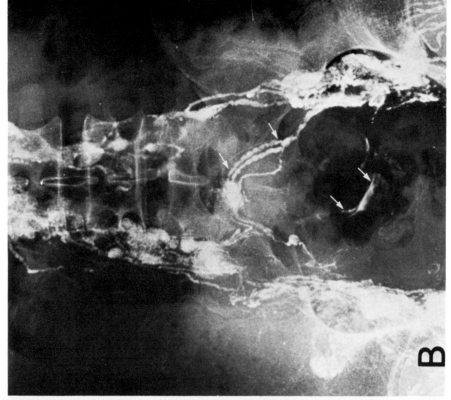

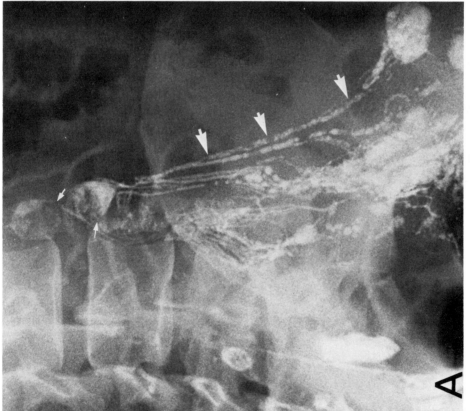

FIG. 8.20. PERSISTENT FILLING OF LYMPHATICS ON 24-HR FILMS

A: Hodgkin's disease. Large defects are seen in the nodes at the L3-L4 level (*small arrows*). Multiple channels extending from the inguinal, iliac, and para-aortic nodes remain densely filled with contrast material (*large arrows*). *B*: Reticulum cell sarcoma. There are multiple nodes which are slightly enlarged, foamy, and contain filling defects. Collateral lymphatic flow is noted via perivesical and retroperitoneal lymphatics (*arrows*). Common iliac and para-aortic channels are opacified at 24 hr.

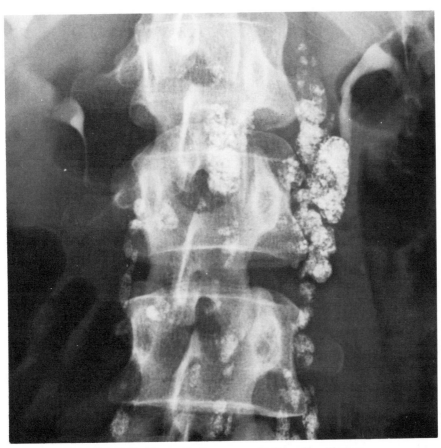

FIG. 8.21. HODGKIN'S DISEASE IN 34-YEAR-OLD WOMAN

Note grade 2 foaminess of nodes adjacent to second lumbar vertebral body. At laparotomy, lymphoid hyperplasia was found.

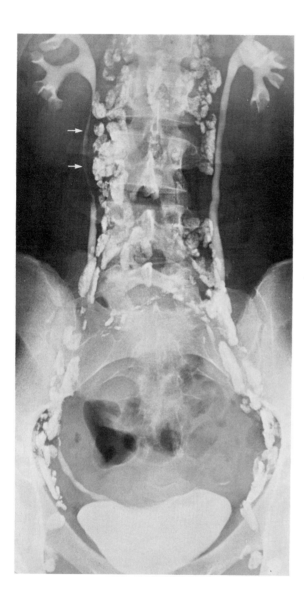

FIG. 8.22. HODGKIN'S DISEASE IN 18-YEAR-OLD WOMAN
There are many para-aortic nodes. There is lateral deviation of the proximal right ureter (*arrows*). Nodal biopsy
showed only hyperplasia with no evidence of Hodgkin's
disease in these nodes.

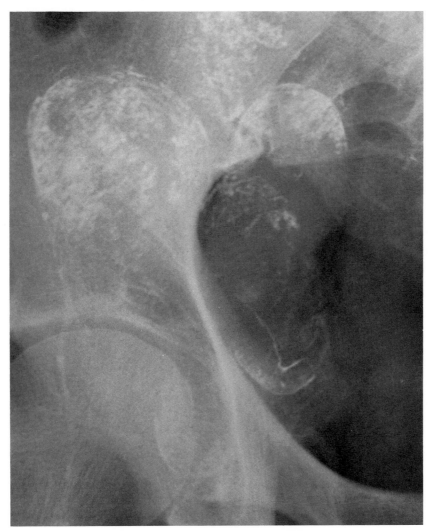

Fig. 8.23. Giant Follicular Lymphoma
Extensive enlargement and reticular appearance of external iliac and femoral nodes are noted.

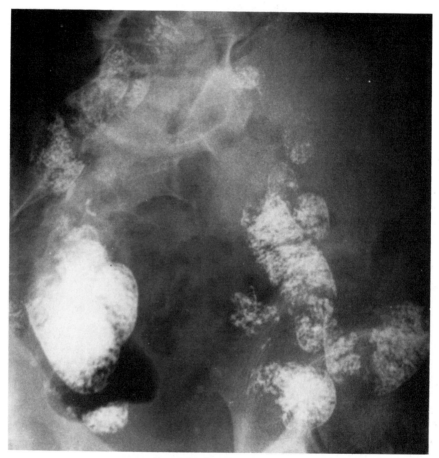

FIG. 8.24. LYMPHOSARCOMA
Extensive enlargement of all visualized nodes with foamy and reticular appearance is seen.

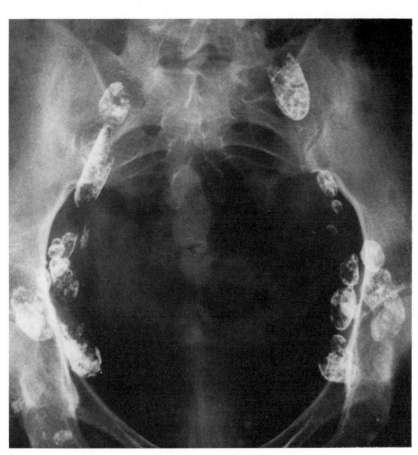

FIG. 8.25. RETICULUM CELL SARCOMA
Multiple nodes show subcapsular sinus filling, filling defects and foaminess.

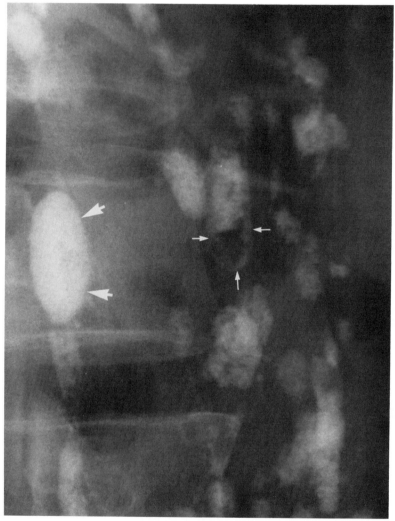

FIG. 8.26. A 36-YEAR-OLD POLICEMAN EVALUATED FOR ASYMPTOMATIC SPLENOMEGALY
There are enlarged nodes (*large arrows*), one with an obvious filling defect (*small arrow*). Biopsy showed noncaseating granulomata consistent with sarcoidosis.

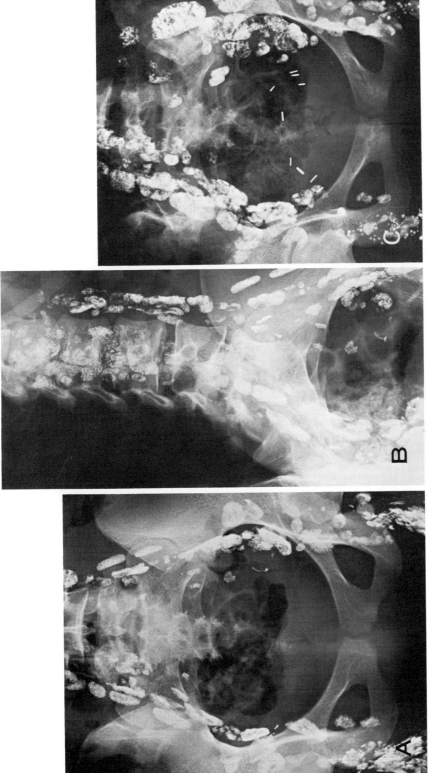

Fig. 8.27. HODGKIN'S DISEASE IN 17-YEAR-OLD WOMAN

A: Normal iliac nodes. B: Extensive grade 2 foaminess and filling defects in para-aortic nodes on the oblique film. The patient received iliac and para-aortic irradiation, but had incomplete pelvic irradiation because of GI symptoms. C: Three years later a second look lymphangiogram demonstrated recurrent disease in the incompletely irradiated pelvic nodes. This responded to combination chemotherapy and radiation therapy.

Acknowledgments

We wish to thank *Radiology* and Dr. Herbert L. Abrams for permission to use Figures 8.15, 8.16, 8.18, 8.20, 8.23, 8.24, and 8.25. Dr. Melvin Clouse assisted us by providing data on lymph-ography from the New England Deaconess Hospital. Our appreciation is also expressed to Ms. Susan Lucker for editorial assistance and to Ms. Laura Weitzler and Ms. Barbara Stock for typing this manuscript.

REFERENCES

Castellino, R. A., Billingham, M. and Dorfman, R. F.: Lymphographic accuracy in Hodgkin's disease and malignant lymphoma with a note on the "reactive" lymph node as a cause of most false-positive lymphograms. Invest. Radiol., *9:* 155–165, 1974a.

Castellino, R. A., Goffinet, D. R., Blank, N. et al.: The role of radiology in the staging of non-Hodgkin's lymphoma with laparotomy correlation. Radiology, *110:* 329–338, 1974b.

Davidson, J. W., Saini, M. and Peters, M. V.: Lymphography in lymphoma with particular reference to Hodgkin's disease. Radiology, *88:* 281–286, 1967.

De Jesus, F. N. Lymphography. Bol. Asoc. Med. P. R., *62:* 239–244, 1970.

Dhawan, I. K., Gandhi, M. G., Haldar, P. K. et al.: Unopacified areas on lymphadenography-their sizes as an index of response to therapy. Indian J. Cancer, *11:* 143–150, 1974.

Fabian, C. E., Nudelman, E. J. and Abrams, H. L.: Post-lymphangiogram film as an indicator of tumor activity in lymphoma. Invest. Radiol., *1:* 386–393, 1966.

Farrell, W. J.: Lymphangiography in the diagnosis and management of lymphoma and metastatic disease. Surg. Clin. North Am., *47:* 565–578, 1967.

Glatstein, E., Trueblood, H. W., Enright, L. P., Rosenberg, S. A. and Kaplan, H. S.: Surgical staging of abdominal involvement in unselected patients with Hodgkin's disease. Radiology, *97:* 425–432, 1970.

Greening, R. R. and Wallace, S.: Further observations in lymphangiography. Radiol. Clin. North Am., *1:* 157–173, 1963.

Gregl, A., Kienle, J. and Eydt, M.: Second- and third-look lymphangiography. Radiology, *95:* 149–156, 1970.

Hass, A. C., Brunk, S. F., Gulesserian, H. P. and Givler, R. L.: The value of exploratory laparotomy in malignant lymphoma. Radiology, *101:* 157–165, 1971.

Juttner, H. U., Miller, W. E., Kiely, J. M. et al.: Influence of lymphography in determining extent of disease in patients with lymphoma. Mayo Clin. Proc., *48:* 249–254, 1973.

Kaplan, H. S.: Role of intensive radiotherapy in the management of Hodgkin's disease. Cancer, *19:* 356–367, 1966.

Kiely, J. M., Miller, W. E. and Scanlon, P. W.: Lymphography in management of lymphoma. Med. Clin. North Am., *54:* 939–949, 1970.

Koehler, P. R. and Salmon, R. B.: Lymphographic patterns in lymphoma, with emphasis on the atypical forms. Radiology, *87:* 623–629, 1966.

Parker, B. R., Blank, N. and Castellino, R. A.: Lymphographic appearance of benign conditions simulating lymphoma. Radiology, *111:* 267–274, 1974.

Peters, M. V.: Prophylactic treatment of adjacent areas in Hodgkin's disease. Cancer Res., *26:* 1232–1243, 1966.

Roxin, T. and Bujar, H.: Lymphographic visualization of lymphaticovenous communications and their significance in malignant hemolymphopathies. Lymphology, *3:* 127–135, 1970.

Schwarz, G., Lee, B. J. and Nelson, J. H.: Lymphography, cavography and urography in the evaluation of malignant lymphomas. Acta, Radiol. [Diagn.] (Stockh.), *3:* 138–144, 1965.

Takahashi, M. and Abrams, H. L.: The accuracy of lymphangiographic diagnosis in malignant lymphoma. Radiology, *89:* 448–460, 1967.

Viamonte, M., Jr., Altman, D., Parks, R. et al: Radiographic-pathologic correlation in the interpretation of lymphangioadenograms. Radiology, *80:* 903–916, 1963.

9

Carcinoma

SIDNEY WALLACE, M.D., AND BAO-SHAN JING, M.D.

LYMPHANGIOGRAPHY IN CARCINOMA

A thorough assessment of the extent of neoplastic disease is a prerequisite to the intelligent management of any patient with cancer. Any technique which contributes to the accuracy of this evaluation is justifiable as long as the rewards warrant the risks and expenses.

Lymphangiography has become an integral part of the pretreatment determination of the extent of involvement in patients with lymphomatous diseases. At M. D. Anderson Hospital and Tumor Institute, lymphangiography has also been utilized to great advantage in the diagnosis and management of patients with epithelial neoplasms. Of the approximately 800 lymphangiograms performed each year at this hospital, one-half were in search of metastatic carcinoma.

In the evaluation of a patient with carcinoma, the nodes involved by metastases should be along the primary and secondary echelons of the lymphatic drainage. Variations in normal lymphatic anatomy are frequent, and assessment of the lymphatic phase is essential in determining the pre-existing anomalous channels which will significantly affect the distribution of metastases. Changes at a distance from the primary site without evidence of bypassing channels or lymphatic obstruction with collateral circulation should be viewed with great caution. Carcinomatous spread at the time of most examinations is usually local in contrast to that seen in lymphomas which is frequently more diffuse by the time the patient reaches the physician.

Tumor emboli from a primary carcinoma travel along the lymphatic channels and gain access to the marginal sinus of the node. At this point their progress is impeded; they enlarge and obstruct the marginal sinus. Lymphatics do not traverse the area replaced by carcinoma but rather are obstructed, distorted, and displaced

(Fig. 9.1). This may also be manifested by stasis of contrast material in channels on the delayed or 24-hr study. Abnormalities in the lymphatics and in the marginal sinus and therefore in the contour of the node usually occur early in carcinomatous appearance. Eventually, alterations also take place in the body of the node. This differs from lymphoma in which the internal architecture is disrupted early in the course of the disease; marginal defects usually are later manifestations. The major differential diagnosis is not usually between carcinoma and lymphoma but carcinoma versus a false positive defect produced by fatty replacement, fibrosis, superimposition of nodes, etc.

The node involved by metastatic carcinoma may be normal in size or enlarged; the shape tends to be more rounded than normal. Metastases most frequently result in a crescent-shaped configuration with the lymphatics (during the vascular phase) absent in the sharply defined marginal concavity. The single most reliable criterion for the lymphangiographic diagnosis of metastatic carcinoma to a lymph node is *a defect which is not traversed by lymphatics*.

The remaining functioning portion of the node is crescent-shaped. The lymphatics leading to the defect are disrupted by the destructive process. It is important to view the lymphatics and nodal defect in multiple projections. If in any one projection the defect is not traversed by the lymphatic channels, the finding is real. This assists in the differentiation from superimposition of vessels. This appearance can be simulated by an abscess formation, caseation necrosis, and fibrosis. In the presence of a known primary malignancy, metastasis is by far the most likely diagnosis.

185

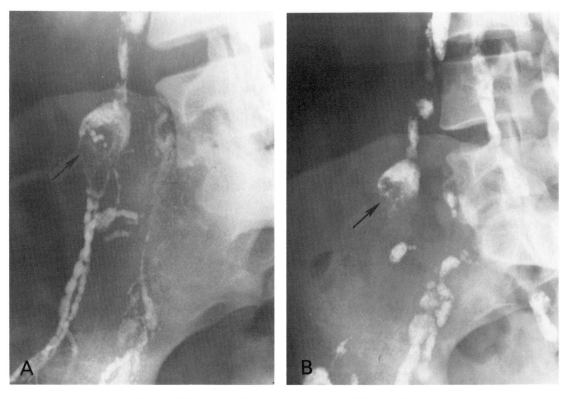

FIG. 9.1. METASTATIC CARCINOMA FROM THE UTERINE CERVIX

A: Lymphatic phase. The lymphatics do not permeate the areas of replacement (*arrow*) by metastatic carcinoma. *B:* Nodal phase. The defects in the margin of the nodes are areas of tumor deposition (*arrow*). The remaining functioning portion of the node is opacified producing a crescent configuration. This represents partial replacement of the nodes by metastatic carcinoma.

As the carcinoma progresses the nodes become totally replaced. The lymphatics may be obstructed or distorted by the carcinomatous focus. Collateral circulation, lymphatic to lymphatic, lymphatic to pre- or paralymphatic, and lymphatic to venous, may be opacified which might be the only evidence of replacement of nodal tissue. Lymphatic obstruction may not be accompanied by collateral channels but may result in a decrease in the number of lymphatics and nodes opacified. Filling of only two of the three major iliac trunks could be of great significance (Fig. 9.2).

Interference in lymphatic flow in itself is secondary evidence of metastases. Confirmation is necessary before a conclusive diagnosis can be made. Complete replacement of lymph nodes with associated lymphatic abnormalities must be further evaluated by complementary procedures such as intravenous urography, inferior vena cavography, pelvic venography, computed tomography, and ultrasound to establish the presence of a mass.

Urography is a complementary examination in the evaluation of the retroperitoneal area in that it may confirm the existence of totally replaced nodes by displacement or obstruction of the urinary tract. Asymmetry of ureters is a common occurrence in the normal. Enlarged nodes usually displace the upper ureters laterally, and the lower portions of the ureters medially. In conjunction with lymphangiography, obstructed or distorted lymphatics and abnormal nodes can be more definitely implicated if they produce an associated change in the urinary tract. This occurred in a patient with carcinoma of the cervix, clinically Stage II, whose lymphangiogram revealed small abnormal iliac nodes in the junctional area between the common and external iliac lymph nodes. Intravenous urography demonstrated nonvisualization of the right kidney presumably due to obstruc-

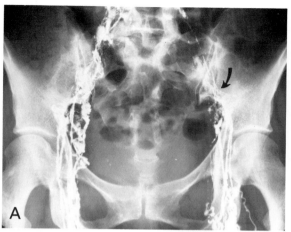
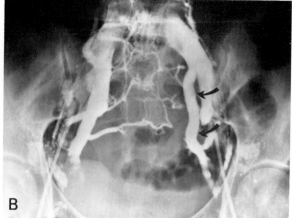

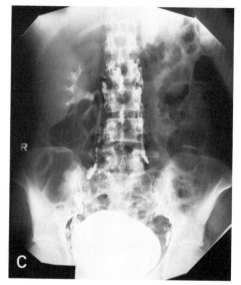

FIG. 9.2. METASTATIC CARCINOMA FROM THE UTERINE
CERVIX

A: There is a decrease in the number of left iliac lymphatics opacified (*arrow*). *B:* Compression venography demonstrates distortion of the left internal iliac vein (*arrows*). The changes in the lymphatics and veins are due to totally replaced lymph nodes. *C:* Intravenous urogram. The left kidney was not visualized due to obstruction of the ureter by metastatic disease.

tion of the right ureter supporting the diagnosis of metastases (Fig. 9.3). In patients with carcinoma of the cervix previously treated by radiation therapy, the obstruction of a ureter is most likely due to recurrent neoplasm.

Venography may be of considerable assistance in establishing the etiology of lymphatic obstruction by demonstrating masses distorting or obstructing the adjacent veins. The limitations of venography depend upon the size and position of the involved nodes in relationship to the opacified veins. The studies available include (1) bilateral iliac venography, (2) inferior vena cavography, (3) compression inferior vena cavography for retrograde opacification of the internal iliac and sacral veins, and (4) selective renal, ovarian, or testicular venography. Selective catheterization of either ovarian vein, usu-

ally the left, will opacify the ovarian, adnexal, and uterine veins bilaterally. Inferior vena cavography can only evaluate the right side of the retroperitoneal space. In the region of L2 where the lumbar trunks usually drain into the cisterna chyli, vena cavography is of utmost importance. It may also assist in establishing the extent of involvement above the point of lymphatic obstruction as well as in the detection of enlarged nodes not ordinarily opacified by lymphangiography. Distortion and obstruction of veins are nonspecific as to etiology. Invasion of veins is usually neoplastic in origin (Fig. 9.4). Difficulties may be encountered by the presence of thrombophlebitis.

Pelvic and retroperitoneal surgery may interrupt lymphatic trunks and remove lymph nodes. This may result in obstruction of lym-

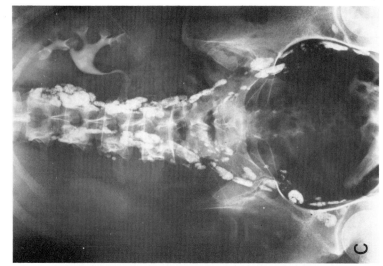

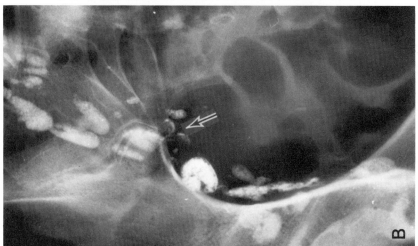

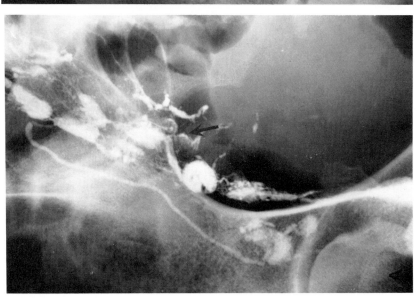

Fig. 9.3. Metastatic Carcinoma from the Uterine Cervix

A: Lymphatic phase. Two small nodes in the right iliac chain at the junctional position (*arrow*) demonstrate the failure of the lymphatics to traverse these nodes. *B:* Nodal phase. The two small nodes containing metastatic carcinoma are crescent in configuration (*arrow*). *C:* Intravenous urogram. The right kidney does not visualize. The obstruction of the ureter may be due to other totally replaced nodes not opacified or from extension of the primary carcinoma into the parametrium.

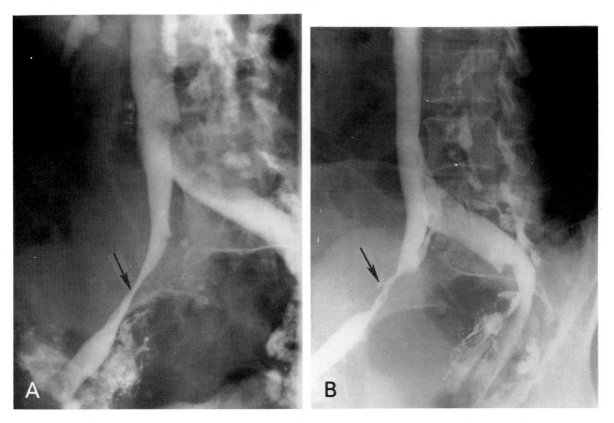

FIG. 9.4. VENOUS INVOLVEMENT BY METASTATIC CARCINOMA FROM THE UTERINE CERVIX

A: Compression of the right external iliac vein (*arrow*) by lymph nodes partially replaced by metastatic carcinoma. Compression can be produced by a mass of any etiology. B: Invasion of the right common iliac vein (*arrow*) by metastatic carcinoma totally replacing the lymph nodes.

phatic channels or lymphocyst formation. These findings are difficult to differentiate even with venography unless appreciated shortly after the surgical procedure. Lymphangiography may assist in the differentiation if the lymphatics opacified from the lower extremities are in continuity with the lymphocyst (Fig. 9.5).

Following radiotherapy and/or chemotherapy the problem in differentiation becomes more difficult. These therapeutic approaches reduce the size and number of nodes with usually little effect on the lymphatic vessels. Irradiation decreases lymphoid tissue but seldom results in obstruction unless associated with extensive fibrosis. It may also decrease the regenerative capacity of lymphatics and nodes. Following radiation therapy, lymphangiography has been of value in establishing the presence of metastatic disease (Fig. 9.6). The extent of previous radio-

therapy can be accurately estimated because of the decreased size of the treated lymph nodes. Under normal circumstances the pelvic nodes are usually larger than the para-aortic nodes.

Successful treatment does not necessarily alleviate an obstruction secondary to metastatic disease. The paucity of nodes visualized as the result of these modes of therapy must be differentiated from total replacement by the malignant disease. Venography could confirm the presence of a mass which would most probably represent neoplastic disease replacing the nodes. However, when the lymphatics are normal in number and distribution in the absence of opacified lymphoid tissue, the possibility of extensive replacement is minimal. Nodal involvement is usually associated with distortion or obstruction of lymphatic pathways. Occasionally an apparently normal individual, without

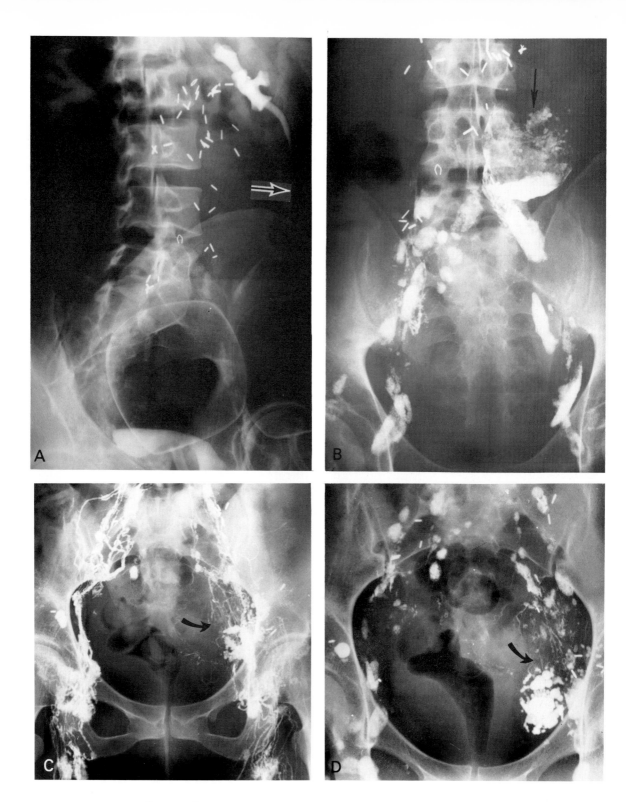

FIG. 9.5. POSTOPERATIVE LYMPHOCYST VERSUS METASTATIC CARCINOMA

A: Intravenous urogram revealed the left ureter displaced by a retroperitoneal mass (*arrow*) in a patient with a left testicular carcinoma previously treated by a retroperitoneal node dissection. *B:* The lymphangiogram opacifies the retroperitoneal lymphocyst (*arrow*). *C:* Pelvic lymphocyst in a patient with carcinoma of the cervix. This occurred following node biopsy for staging laparotomy. Lymphangiography confirmed the presence of a lymphocyst, a collection of contrast material accumulated in the left iliac area (*arrow*). *D:* Nodal phase demonstrated the collection of contrast in the lymphocyst (*arrow*). When the patient was placed in a dependent position, a fluid level was seen.

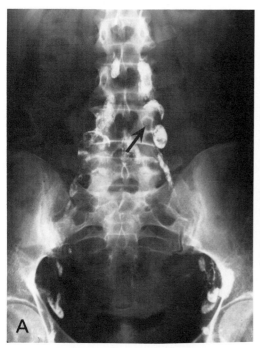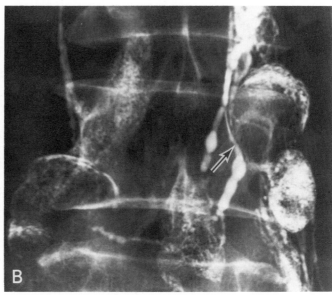

FIG. 9.6. METASTATIC CARCINOMA OF THE CERVIX FOLLOWING RADIATION THERAPY

A: The pelvic nodes are small up to the top of L5. This was the level of the treatment portal. The lymph nodes in the para-aortic area are enlarged and involved by metastatic carcinoma (*arrow*). *B:* The lymphatic phase reveals crescentic configuration of the metastatic nodes and the lymphatics which fail to traverse the defects (*arrow*).

any previous therapy, may have relatively few nodes in the retroperitoneal area, but the lymphatic distribution is normal (Fig. 9.7).

Modes of Metastases

The modes of lymph node metastases are in part governed by (1) the normal distribution of lymphatic drainage, (2) the variations in normal drainage, and (3) the collateral pathways available in the event of obstruction.

In the evaluation of a patient with carcinoma, the nodes involved by metastases should be along the primary and secondary echelons of the lymphatic drainage. In the interpretation of the lymphangiogram it is essential to be thoroughly acquainted with the normal lymphatic drainage from the involved viscera. From the pelvic viscera the lymphatic drainage is primarily to the lymph nodes of the internal, external, and common iliac chains as well as to the presacral area. Bilateral pedal lymphangiography opacifies most but not all of these lymph nodes. The external and common iliac pathways consist of three major trunks: the medial, the middle, and the lateral (Fig. 9.8). The obturator nodes or the principal nodes of drainage from some of the

pelvic viscera are usually considered to be part of the medial group of the external iliac chain. These nodes are almost invariably opacified. Nodes in the obturator fossa when present (7%) are seldom visualized. The internal iliac and presacral nodes are not consistently opacified. Changes in lymph nodes at a distance from the sites of usual drainage and in the absence of lymphatic variation or obstruction must be viewed with great caution.

Variations in normal lymphatic anatomy are frequent, and assessment of the lymphatic phase is essential in determining the pre-existing anomalous channels which will significantly affect the distribution (Fig. 9.9). The many variations of the normal can be best illustrated by the examination of the thoracic duct (Figs. 9.10 and 9.11). The classical distribution of the thoracic duct as described by Bartels (1909) is found in approximately 50% of patients. Opacification of the mediastinal, hilar, paratracheal, and bilateral supraclavicular nodes depends upon the numerous variations of normal (Fig. 9.12). At times lower cervical and axillary node visualization may be a manifestation of these anomalous pathways.

Metastases are usually logical and orderly in

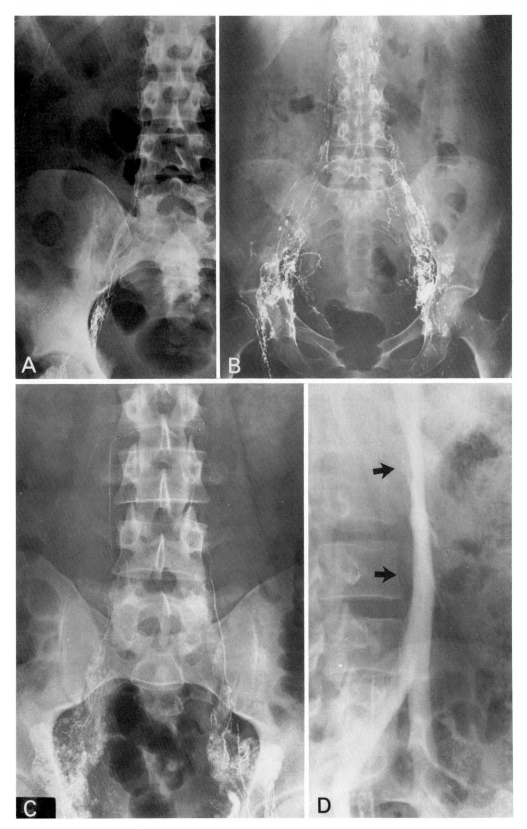

FIG. 9.7. PAUCITY OF OPACIFIED LYMPHOID TISSUE

A: Postchemotherapy. The number and distribution of channels opacified in the right lumbar area are normal. The absence of nodes is related to treatment for lymphoma. *B:* The number and distribution of channels in the lumbar region is within the normal range. The lack of lymphoid tissue had no obvious etiology. *C:* Hodgkin's disease. The number of lymphatics and the distribution of those opacified are abnormal. *D:* An inferior vena cavogram reveals extrinsic compression by nodes (*arrows*) totally replaced by Hodgkin's disease.

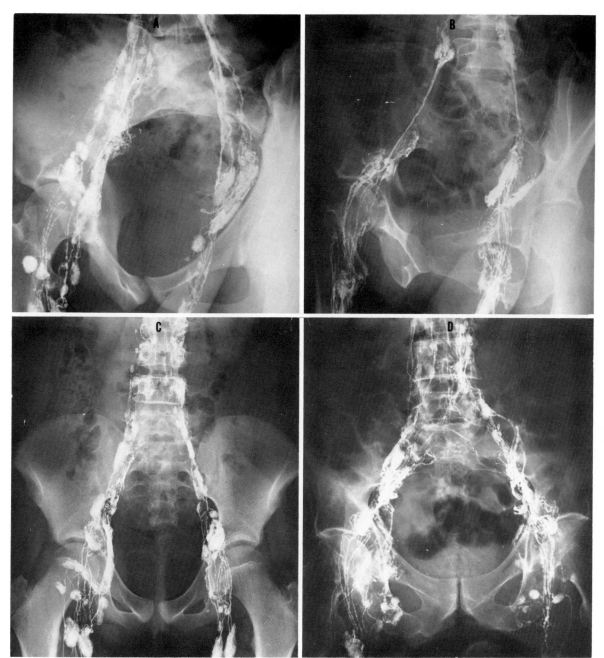

FIG. 9.8. NORMAL PELVIC LYMPHATICS AND NODES

A: Oblique view. Three major trunks, similar bilaterally. *B:* Only one major common iliac trunk opacifies bilaterally as a variation of normal. *C:* Normal distribution of lymphatics and nodes opacified in a child. *D:* Normal distribution in a patient 65 years of age. The distortion of the left common iliac lymphatics is due to a dilated tortuous iliac artery.

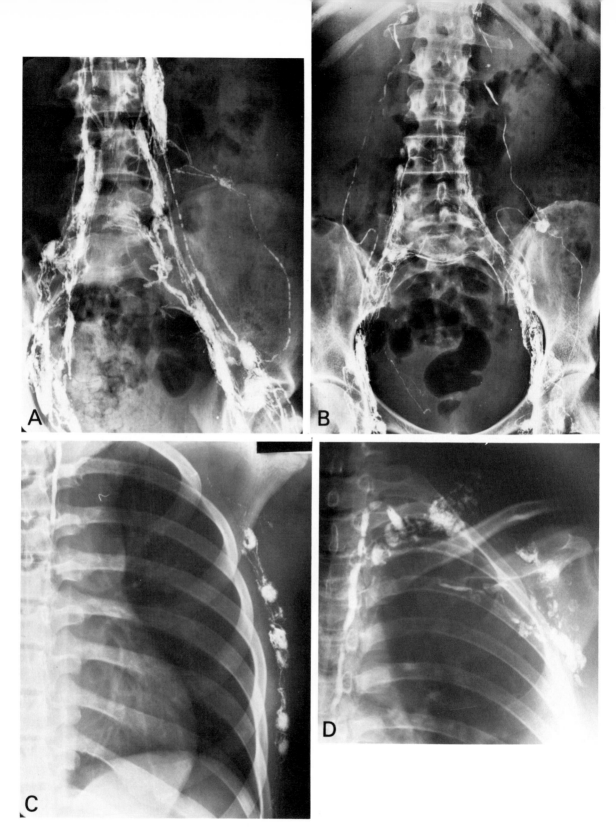

FIG. 9.9. VARIATIONS IN THE NORMAL LYMPHATIC DISTRIBUTION

A: Abdominal lymphatic variations of circumflex iliac lymphatics and nodes. Usually one node is opacified at the iliac. *B:* Retroperitoneal bypass as an unusual variation of the normal. The normal lumbar lymphatics and nodes are also opacified. *C:* Opacification of a bypass from the external iliac lymphatics to the anterior abdominal wall eventually draining into the inferior aspect of the axilla. *D:* Opacification of the lymphatic from the thoracic duct to the superior aspect of the axilla as a variation of the normal.

194

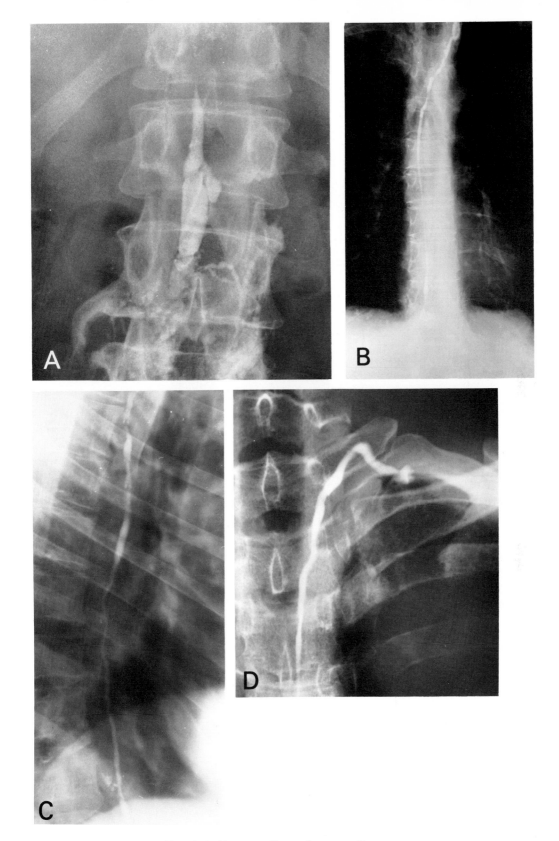

FIG. 9.10. THORACIC DUCT, CLASSICAL DISTRIBUTION

A: Cisterna chyli; *B:* thoracic duct, anteroposterior view; *C:* thoracic duct, lateral view; and *D:* terminal portion emptying into the venous angle in the left neck.

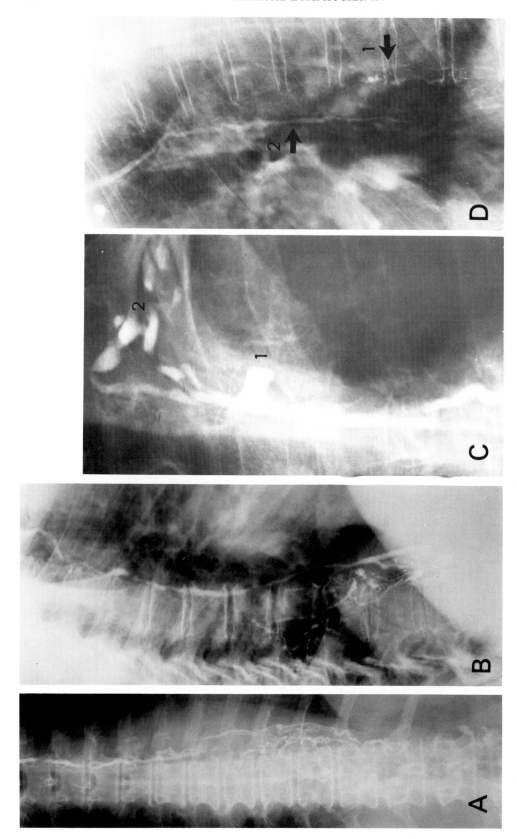

FIG. 9.11. THORACIC DUCT, VARIATIONS OF NORMAL

A: Plexiform origin of the thoracic duct, anteroposterior view; B: plexiform origin of the thoracic duct, lateral view; C: double thoracic duct, anteroposterior view; D: double thoracic duct, lateral view; E: bilateral termination; F: right-sided termination; and G: communication with lower cervical lymphatics and nodes.

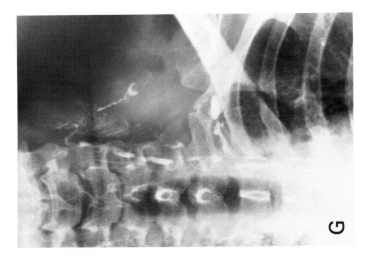

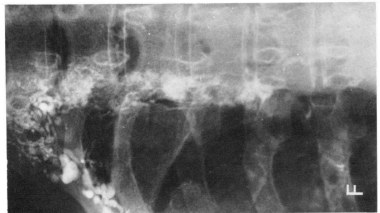

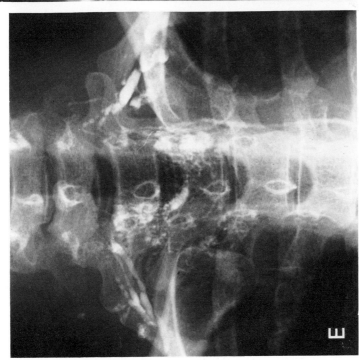

Fig. 9.11. E–G

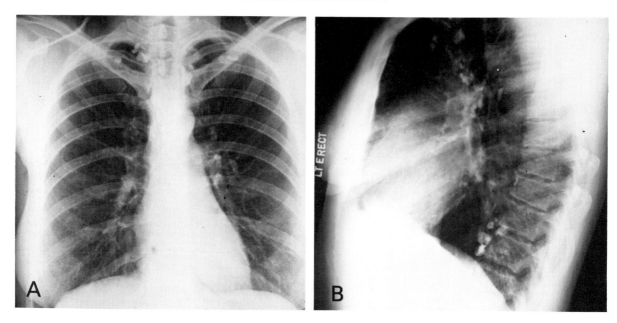

FIG. 9.12. VARIATIONS OF NORMAL

A: Opacification of bilateral supraclavicular and paratracheal nodes. *B:* Mediastinal lymph node opacification as a manifestation of the variations of normal.

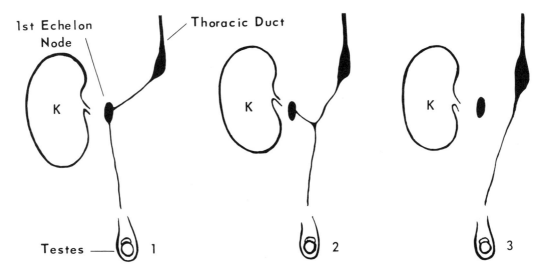

FIG. 9.13. VARIATIONS IN LYMPHATIC DISTRIBUTION IN PART DETERMINE MODES OF METASTASES

From Engeset, A.: An experimental study of the lymph node barrier—injection of Walker carcinoma 256 in the lymph vessels. Extrait de Acta Union Internationale le Centre Le Cancer, Vol. 15, No. 3-4, 1959.

distribution and are, in part, determined by normal lymphatic drainage and individual variations as long as these vessels are present and patent. Engeset (1959) verified this concept by the injection of tumor cells and mercury into the testicular lymphatics of rats demonstrating these basic patterns (Fig. 9.13), as follows: (1) metastases to the sentinel node (primary or first echelon draining node frequently at the renal hilar area) preceded lung metastases; (2) sentinel node and lung metastases occurred simultaneously; and (3) lung metastases existed prior to, or in the absence of, sentinel node metastases.

The alteration in lymphatic dynamics results in the utilization of patent collateral pathways that are immediately available at the site of obstruction. The significance of this altered dynamic environment is illustrated by the following case of a patient with melanoma of the right lower extremity treated by a local excision and an inguinal node dissection (Fig. 9.14). Progressive edema of the right lower extremity ensued. Lymphangiography demonstrated an increase in opacified dermal and subcutaneous lymphatic pathways, a manifestation of the obstruction. The normal left inguinal, pelvic, and retroperitoneal areas can be used for comparison. Following the dissection, an entirely new environment was created for subsequent lymphatic flow. The nodes in the right iliac and para-aortic areas were bypassed by collateral channels. Subsequent metastases would progress along these alternate pathways. Any surgical procedures performed in an attempt to eradicate metastases must appreciate this new dynamic environment.

Another case (Fig. 9.15) demonstrates the importance of this knowledge prior to the proposed surgical procedure. This patient with a carcinoma of the cervix was to be treated by a pelvic node dissection. The left iliac lymphatic pathways were obstructed by metastases with collateral channels, opacified in the abdominal and chest walls, eventually filling metastatic left axillary nodes. Any attempt to surgically remove the tumor and its metastases would surely fail since the metastases had progressed far beyond the local site. Axillary metastases from a carcinoma of the cervix may also occur if anomalous pathways exist from the thoracic duct to the axillary lymphatics.

Thoracic duct obstruction will also result in the utilization and opacification of collateral channels (Fig. 9.16).

Paralymphatic Pathways

Pathways, other than the endothelial lined lymphatic channels, are available in the event of obstruction. These include the body's potential cavities (pleural, pericardial, and peritoneal), the interstitial spaces, the perineural and perivascular spaces, etc., which, for the sake of simplicity, can be termed the pre- or paralymphatic system. These avenues are available for fluid transport and therefore could function as routes for dispersion of metastases.

Occasionally, with obstruction of the lymphatic pathways, there is reflux of contrast material into the visceral pathways and eventually into the wall of the viscera. This may explain the mechanism of mural metastases via the lymphatic system (Fig. 9.17A–C). In the presence of obstruction, it is essential to follow the lymphangiographic pattern for days or perhaps weeks by serial roentgenograms to appreciate the complexity of this alternate circulation.

The perineural and perivascular sheaths may also function for lymph flow. The potential space is probably the route of metastases for perineural spread of carcinoma encircling nerves. A perivascular cuff has been demonstrated as a collateral channel opacified as the result of obstruction of iliac channels by a metastatic carcinoma of the cervix (Fig. 9.17D).

Lymphaticovenous Anastomoses

Another fascinating alternate pathway available in the event of obstruction is lymphaticovenous anastomosis which is a direct communication between these two vascular systems. Such communications are best recorded during the injection of the contrast material when there is a forward head of pressure. The difference in velocity of flow makes the event difficult to capture, for once the oil droplet enters the venous system, it is caught in the relatively rapid current of venous flow. The transient appearance of radiopaque droplets along the distribution of the veins is evidence of the presence of these communications (Fig. 9.18A and B). Probably relatively dormant under normal circumstances, these channels can be utilized in the event of an imbalance of pressures in the two systems. This imbalance is most frequently precipitated by malignant involvement or postsurgical obstruction of lymphatic pathways. Opacification of the inferior vena cava was observed in a patient with metastases to the retroperitoneal nodes from a seminoma of the testicle (Fig. 9.18C). The intrahepatic branches of the portal vein were filled during lymphangiography in another patient with obstruction of the major lymphatic pathways (Fig. 9.18D and E).

In summary the modes of lymphatic metastases depend upon the normal distribution of lymphatic drainage, the variations of the norm, and the collateral pathways in the event of obstruction of normal channels which include lymphatic to lymphatic, lymphatic to paralymphatic, and lymphatic to venous.

Utilizing the described criteria the positive diagnosis of nodal metastatic disease by lymphangiography with the assistance of venography

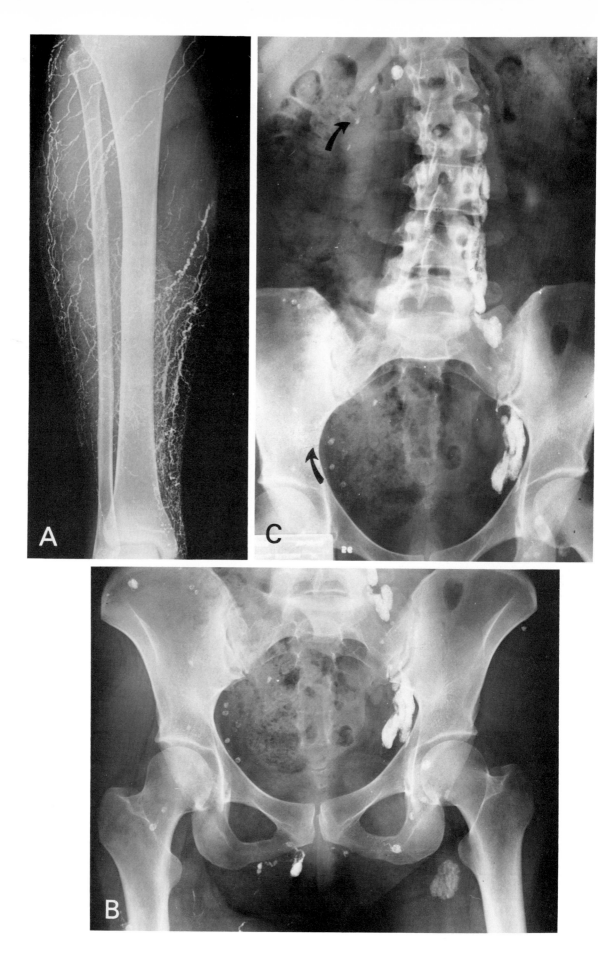

FIG. 9.14. ALTERED LYMPHATIC DYNAMICS INFLUENCE MODES OF METASTASES

A: Edema of the right lower extremity 6 months after a radical inguinal node dissection for melanoma. Opacified dermal and subcutaneous lymphatics are manifestations of lymphatic obstruction. *B:* The right inguinal nodes are still present and are not opacified. The left side can be considered the normal. *C:* The right ascending lumbar nodes were also bypassed as a manifestation of collateral flow (*arrow*).

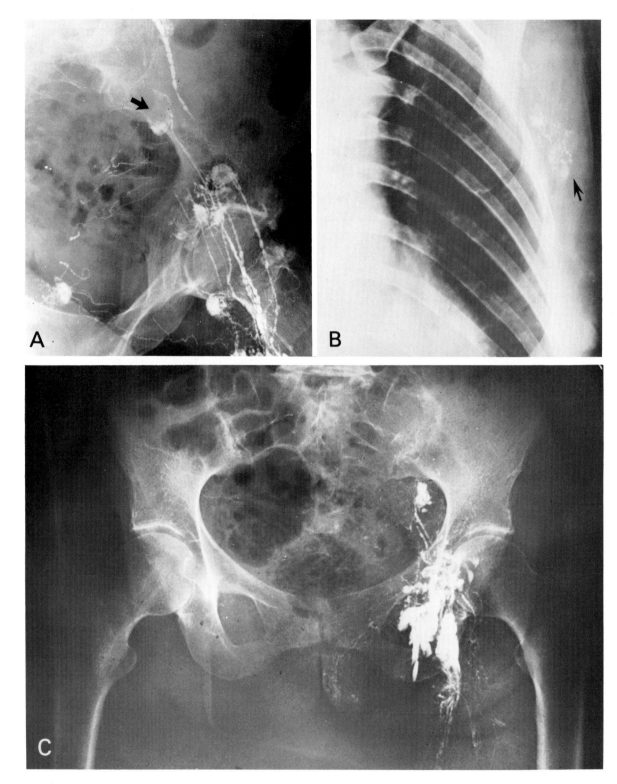

FIG. 9.15. METASTASIS TO AXILLARY LYMPH NODES FROM CARCINOMA OF THE CERVIX

A and B: The left iliac nodes show evidence of metastasis. There is obstruction of the iliac lymphatics (*arrow*). The lower axillary nodes are opacified. *C, D, and E:* Another patient with carcinoma of the cervix, with obstruction of the left iliac lymphatics by metastases, demonstrated the lymphatics of the anterior abdominal wall and chest wall (*arrows*) as collateral pathways to the axilla (Wohlgemuth). *F and G:* Metastases to axillary nodes were also demonstrated in still another patient with obstruction of the left common iliac lymphatics (*arrow*). Tomograms through the axillary nodes verified the metastasis.

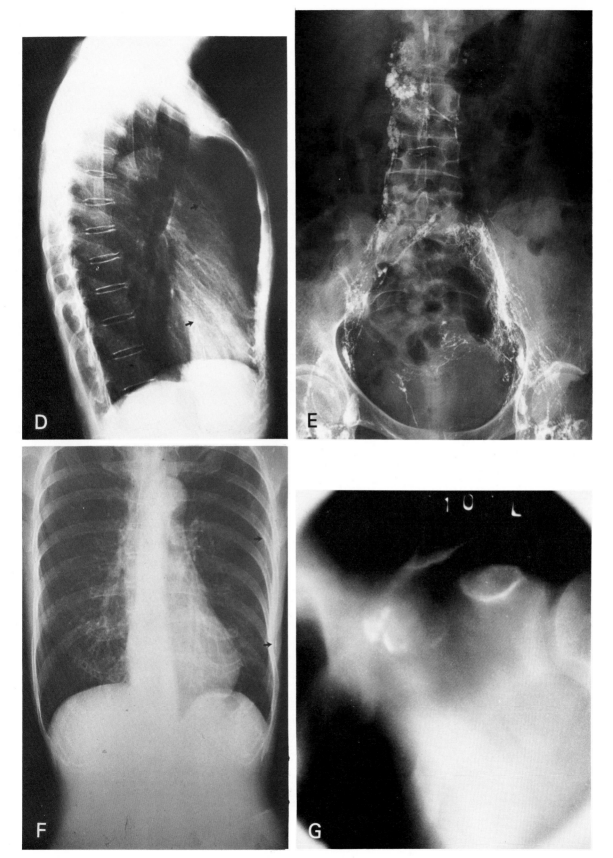

F‌ɪɢ. 9.15. D–G

203

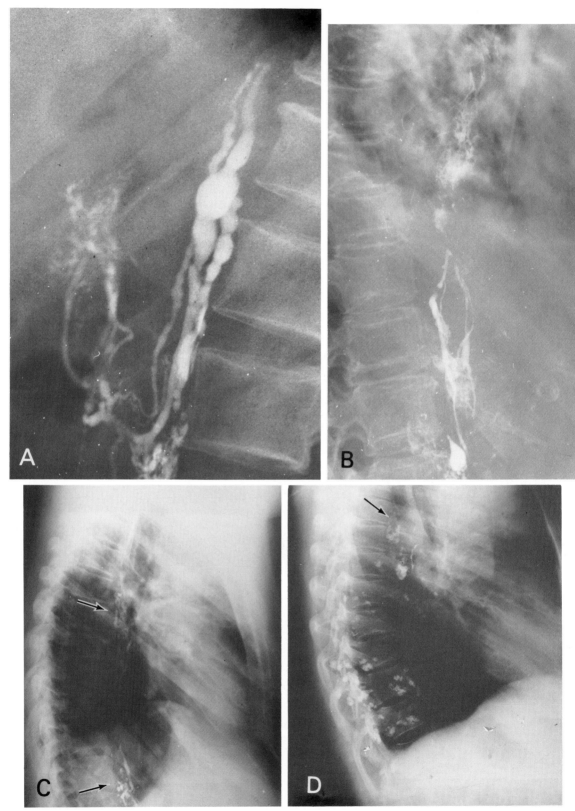

FIG. 9.16. THORACIC DUCT OBSTRUCTION

A: Retrograde visualization of the gastrointestinal lymphatics as the result of thoracic duct obstruction. *B:* Carcinoma of the pancreas obstructing the thoracic duct with opacification of collateral channels. *C and D:* Obstruction of the thoracic duct by a carcinoma of the lung resulted in opacification of mediastinal lymphatics and nodes (*arrows*).

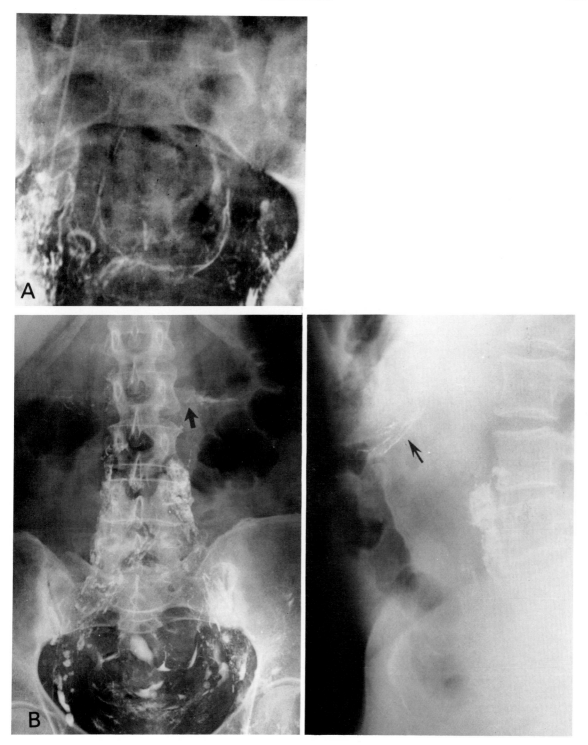

FIG. 9.17. PARALYMPHATIC PATHWAYS

A: Visceral lymphatics opacified in the wall of the rectum. *B:* Contrast material in the wall of the stomach (*arrows*). *C:* The bladder wall lymphatics are delineated (*arrows*). *D:* Perivascular channels demarcate the right iliac artery (*top arrow*). There is apparent continuity with the lymphatics above the kidney (*bottom arrow*).

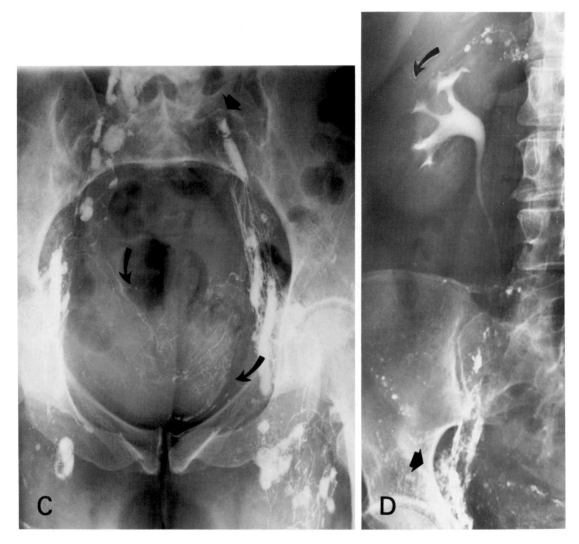

Fig. 9.17. C–D

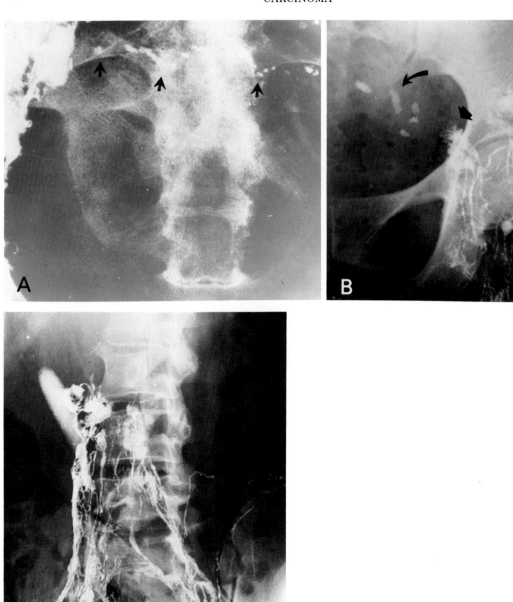

FIG. 9.18. LYMPHATICOVENOUS ANASTOMOSES

A: Droplets of contrast material in the distribution of sacral veins (*arrows*). *B:* Lymphaticovenous anastomoses secondary to lymphatic obstruction by metastatic carcinoma of the cervix (*arrows*). *C:* Lymphaticoinferior vena caval anastomoses, as described by Wolfel. *D and E:* Lymphaticoportal anastomoses (*arrow*) in a patient with carcinoma of the testis with extensive retroperitoneal nodal involvement.

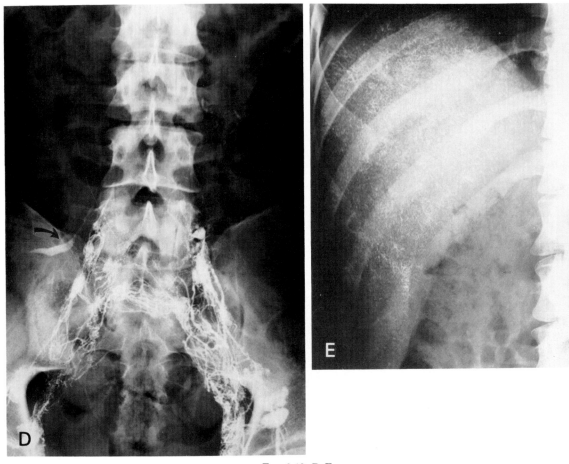

FIG. 9.18. D–E

and pyelography can yield a positive pathologic correlation of 90–95%. Suspicious or negative findings do not influence the management of the patient. False negative examinations are due to metastases too small to detect and failure of opacification of the involved nodes.

UTERINE CERVIX

The survival rate of patients with advanced carcinoma of the cervix has increased only slightly despite improved control of tumor in the irradiated area with megavoltage radiotherapy. At M. D. Anderson Hospital the survival rate in Stage IIIA cervical carcinoma has gone from 41–45% and in Stage IIIB from 31–36% in the kilovoltage and megavoltage areas respectively. A prime reason for this is the high incidence of lymph node metastases in advanced cervical cancer, many of which are outside the pelvic portals utilized. Improved results with extended radiation fields may be possible with accurate assessment of the extent of disease.

Usually the earlier and smaller the primary neoplasm, the smaller and fewer the metastases. Therefore, the yield of lymphangiography in the detection of metastases in patients with carcinoma of the cervix Stage I is small. The metastases when present in this group are usually in the pelvis and most likely included within the usual radiation treatment portal. However, with the more advanced tumors (the bulky or barrel-shaped Stage I and above) bilateral pedal lymphangiography can be of considerable assistance in determining the extent of involvement because of the relatively high incidence of lymph node metastases.

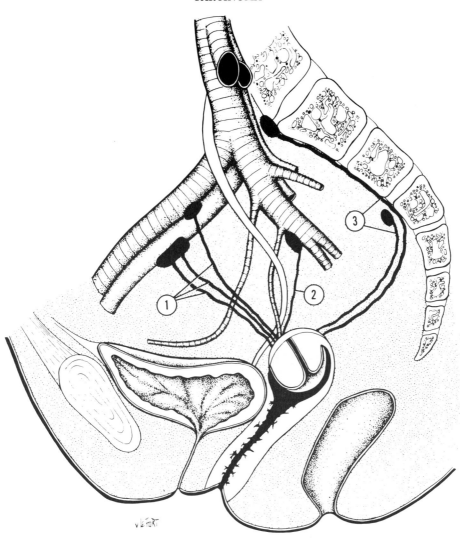

FIG. 9.19. LYMPHATICS OF THE UTERINE CERVIX

1, External iliac pedicle; *2*, hypogastric pedicle; and *3*, posterior pedicle.

The Lymphatics of the Uterine Cervix

The lymphatics of the uterine cervix (Fig. 9.19) form a rich plexus. From this plexus, the collecting trunks leave the lateral border of the cervix and gather into three main pedicles and the intercalated lymph nodes:

1. *External Iliac Pedicle*. This pedicle consists of two to three collecting trunks which follow the course of the uterine artery and pass in front of the uterine artery and in front of the ureter. The trunks then cross the medial aspect of the umbilical artery and terminate in the superior and middle nodes of the middle or medial chain of the external iliac group. This pedi-

cle is designated as the principal chain of the external iliac group.

2. *Hypogastric Pedicle*. This pedicle consists of one to three collecting trunks which follow the course of the uterine vein, pass behind the ureter, and terminate in one of the hypogastric nodes near the uterine artery. Occasionally, a lymphatic trunk passes the hypogastric station and ascends along the common iliac artery to a node of promontory.

3. *Posterior Pedicle*. The posterior pedicle is formed by two to four collecting trunks which are less rich and less constant than those in the other two pedicles. The trunks run in an antero-posterior direction following the lateral wall of

the rectum and later ascend in front of the sacrum; they then terminate in the lateral sacral nodes and in the nodes of the promontory.

4. *The Intercalated Lymph Nodes.* This group of intercalated nodes includes parametrial nodes and paracervical nodes. In the parametrium, small lymph nodules are often found along the major lymphatic trunks transversing the parametrium. The paracervical nodes are located near the crossing of the uterine artery and the ureter. The collecting trunks of the external iliac pedicle are frequently interrupted by this group of nodes.

In general the lymphatics of the uterine cervix are drained by the middle and superior nodes of the middle and medial chains of the external iliac group and sometimes also by the hypogastric nodes of the promontory.

In the evaluation of 103 patients with advanced cancers of the cervix including bulky or barrel-shaped Stage I lesions and postirradiation recurrences, 42 were diagnosed as positive for metastatic disease, later confirmed by biopsy. As shown in Table 9.1, only 1 lymphangiogram was diagnosed as positive with the subsequent biopsy proving negative; 49 were negative on both roentgenographic evaluation and histologic study; and another 12 had negative interpretation on lymphangiography but proved to be positive on biopsy. When a definite positive diagnosis was made, the accuracy was 97.6% (41 of 42). Therefore on a roentgenographic basis, at least 40% of this group (41 of 103) had definitely positive lymph node disease that could not be deduced from palpatory findings. As seen in Table 9.2, of the 53 patients with positive biopsy specimens, we were able to diagnose 41 (77.7%) by lymphangiography.

Table 9.3 lists the groups of lymph nodes biopsied. In the group with positive roentgenographic and biopsy evidence of malignancy, there were 14 with positive aortic lymph nodes and 10 with disease in the common iliac area. Most of these were beyond the usual field of pelvic irradiation for cervical carcinoma.

Only 1 patient in this series had had a pelvic lymph node biopsy prior to the lymphangiography; however, 34 women had had previous pelvic irradiation (Table 9.4). It is stressed that, even in the 15 patients with previous irradiation who had both roentgenographic and histologic proof of recurrence, previous irradiation did not invalidate the interpretation of the subsequent lymphangiogram.

Eight patients were excluded from the study because the abnormal lymph node seen on

TABLE 9.1
CORRELATION OF LYMPHANGIOGRAMS AND BIOPSIES

Lymphangiogram	Biopsy	No.
Positive	Positive	41
Positive	Negative	1
Negative	Negative	49
Negative	Positive	12
Total		103

TABLE 9.2
POSITIVE BIOPSIES

Lymphangiogram and biopsy positive	41
Lymphangiogram negative-biopsy positive	12
Total positive biopsies	53

TABLE 9.3
GROUPS OF LYMPH NODES BIOPSIED[a]

Lymph Node Group	Pos.[b]-Pos.[c, d]	Neg.[b]-Neg.[d]	Neg.[d]-Pos.[c, d]
Aortic	14	69	6
Common iliac	10	41	0
External iliac	20	45	7
Internal iliac	1	37	0
Obturator	0	36	3
Inguinal	2	0	0
Supraclavicular	1	0	0

[a] Does not include actual numbers of lymph nodes, only groups.
[b] Lymphangiogram diagnosis.
[c] Does not include negative lymph nodes removed at the same time.
[d] Biopsy diagnosis.

TABLE 9.4
PREVIOUS IRRADIATION

Pos.[a]-Pos.[b]	Neg.[a]-Neg.[b]	Neg.[a]-Pos.[b]
15	14	5
	Previous lymph nodal biopsy	
0	1	0

[a] Lymphangiogram diagnosis.
[b] Biopsy diagnosis.

lymphangiography was still present on follow-up roentgenograms obtained shortly after surgical exploration.

To insure biopsy of the suspected nodes, radiographs should be taken during and after laparotomy. At times during surgery nodes are difficult to find or impossible to reach (Fig. 9.20). The removed nodes are placed in the ana-

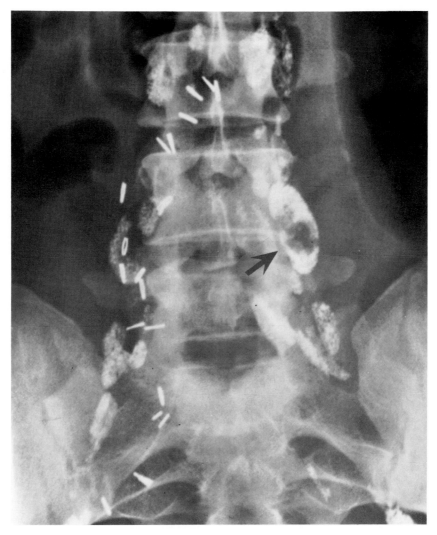

FIG. 9.20. CARCINOMA OF THE CERVIX

The single metastatic node (*arrow*) was beyond the reach of the surgeon. Postoperative radiographs were necessary to confirm the biopsy of the nodes in question.

tomic position on a Plexiglas template which has the outline of the inferior vena cava and the aorta (Fig. 9.21). Specimen radiographs are correlated with the preoperative and postoperative lymphangiogram. The template and specimen radiographs are also of assistance in separating fatty tissue from nonopacified nodes.

The use of lymphangiography and exploratory laparotomy in the staging of patients with carcinoma of the cervix is still under investigation. This surgical procedure is used to assist in establishing the extent of disease as well as to remove large metastatic deposits so that irra-

diation might be more effective. If metastases are found in the external iliac nodes, the irradiation portals are extended to the level of L4. When the disease involves the common iliac nodes and above, the treatment is extended to the level of the diaphragm. At present the combination of retroperitoneal node biopsy and extended field irradiation has been associated with complications necessitating re-evaluation of the approach. Percutaneous transperitoneal lymph node biopsy has been employed to verify the lymphangiographic findings.

The lymphangiographic information can be

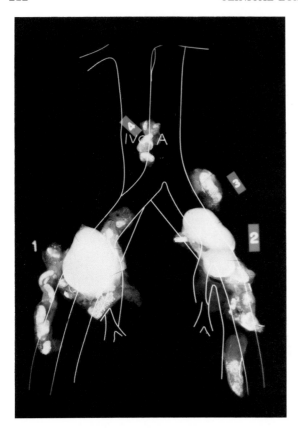

FIG. 9.21. TEMPLATE UTILIZED FOR SURGICAL
CONFIRMATION

The nodes are specifically labeled and comparison is
made with the postoperation radiographs. *IVC*, inferior
vena cavogram; *A*, aorta; *1*, right external iliac nodes; *2*,
left external iliac nodes; *3*, left common iliac nodes.

followed at regular intervals of every 3 months
by roentgenograms of the abdomen. Changes in
the nodes, such as localized areas of destruction
or enlargement, might indicate progression of
disease. The lymphangiographic examination
can be repeated, if necessary, to establish the
presence of metastases especially if the patient
was treated by radiation alone.

UTERINE CORPUS

The uterus has four intercommunicating lymphatic networks which run in the mucosa, muscularis, serosa, and subserosal areas. The collecting trunks originate in the lateral borders of
the wall as well as in the superior angles of the
uterus. They form three main pedicles (Fig.
9.22):

1). The Principal or Utero-ovarian Pedicle.
This pedicle is composed of four to six collecting
trunks. It leaves the wall below the cornua of
the uterus and travels in the broad ligament
until it reaches the hilum of the ovary. Here,
the trunks anastomose and join with the ovarian lymphatics. The uterine trunks, therefore,
ascend with those of the ovary along the ovarian
blood vessels and having arrived at the level of
the lower pole of the kidney, they bend medially
and terminate, on the right side, in the precaval
and lateroaortic nodes, particularly in the precaval node near the origin of the inferior mesenteric artery.

2). External Iliac Pedicle. This pedicle contains fewer trunks than the utero-ovarian pedicle. The trunks follow a transverse direction
outward across the medial site of the umbilical
artery and end in the lymph nodes of the middle
chain of the external iliac group, usually in the
uppermost node of this chain.

3). Round Ligament Pedicle. This pedicle is
formed by a single trunk which follows the
round ligament from its insertion in the uterine
fundus to the inguinal canal and ends in the
superficial inguinal nodes.

In summary, the lymphatics of the uterine

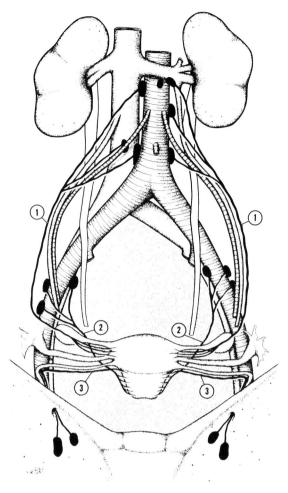

Fig. 9.22. Lymphatic Drainage from Uterine Corpus

1, Principal or utero-ovarian trunks; *2*, external iliac trunks; and *3*, round ligament trunks.

corpus terminate in the lateroaortic nodes and the preaortic nodes in the vicinity of the origin of the inferior mesenteric artery, in the nodes of the middle group of the external iliac chain, and sometimes also in the superomedial superficial inguinal nodes.

In patients with carcinoma of the endometrium, metastases to the regional lymph nodes occur relatively infrequently. In a group of 233 patients with adenocarcinoma of the corpus treated at M. D. Anderson Hospital between 1948 and 1964 with irradiation followed by hysterectomy, only 1 patient was found to have disease in the pelvic lymph nodes, and 6 patients (3%) had tumor in the para-aortic nodes. Of 82 patients with adenocarcinoma involving the corpus and cervix (corpus et collum) treated

during the same period of time, the incidence of positive disease was 6% (5 of 82 patients). Metastasis to the para-aortic nodes was also seen in 5 patients (6%).

In studies employing lymphangiography prior to any treatment, the yield of positive disease was considerably higher. Douglas et al. (1972) reported an overall incidence of lymph node metastases of 19%. Para-aortic lymph node metastases in that study was 9% in contrast to an incidence of 16% found by Gerteis (1967).

In view of these statistics, the yield from lymphangiography is small but of value in selected cases, especially in the larger lesions. The criteria for the diagnosis of metastatic disease are the same as those already discussed, as illustrated in Figures 9.23–9.25.

214 CLINICAL LYMPHOGRAPHY

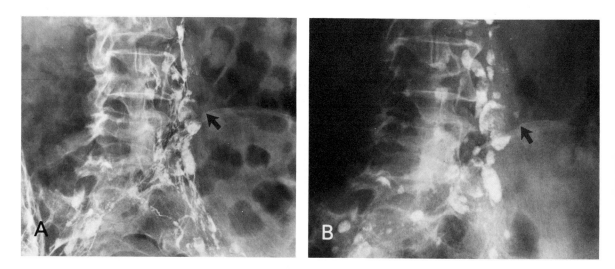

FIG. 9.23. METASTATIC DISEASE TO THE LEFT LOWER LUMBAR LYMPH NODES FROM ADENOCARCINOMA OF THE
UTERINE CORPUS

A: Lymphatic phase (*arrow*); B: nodal phase (*arrow*).

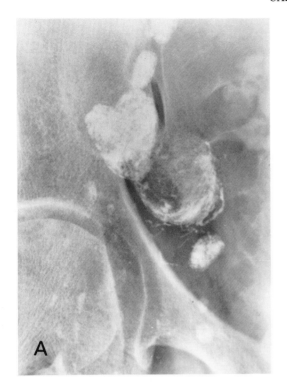

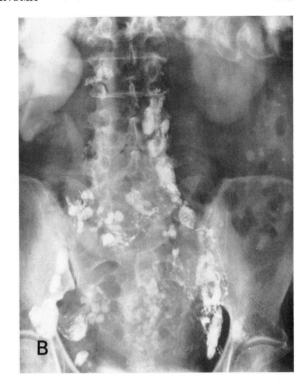

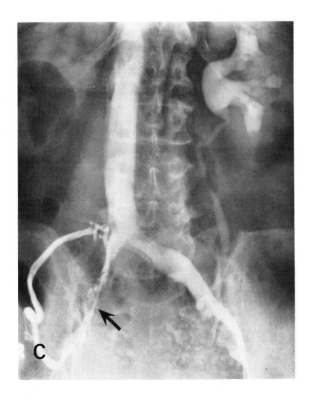

FIG. 9.24. METASTASES FROM ADENOCARCINOMA OF THE
UTERINE CORPUS TO THE RIGHT ILIAC LYMPH NODES

A: Crescentic configuration of a right external iliac
lymph node due to metastatic carcinoma. *B:* Obstruction of
the right ureter by metastatic disease. Calcifications are
noted in a uterine leiomyoma. *C:* Compression and invasion into the right external and common iliac veins (*arrow*)
due to the lymph node metastases. The extent of involvement is more completely delineated with the help of venography.

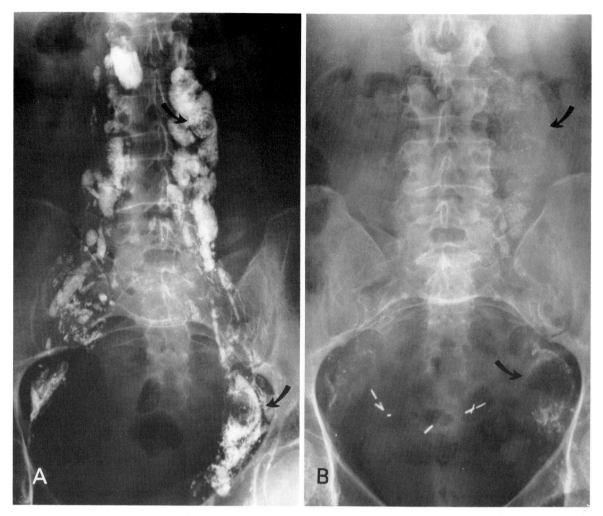

FIG. 9.25. ADENOCARCINOMA OF THE ENDOMETRIUM

A: Metastatic disease (*arrow*) to the external iliac and para-aortic nodes demonstrated in the initial lymphangiogram.
B: Follow-up roentgenograms 7 months later reveal progression of the disease (*arrows*).

OVARY

Carcinoma of the ovary is the fourth most frequent cause of female cancer deaths in the United States and the leading cause of death among gynecologic cancers, accounting for 100,000 deaths in the last 10 years. The 5-year survival rates range from 6–51%. These disappointing statistics are in part due to the late stage at which many ovarian cancers are usually discovered.

The importance of lymph node metastases arising from ovarian neoplasms has been virtually ignored except in the case of dysgerminoma. Little is known about the incidence of lymph node metastases in patients with epithelial cancers of the ovary, and little attention is paid to this factor when planning treatment. Bilateral pedal lymphangiography, by demonstrating lymph node metastases, may prove of value in the more thorough assessment of the extent of disease—a prerequisite for intelligent management of any patient with cancer.

Lymphatic Drainage from the Ovary (Fig. 9.26).

The parenchyma of the ovary contains a rich capillary network of lymphatics, chiefly in the

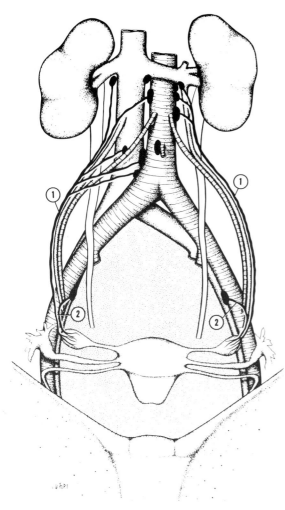

FIG. 9.26. LYMPHATICS OF THE OVARY

Normal ovarian lymphatic drainage. *1*, Para-aortic lymphatic pedicle; *2*, external iliac lymphatic pedicle.

theca externa of the follicles and corpora lutea. Lymphatics are absent in the tunica albuginea. Six to eight large lymphatic collecting trunks emerge from the hilum, converging in the mesovarium with the efferent lymph vessels from the uterine fundus and fallopian tube to form the subovarian plexus. In the ovarian suspensory ligament, the lymphatics, with the ovarian blood vessels, cross the ureter and external iliac vessels and travel upward along the lateral aspect of the ureter to the level of the inferior pole of the kidney. Here the lymphatics turn medially, leaving the ovarian blood vessels, and cross the ureter again to reach its medial aspect. This crossing occurs at a higher point on the left than on the right. On the right, the collecting

trunks diverge and drain into the precaval and lateral caval nodes which lie along the inferior vena cava from its bifurcation to the renal pedicle. On the left, these trunks diverge to a lesser extent and at a higher level than on the right and end in the lateroaortic and preaortic nodes which are placed one above another below the left renal pedicle.

In 3 of 14 cases, Marcille (1902) discovered an accessory lymphatic pedicle from the ovary. The ovarian collecting trunks traveled in the broad ligament from the hilar plexus and then passed posteriorly under the peritoneum to end in a node of the middle chain of the external iliac group. Anastomoses also occur between the ovarian lymph vessels and those of the uterus and the fallopian tubes, so that other variations might exist. In addition, the presence of a malignant neoplasm extending beyond the ovary with invasion of adjacent pelvic viscera and peritoneum may allow direct lymphatic continuity with the inguinal nodes and with external and common iliac nodes.

Seventy-two lymphangiograms were performed on 66 patients with 6 patients examined twice. Of these 72 lymphangiograms 33 (46%) revealed lymph node metastases, which are presented in Table 9.5, according to the histologic classification utilized at M. D. Anderson Hospital.

Of the 33 positive examinations, the distribution of lymph node metastases was para-aortic, 23 (70%) (Fig. 9.27); iliac, 19 (58%); inguinal, 9 (27%); and supraclavicular, 2 (6%). Para-aortic nodal involvement alone was seen in 14, and iliac lymph node metastases alone were demonstrated in 4. The combination of iliac and para-aortic nodal metastases was diagnosed by lymphangiography in 9 (Figs. 9.28–9.30). In each of the 9 patients with inguinal node metastases, there was concomitant iliac lymph node involvement. Three of these patients also had para-aortic lymph node metastases. The 2 patients with supraclavicular lymph node metastases also had iliac node involvement (Fig. 9.31).

The relationship between lymph node metastases and histologic classification is shown in Table 9.6. Of the 10 patients with nodal metastases from cancers of germ cell origin, para-aortic nodal involvement was found in 9, and iliac metastases in 3. Lymph node metastases from ovarian epithelial cancers (Müllerian derivatives and carcinomas not otherwise specified) were found in 22 lymphangiograms, the para-aortic lymph nodes were involved in 13,

TABLE 9.5
SUMMARY OF CASES

Histologic Classification	Lymphangiogram		Confirmation of Positive Finding		
	Pos.	Neg.	Surgical	Clinical	None
I.Malignant neoplasm, NOS[a]	0	3			
II.Carcinoma, NOS	4	2	4		
III.Müllerian derivative carcinomas					
A. Serous	14	21	10	4	
B. Mucinous	1	1		1	
C. Endometroid	3	4	3		
IV.Germ cell tumors					
A. Dysgerminoma	8	3	5	1	2[b]
B. Embryonal carcinoma	0	2			
C. Teratoma, malignant	0	1			
D. Mixed germ cell tumor	2	0	2		
V.Sex cord tumors					
A. Granulosa-theca cell	0	0			
B. Sertoli-Leydig	1	2	1		
Total	33	39	25	6	2

[a] NOS, not otherwise specified.

[b] In 2 cases, no laparotomy was performed.

and the iliac nodes in 16. Of these, para-aortic nodal involvement alone was seen in 6 and combined iliac and para-aortic in 7.

Clinical staging was determined by abdominal exploration. Lymphangiography was usually performed following this staging procedure. The distribution of the stages in 66 patients was Stage I, 5; II, 9; III, 35; and IV, 17 (Table 9.7).

Seven patients with ovarian carcinoma and ascites were studied by lymphangiography to determine whether there was a relationship between lymph node metastases and ascites. Only 1 of these 7 patients had lymph node metastases. Peritoneal implants were found in all 7 patients with ascites. In one of these patients, the liver was small with extensive fatty infiltration. Conversely, of the 33 with lymph node metastases, only 1 had ascites. The histologic classification of these 7 patients with ovarian carcinoma and ascites was epithelial neoplasm in 6 and germ cell tumors in 1, a malignant teratoma.

Lymph node metastases from cancer of the ovary have been demonstrated by lymphangiography. Douglas et al. (1971) found para-aortic nodal metastases in 8 (18%) of 44 patients with ovarian cancer. The high incidence (46%) of positive lymphangiograms in our series certainly does not reflect the true frequency of nodal metastases in cancer of the ovary. It does, however,

emphasize that nodal metastases do occur in both epithelial and germ cell neoplasms of the ovary more frequently than is commonly recognized.

Lymphatic drainage from the ovary is primarily to the para-aortic nodes. This distribution was confirmed by the 70% incidence of para-aortic lymph node metastases in the 33 lymphangiograms with evidence of nodal metastases. However, iliac lymph node metastases were found in 58% and inguinal node involvement was seen in 27%. This is somewhat higher than might be expected based on Marcille's investigation revealing approximately 20% of 14 cases with an accessory lymphatic pedicle from the ovary which drained to the external iliac lymph nodes. Inguinal lymph node metastases were almost always associated with iliac node disease. This could be due to direct drainage to the inguinal area, as might be expected if the uterus or fallopian tubes were invaded, or due to obstruction of iliac lymphatics with retrograde spread.

The distribution of lymph node metastases was further related to the histologic types of ovarian neoplasm. The germ cell tumors almost invariably metastasized to the para-aortic nodes (90%) and to a lesser extent to the iliac nodes (30%). On the other hand, the ovarian cancers of epithelial cell origin metastasized to the iliac

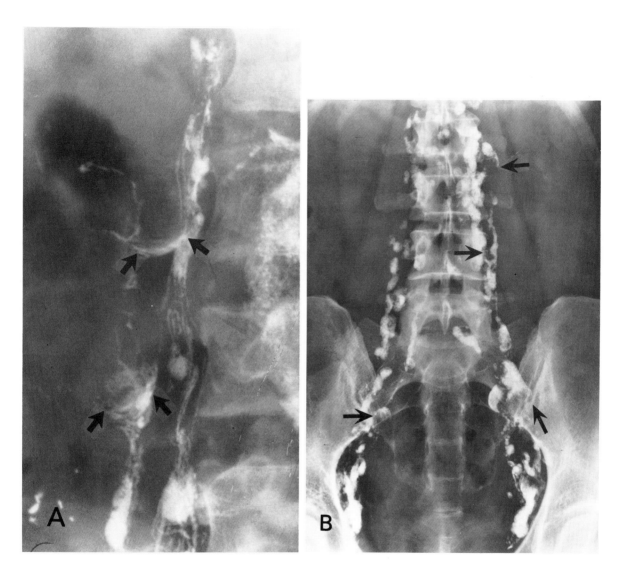

FIG. 9.27. METASTATIC DYSGERMINOMA FROM THE RIGHT OVARY

A: The lymphatics do not traverse the filling defects in the right lumbar lymph nodes in the lymphatic phase (*arrows*).
B: Crescent configuration (*arrows*) of the residual functioning portion of these nodes involved by metastases.

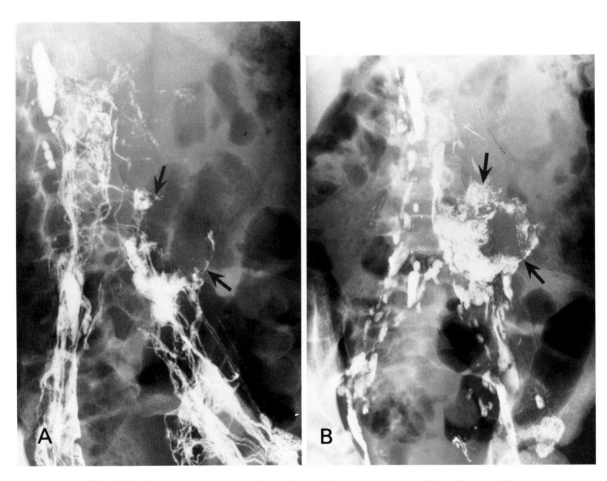

FIG. 9.28. DYSGERMINOMA OF THE LEFT OVARY, METASTASES TO THE LEFT COMMON ILIAC
A: Lymphatic phase (*arrows*); *B:* nodal phase (*arrows*).

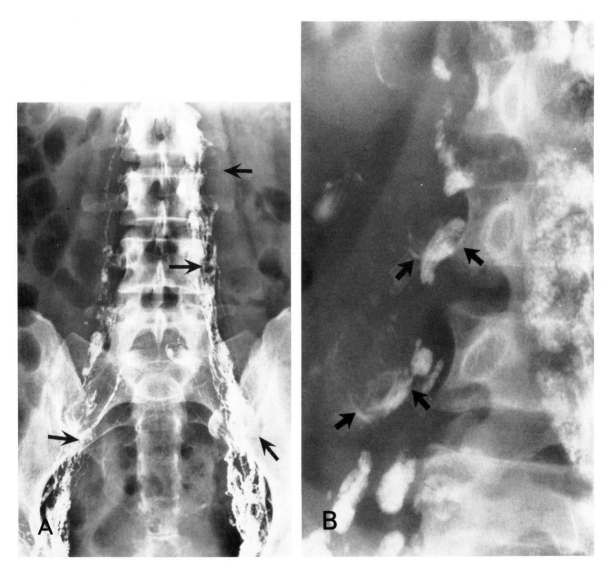

FIG. 9.29. EPITHELIAL CARCINOMA OF THE OVARY

A: Lymphatic phase. The lymphatics do not traverse filling defects in the iliac and para-aortic lymph nodes (*arrows*).
B: Nodal phase. Note the crescentic configuration of nodes containing metastases (*arrows*).

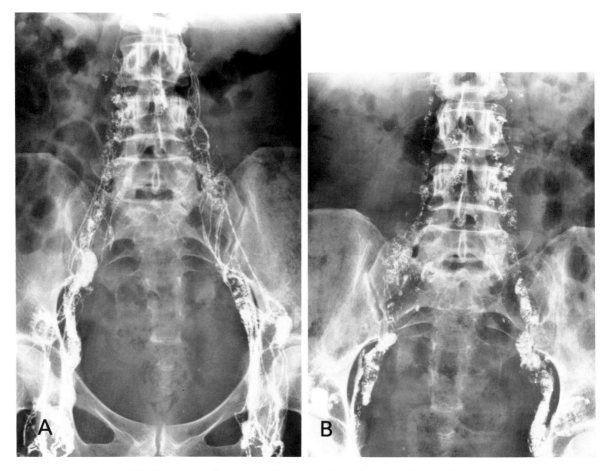

FIG. 9.30. EPITHELIAL CARCINOMA INVOLVING BOTH OVARIES—SEROUS CYST ADENOCARCINOMA

A: Lymphatic phase; *B:* nodal phase, the "lymphoma" pattern in metastatic ovarian carcinoma.

nodes in 41%. This suggests that the neoplasms of germ cell origin are usually confined to the ovary and spread along the anatomically defined lymphatic drainage. Epithelial cell malignancies are more likely to extend through the capsule to involve adjacent pelvic viscera, which may account for the frequency of pelvic nodal metastases, both to inguinal and iliac lymph nodes. In many instances the ovarian lesion was huge and was described as adhering to the pelvic walls. The iliac nodes may be involved by contiguity. The demonstration of para-aortic in addition to iliac and inguinal nodal metastases in some of these cases may be spread by contiguity.

Mediastinal and supraclavicular nodal metastases are most probably a manifestation of variations in normal lymphatic distribution of the thoracic duct. This would explain the apparent continuity of metastases in the pelvic, para-aortic, and supraclavicular lymph nodes in 2 cases in this series.

Hanks and Bagshaw (1969) describe the use of lymphangiography as an aid in staging and planning therapy. Para-aortic lymph node metastases were demonstrated in 7 of 20 patients even though these areas were palpably normal at surgical exploration. As the result of the lymphangiographic findings, the stage was changed in 6 of these patients and the therapy altered.

Ascites, although a frequent finding in patients with ovarian cancer, was found in only 7 patients in our series. This may have been a product of the nonrandomized selection. The mechanisms underlying the development of ascites in patients with peritoneal carcinomatosis

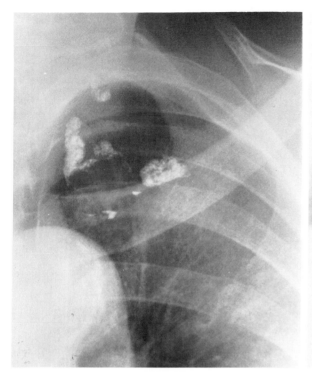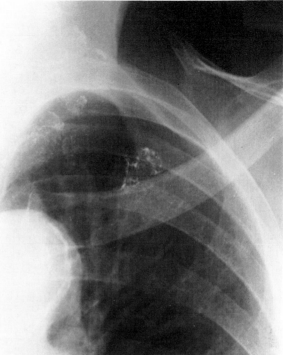

FIG. 9.31. SUPRACLAVICULAR LYMPH NODE METASTASES FROM OVARIAN CARCINOMA

Progression of supraclavicular metastases over a 6-month period.

TABLE 9.6
OVARIAN CANCER AND LYMPHANGIOGRAPHY

	Distribution of Lymph Node Metastases[a]						
	P	I	P, I	I, In	P, I, In	P, I, S	P, I, In, S
Epithelial	6	3	3	6	2	1	1
Germ cell	7	1	2				
Sex cord tumor	1						

[a] P, para-aortic; I, iliac; In, inguinal; S, supraclavicular.

TABLE 9.7
STAGE-GROUPING FOR PRIMARY CARCINOMA OF
THE OVARY

Stage   I. Growth limited to the ovaries
Stage II. Growth involving one or both ovaries with pelvic extension
Stage III. Growth involving one or both ovaries with widespread intraperitoneal metastases
Stage IV. Growth involving one or both ovaries with distant metastases

are still obscure. Ascites may be the result of either an increased inflow or obstruction to outflow of fluid from the peritoneal cavity. Lymphangiography was performed in these patients to determine if there was a relationship between lymph node metastases producing lymphatic obstruction, lymphatic fistulae, and ascites. Only 1 of 33 with lymph node metastases had ascites. On the other hand, each of the 7 patients with ascites was found to have peritoneal implants of ovarian cancer. Increased production of fluid has been attributed to an increased capillary permeability to protein especially at the peritoneal tumor implants. Perhaps peritoneal implants encroach upon the available surface for fluid absorption by interfering with the lymphatic network draining the peritoneal cavity. Tumor cells were found obstructing diaphragmatic lymphatics in experimentally produced ascites due to peritoneal carcinomatosis. Another etiologic agent to be considered in the presence of ascites in patients with ovarian cancer treated by total abdominal irradiation is radiation hepatitis.

VULVA

The vulva is supplied by a particularly rich capillary network of lymphatics. The collecting trunks are drained into the superficial and deep inguinal nodes. There may be drainage to the hypogastric nodes through the lymphatic network of the urethra and to external iliac nodes. Free anastomoses exist between the lymphatics of both sides of the vulva (Fig. 9.32).

Bilateral pedal lymphangiography opacifies many of these nodes. Although there are added difficulties in the interpretation of changes in the inguinal nodes because of the common occurrence of chronic inflammatory disease, a diagnosis of metastases can be made if the criteria previously discussed are present.

Metastases are frequently observed in the inguinal nodes; one third of the patients seen with carcinoma of the vulva are found to have metastases. When radical vulvectomy and bilateral inguinal node dissection are planned, preoperative evaluation of the iliac nodes is essential (Fig. 9.33 and 9.34).

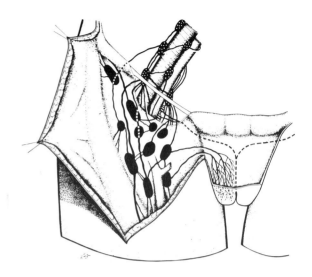

FIG. 9.32. LYMPHATIC DRAINAGE FROM THE VULVA

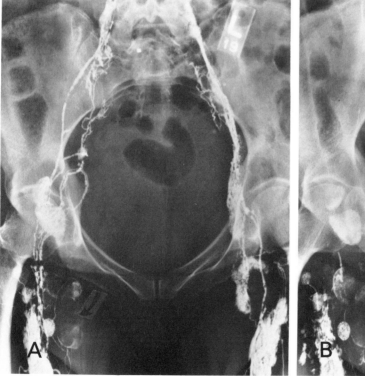
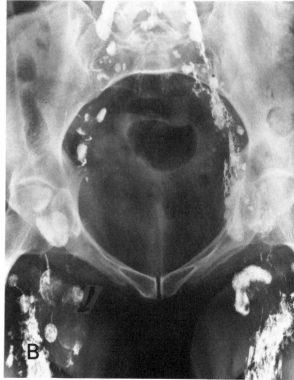

FIG. 9.33. METASTATIC CARCINOMA TO THE RIGHT INGUINAL NODES FROM A CARCINOMA OF THE VULVA

A: Lymphatic phase, the lymphatics do not traverse the defect in the nodes. *B:* Nodal phase, inguinal nodes involved by metastatic disease can be detected by lymphangiography (*arrow*).

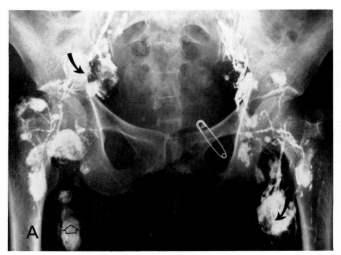
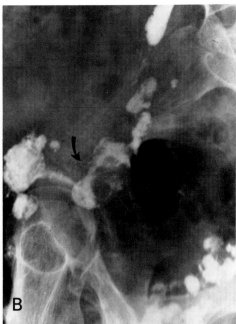

FIG. 9.34. CARCINOMA OF VULVA

A: Metastases in each inguinal area as well as a right external iliac lymph node *(arrows)*. *B:* Oblique projection of the right external iliac nodal metastases *(arrows)*.

TESTES

In preparation for a discussion of our experience with lymphangiographic diagnosis in testicular malignancies, a description of the embryology and anatomy of the testicle and its lymphatic drainage is of value.

Embryology

The urogenital fold ultimately extends from C6 to S2. The ridge divides into a lateral mesonephric fold and a median genital fold, the anlage of the genital gland. The testicle descends from the para-aortic region to the scrotum. Gonadal tissue may exist anywhere along this distribution.

Lymphatic Drainage (Fig. 9.35)

Testicular lymphatics accompany the internal spermatic artery and vein and drain into the lumbar nodes. The right trunks terminate in the right lumbar glands which lie between the level of the aortic bifurcation and the renal vein. In 10%, these trunks end in a node in the angle between the right renal vein and the inferior vena cava (Rouviere, 1938). The left testicular lymphatics drain into the para-aortic nodes near the left renal vein in approximately two-thirds of the cases. They may also end in glands at the level of the bifurcation of the aorta or into the common iliac nodes (Cuneo, 1901).

Lymphatics from the epididymis may accompany the testicular lymphatics to the lumbar nodes or terminate in the external iliac nodes.

Clinical investigation utilizing direct testicular lymphangiography by Busch et al. (1965), Chiappa et al. (1966a, b), Cook et al. (1965), and others have confirmed Rouviere's findings (Figs. 9.36 and 9.37). They demonstrate testicular lymphatic channels terminating in a sentinel node at the level of L1/L2 on the left and L1/L3 on the right slightly lateral to the lumbar nodes usually opacified by pedal lymphangiography. From the right testis there may be direct filling of the right lateral nodes, above or below the renal vein, or directly to the left lateral nodes. There may be immediate cross-over of the right testicular lymphatics to the contralateral nodes, while the left testicular vessels cross over after permeating the sentinel nodes. Cross-over from

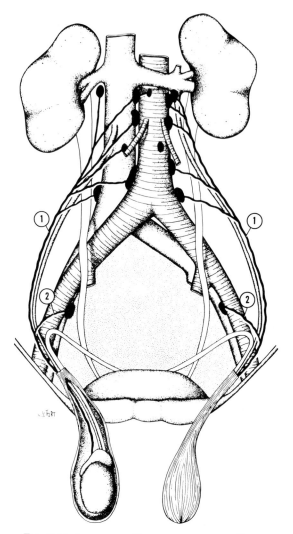

FIG. 9.35. LYMPHATIC DRAINAGE FROM THE TESTICLE

1, The major draining trunks empty into the lumbar lymph nodes from the level of the renal hilum to the bifurcation of the aorta. *2*, The external iliac nodes may occasionally drain the testicles.

left to right is most unusual. From the lumbar nodes, continuity of the lymphatic system is usually maintained through the thoracic duct. In the final analysis, important nodes are filled by testicular lymphangiography that are not opacified by the pedal route necessitating the combined approach whenever possible (Figs. 9.38–9.40). Thus far in human testicular lymphangiography with the injection of one or perhaps two testicular lymphatic trunks, analogous categories to those demonstrated by Engeset (see

Fig. 9.16) in his animal experiments, have only in part been found. However, the clinical distribution of metastases from carcinoma of the testicle has paralleled Engeset's findings. On rare occasions pulmonary metastases are discovered in the absence of retroperitoneal disease.

Nodal metastases from testicular malignant disease show several different architectural patterns. Involved nodes are more spherical than normal and may have a crescent deformity with the lymphatics failing to penetrate the marginal defects (carcinoma pattern) (Figs. 9.41–9.43). Occasionally, they may have an abnormal internal architecture with a relatively intact marginal sinus (lymphoma pattern). The latter picture is more frequently seen in some seminomas, lymphomas, and rhabdomyosarcomas of the testicle (Figs. 9.44–9.46). At times the metastatic nodes show both carcinoma and lymphoma type patterns, a mixed variety. Perhaps this mixed pattern reflects the varied components that are present at times in a testicular neoplasm.

By determining the nature, location, and extent of disease in testicular malignancies, the lymphangiogram facilitates the accurate placement of the radiation therapy portal. The contrast material retained in the lymph nodes can be followed during the course of the disease by roentgenograms of the abdomen to evaluate the effectiveness of the treatment.

In the presence of widespread disease, Stage III, where chemotherapy is the initial therapeutic approach, lymphangiography is of assistance in determining the status of the retroperitoneal lymph nodes. After a favorable response to chemotherapy, e.g., resolution of pulmonary metastases, the patient is then managed as if a Stage II with the primary treatment by radiation therapy to the retroperitoneal and ipsilateral iliac area followed by lymph node dissection. Changes in size and architecture of the opacified lymph nodes will assist in determining the response to therapy. If there is inadequate residual contrast material, a repeat lymphangiogram should be performed. We have repeated the study on many patients with a maximum of five lymphangiograms in a patient over a 7-year period. The same basic criteria are operative for the establishment of metastatic disease.

Lymphangiography can also be utilized as a guide to the surgeon prior to retroperitoneal lymphadenectomy. Node dissections regardless of the thoroughness or talents of the surgeon are

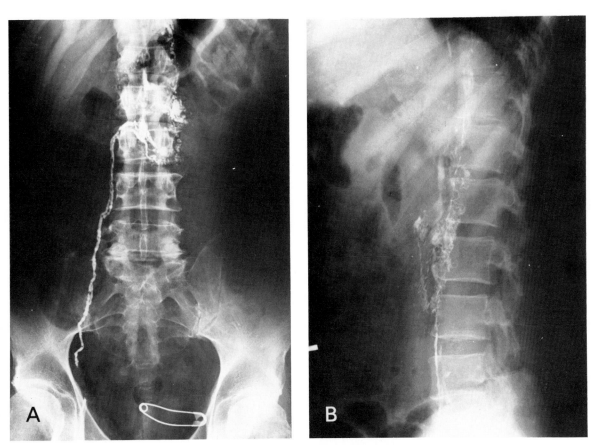

FIG. 9.36. TESTICULAR LYMPHATIC DRAINAGE

A: Right testicular lymphangiogram. Note the para-aortic distribution with cross-over to the left side, anteroposterior projection. *B:* Lateral view (Busch and Sayegh).

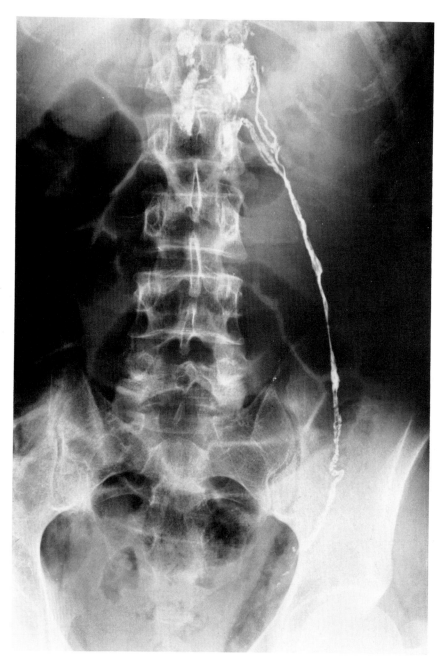

FIG. 9.37. LEFT TESTICULAR LYMPHANGIOGRAM

Opacification of the left lumbar as well as the nodes between the aorta and inferior vena cava (Busch and Sayegh, 1963).

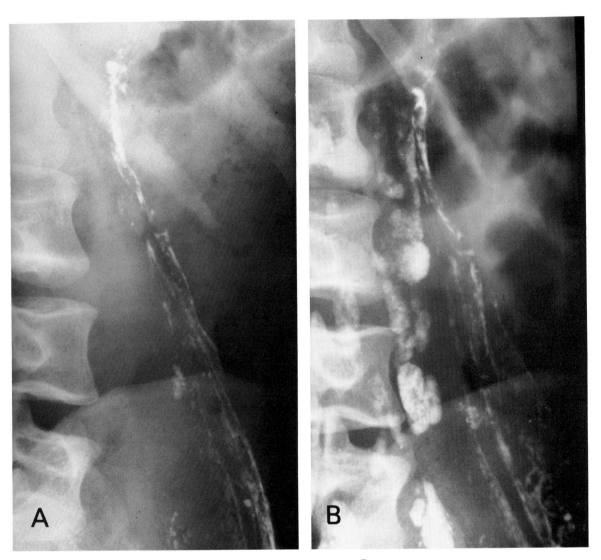

FIG. 9.38. TESTICULAR LYMPHATIC DISTRIBUTION

A: Left testicular lymphangiogram opacifies the first echelon nodes at the level of the renal hilum. These nodes were not visualized by the pedal route, left posterior oblique projection. *B:* Pedal lymphangiogram. The lumbar nodes are opacified, left posterior oblique projection.

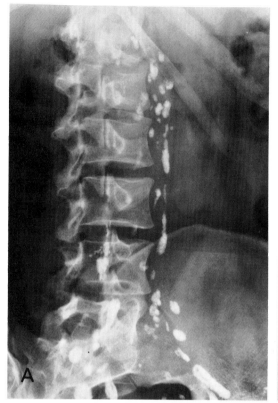

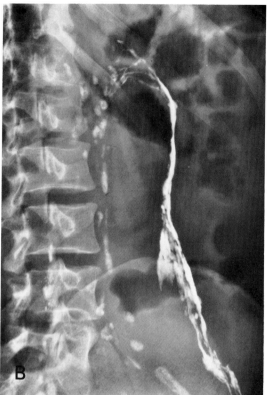

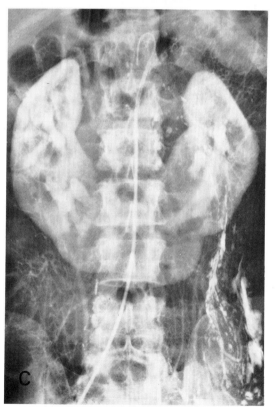

FIG. 9.39. TESTICULAR LYMPHATIC DISTRIBUTION IN A
PATIENT WITH A HORSESHOE KIDNEY

A: Left oblique of the pedal lymphangiogram. B: Left
testicular lymphangiogram. Nodes are opacified by this
pathway that are not seen via the pedal route. C: Aorto-
gram demonstrates the horseshoe kidney and the location
of the lymph nodes opacified by the left testicular lymphangiogram.

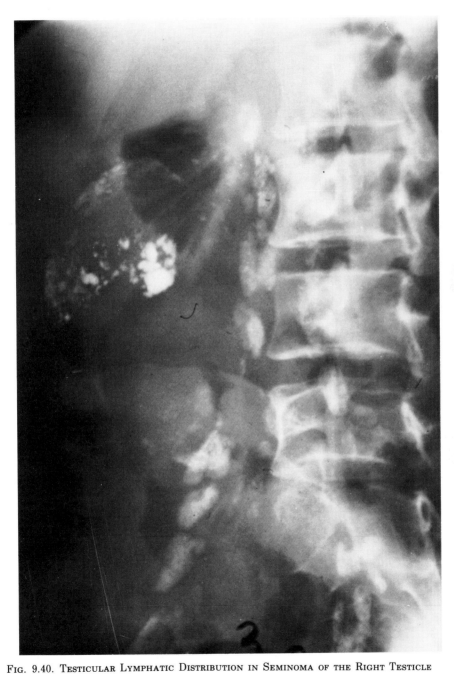

FIG. 9.40. TESTICULAR LYMPHATIC DISTRIBUTION IN SEMINOMA OF THE RIGHT TESTICLE

Seminomatous metastases to the first echelon node demonstrated by testicular lymphangiography. This involved node was not opacified by pedal lymphangiography (Cook et al.).

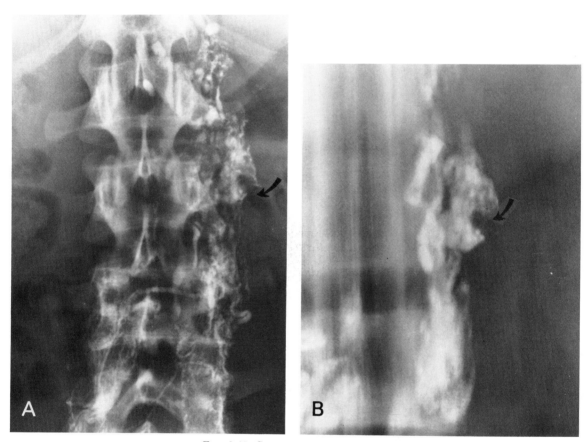

FIG. 9.41. CARCINOMA OF THE TESTICLE

A and B: Carcinoma pattern. The lymphatics do not traverse a small defect in the node at the level of L2 on the left (*arrows*). Tomogram through the retroperitoneal nodes enhances the demonstration of the defect and the residual crescentic configuration in metastatic carcinoma from an embryonal carcinoma of the left testicle.

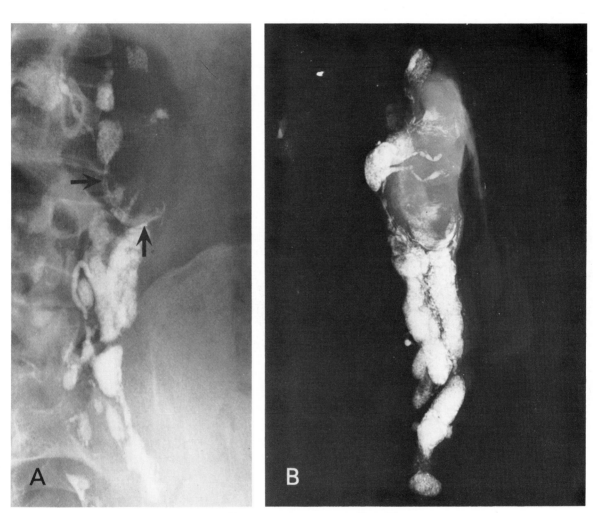

FIG. 9.42. TERATOCARCINOMA OF THE LEFT TESTICLE

A: The crescentic configuration (*arrows*) is the opacification of the residual functioning portion of the node. *B:* The specimen better reveals the extent of the replacement by metastases.

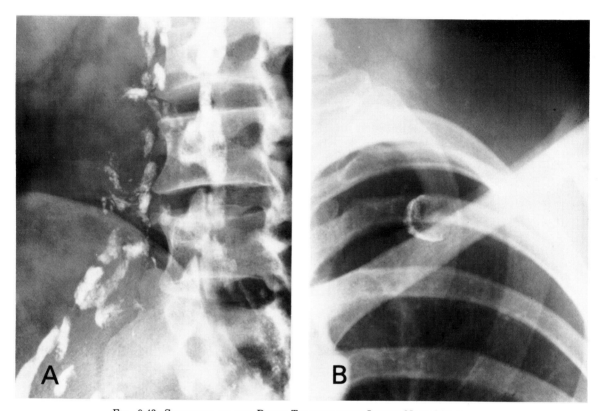

FIG. 9.43. SEMINOMA OF THE RIGHT TESTICLE WITH LYMPH NODE METASTASES

A: The crescentic configuration in the retroperitoneal nodes due to metastases. *B:* Supraclavicular metastases in the same patient.

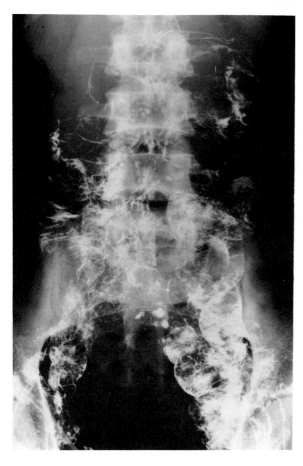

Fig. 9.44. Seminoma of the Left Testicle with Extensive Nodal Metastases

The lymphangiographic pattern simulates that seen in lymphoma.

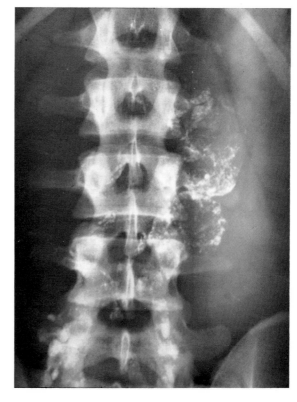

Fig. 9.45. Teratocarcinoma of the Left Testis

"Lymphomatous" pattern in metastatic carcinoma to the left para-aortic nodes.

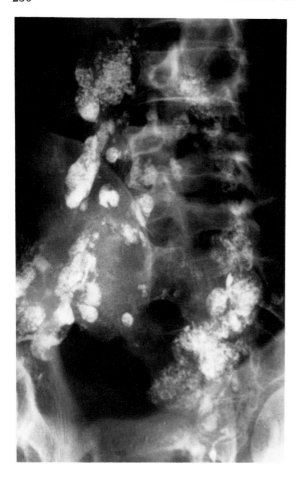

FIG. 9.46. RHABDOMYOSARCOMA OF THE TESTIS

The pattern of metastases simulates that seen in lymphoma.

seldom complete. Roentgenograms of the abdomen obtained in the operating room during the surgical procedure must be undertaken to insure the completeness of the dissection. Radioactive and marker substances such as chlorophyll in Ethiodol have been utilized in an attempt to achieve a more complete dissection but are no longer commercially available. Crossover of the lymphatic drainage between the two sides of the para-aortic region is a normal finding. Contralateral metastases of testicular carcinoma are not uncommon; consequently bilateral node dissection is essential especially if the neoplasm originates in the right testicle (Fig. 9.47). The extent of the dissection should be determined in part by the lymphatic distribution. This depends upon the level at which the testicular and lumbar lymphatic trunks empty into the thoracic duct. At times this continues above the L2 level to T10 or above. Under such circumstances it is somewhat difficult to surgically remove the complete lymphatic drainage from the testis.

In evaluating the patient with testicular malignancy, it is preferable to perform both testicular and pedal lymphangiography. The lymphatic drainage is delineated more completely so that therapy may be tailored to the individual anatomic distribution. If the testicle has been removed pedal lymphangiography should be completed by inferior vena cavography, bilateral renal venography, and pyelography. These studies provide maximal information as to the staging and extent of nodal metastases.

Our experience with 291 cases of testicular malignancies studied by pedal lymphangiography is described in Table 9.8. Patients with seminoma, of whom 24% had abnormal findings by lymphangiography, were treated by radiotherapy alone, making specific nodal correlation impossible. All other testicular malignancies were managed by a combination of surgery

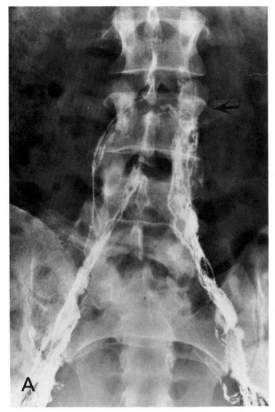

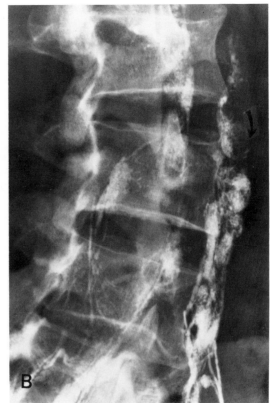

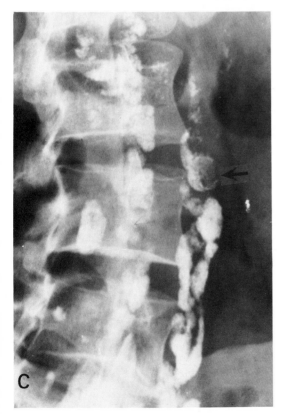

FIG. 9.47. CROSS-OVER METASTASES FROM CARCINOMA OF THE RIGHT TESTICLE TO LEFT PARA-AORTIC LYMPH NODES

A: Anteroposterior view, lymphatic phase (arrow); B: oblique view, lymphatic phase (arrow); and C: oblique view, nodal phase (arrow).

TABLE 9.8
LYMPHANGIOGRAMS OF CARCINOMA OF THE
TESTICLE (291 CASES)

	Pos.	Neg.
Seminoma	28	76
Carcinoma	76	105
Rhabdomyosarcoma	2	4
Total	106	185

TABLE 9.9
LYMPHANGIOGRAPHIC-PATHOLOGIC
CORRELATION IN 121 SURGICAL AND/OR
AUTOPSY CASES[a]

Positive	37	Carcinoma	117
False positive	1	Rhabdomyosarcoma	4
Negative	70		
False negative[b]	13		
Total	121		121

[a] For the purpose of correlation and patient management, all equivocal or suspicious readings are considered negative.

[b] In false negative group, 1 case had 2 nodes positive in 11 central para-aortic group and 45 nodes in right and left para-aortic areas were all negative; 1 case had no evidence of metastasis on lymphangiogram; 8 cases had positive nodes in primary testicular lymphatics; and 3 cases had a microscopic lesion of less than 3 mm.

and radiotherapy, permitting closer scrutiny of the lymphangiographic findings. A normal lymphangiogram and normal findings at surgical exploration negate the necessity of any radiotherapy.

Surgical or autopsy findings or both were correlated with lymphangiographic findings (Table 9.9). Retroperitoneal node dissections were performed at times following radiation therapy. Of the 50 node dissections in which positive nodes were found, 37 patients (74%) were diagnosed preoperatively by pedal lymphangiography. Positive roentgenographic interpretation had excellent correlation (97%). Surgical exploration was not uniformly undertaken especially in patients with more advanced disease. Of a total of 83 considered negative by lymphangiography, 70 (84%) were negative at exploration. Eight of the 13 patients who exhibited false negative findings were found to have metastases in nodes lateral to those usually opacified by pedal lymphangiography; these metastases may have been diagnosed by the testicular route. Routine inferior vena cavography may have been advan-

tageous to decrease the false negative rate; however, the yield of these examinations would be small.

The lymph nodes removed during the retroperitoneal dissection are placed on a Plexiglas template in their in vivo position and a radiograph of the nodes is then done (Fig. 9.48). This is compared with the preoperative and postoperative radiographs especially to verify the presence and removal of abnormal lymph nodes. This is especially important when the node dissection follows the initial course of radiotherapy. At times 2500 rads will produce a dramatic response in the metastatic disease. In 6 cases previously diagnosed as metastatic carcinoma, the initial evaluation of the removed retroperitoneal nodes revealed no evidence of neoplasm. However, with the assistance of specimen radiography to specifically localize the abnormal lymph nodes, re-evaluation established the presence of necrosis and radiation effect in areas previously occupied by metastases or residual neoplasm.

In 11 patients repeat lymphangiography was performed following retroperitoneal node dissection. Ligation of lymphatic channels resulted in utilization of collateral pathways. These collateral pathways resulted in the opacification of nodes beyond the usual drainage from the testicle. Any subsequent metastases might therefore occur along this new route of lymph flow. In another patient a postoperative lymphocyst displaced the ureter and kidney (Fig. 9.49).

Follow-up lymphangiography opacified the large cyst which was treated surgically. Still another effect of para-aortic node lymphadenectomy was the utilization of lymphaticovenous anastomoses as collateral pathways in the face of surgically produced lymphatic obstruction.

The importance of constant monitoring of the disease by lymphangiography is illustrated in a patient with a seminoma of the right testicle (Fig. 9.50). The right testicular lesion invaded the scrotum. The testicle as well as a portion of the scrotum were surgically removed and the right iliac and para-aortic areas were treated by radiation therapy. Follow-up evaluation demonstrated collateral pathways to the lymphatics and nodes in the left inguinal and iliac areas. Metastases subsequently appeared in these nodes.

Lymphangiography should be utilized as a guide in the management of patients with testicular malignancy. In seminomas, when lymphangiography is positive, radiotherapy is given to the ipsilateral iliac and bilateral retro-

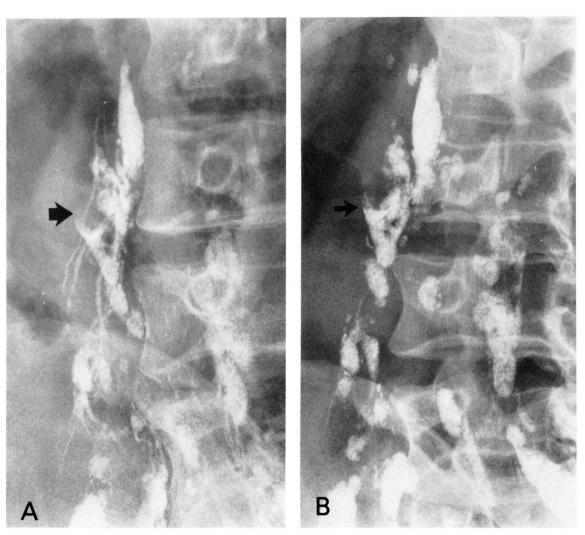

Fig. 9.48. Carcinoma of the Right Testicle

A: The single metastatic node is seen in the right para-aortic group of lymph nodes adjacent to the L2 and L3 interspace (*arrow*). The lymphatics do not traverse the defect. *B:* The crescentic configuration (*arrow*) denotes the residual functioning portion of the lymph node. *C:* The Plexiglas template at the time of the dissection. Specimen radiograph confirms the removal of the involved node. The lymph nodes are smaller because of the effect of the radiation therapy. The reduction in size is also due to the magnification caused by the in vivo position of the node. *IVC,* inferior vena cavogram; *A,* aorta; *1,* left para-aortic nodes; *2,* right para-aortic nodes; *3,* common iliac nodes; *arrow,* abnormal node. *D:* The postoperative examination of the abdomen again verifies the removal of the involved nodes.

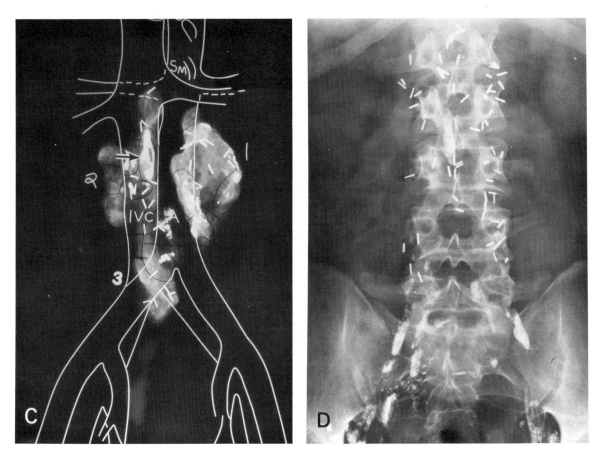

FIG. 9.48. C–D

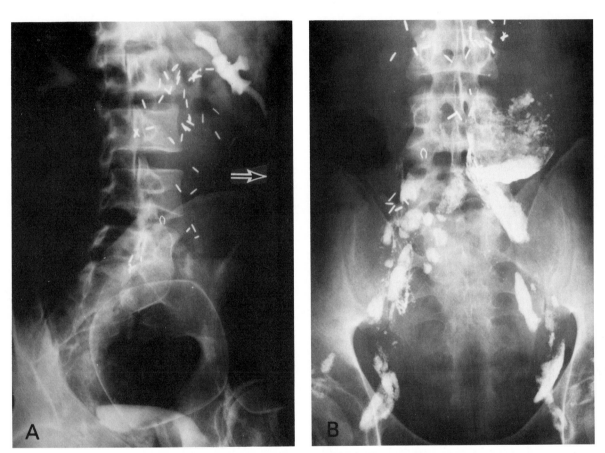

FIG. 9.49. POSTOPERATIVE RETROPERITONEAL LYMPHOCYST

A: The left ureter is displaced anteriorly and laterally (*arrow*). *B:* Repeat lymphangiogram opacifies a large retroperitoneal lymphocyst. The fluid-contrast level is obtained by examining the patient in the erect position.

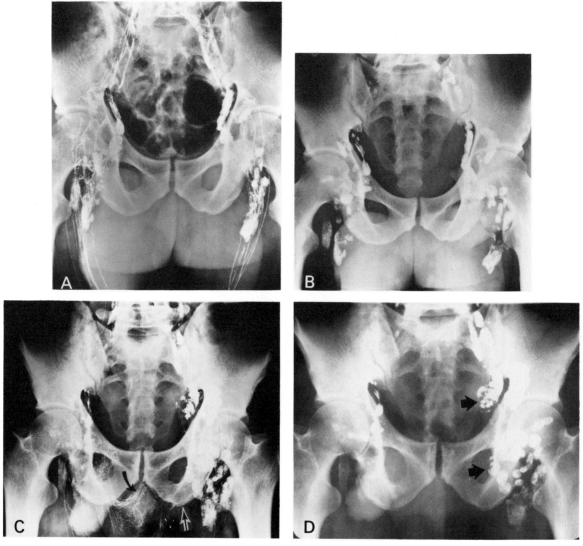

FIG. 9.50. ALTERATION IN THE DISTRIBUTION OF METASTASES SECONDARY TO THE DISEASE AND THE THERAPY IN A PATIENT
WITH SEMINOMA OF THE RIGHT TESTICLE

A: The initial study reveals the lymphatics and nodes to be normal. *B:* Nodal phase. *C:* Repeat lymphangiogram 1 year
later following orchiectomy and radiation demonstrates obstruction of the lymphatics in the right inguinal area (*curved
arrow*) with collateral circulation to the opposite side (*black and white arrow*). *D:* Metastases are noted on the left (*arrows*)
probably due to the alteration in lymphatic flow.

peritoneal nodes to the diaphragm. The mediastinum and both supraclavicular areas are also
treated. In the presence of a negative lymphangiogram radiotherapy is given only to the level
of the diaphragm.

In nonseminomatous malignancies a patient
with a positive lymphangiogram is treated by
radiotherapy to a tumor dose of 2500 rads to the
nodes up to the diaphragm. A retroperitoneal
node dissection is then undertaken to remove

residual tumor tissue with additional radiotherapy, 2500 rads, following the retroperitoneal
node dissection. In the presence of negative lymphangiographic findings, the retroperitoneal
node dissection is undertaken initially. If the
node dissection is negative, no further treatment is instituted. Therefore, lymphangiography has become an essential tool in the evaluation as well as the management of the patient
with testicular malignant disease.

URINARY BLADDER

Carcinoma of the bladder is the most common malignancy of the urinary tract. In spite of all modern advances in diagnosis, treatment, and prevention, the mortality from bladder cancer is rising, especially in young men and in persons from industrial centers.

It is often maintained that carcinoma of the bladder tends to remain localized. Metastases from bladder tumors occur relatively late. At first, they appear in the regional lymph nodes; later, they are seen in the para-aortic nodes, the liver, the lungs, and other organs.

The Lymphatic Drainage of the Bladder

The lymph drainage of the bladder (Fig. 9.51) is by three routes:

1. The Collecting Trunks of the Trigone. These trunks emerge from various points of the bladder wall situated medial to the ureters in the female and to the deferent ducts in the male. They follow the uterine or the ductus deferens artery and terminate in the lymph nodes of the middle or medial group of the external iliac chain.

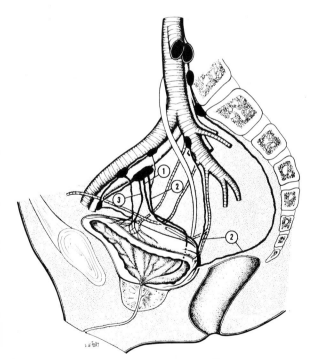

FIG. 9.51. LYMPHATICS OF THE BLADDER

1, The collecting trunks of the trigone; *2*, the collecting trunks of the posterior wall; and *3*, the collecting trunks of the anterior wall.

2. The Collecting Trunks of the Posterior Wall. The lymphatic arising from these trunks may follow different directions: (a) they may reach the posterolateral angle of the bladder, cross the umbilical artery, and terminate in one of the nodes of the middle or medial group of the external iliac chain; (b) less frequently, they may terminate in the retrocrural nodes; (c) they may empty into one of the collecting trunks of the trigone; and (d) occasionally they may terminate in the hypogastric nodes or in the lateral nodes of the common iliac group.

3. The Collecting Trunks of the Anterior Wall. These trunks converge toward the middle third of the lateral border of the bladder, in the region of the middle vesical artery. They descend toward the origin of the middle vesical and umbilical arteries, meet the collecting trunks of the posterior wall, merge with them, and share their nodal connections, i.e., terminate in the same lymph node.

The course of the collecting trunks is frequently interrupted by small intercalating lymph nodules. In the majority of cases, additional small nodules are found on the wall of the bladder—the paravesical nodes. The paravesical nodes can be divided into three groups: anterior, lateral, and posterior. These nodes are situated in the vesical lodge, i.e., under the peritoneum posteriorly and under the vesical fascia anteriorly.

In summary, if all of the small intercalating nodules and paravesical nodules are withdrawn from consideration, the first lymphoid echelon for the lymphatics of the bladder is represented by the external iliac lymph nodes, particularly the middle and medial groups and occasionally by the hypogastric and common iliac nodes.

Lymphangiography will opacify the external and common iliac lymph nodes. In exceptional cases isolated hypogastric nodes (close to the origin of the internal iliac artery) may be demonstrated. Negative findings may result even though the paravesical or hypogastric nodes and the occasional node in the obturator fossa may be affected by metastases for these lymph nodes escape visualization.

The indication for lymphangiography in carcinoma of the bladder is the more accurate staging of the disease which then dictates the management. Prognosis is related to the stage of the disease. The modality of treatment also varies with the extent of the lesion.

Staging of a carcinoma of the bladder is clinical and includes cystoscopy and bimanual rectoabdominal palpation of the anesthetized patient. The classification is based upon the system proposed by Jewett and Strong (1946) and modified by Marshall (1956). Allocations to Stages O, A, and B1 are based entirely on microscopic assessment of the depth of invasion in patients in whom bimanual examination is negative. When bimanual palpation reveals induration or thickening without a definite mass, a Stage B2 classification is assigned. If a distinct mass is palpable, the tumor is labelled Stage C. Stage D1 classification is utilized when there is fixation of the mass to the pelvic or abdominal wall, uterus, or prostate; extension into the vagina, peritoneum, or bowel; or microscopic evidence of invasion or prostatic glandular substance. The presence of pelvic lymph node metastases also places the patient in a Stage D1 classification. Stage D2 is reserved for patients with metastases to lymph nodes at or above the aortic bifurcation and/or to other sites outside the confines of the true pelvis.

The diagnostic criteria for nodal metastasis in carcinoma of the bladder are the same as that described earlier. The single most reliable criterion is a filling defect in a node not traversed by lymphatics (Figs. 9.52 and 9.53). When the node is completely replaced, the lymphatics may be displaced or obstructed (Fig. 9.54 A). Lymphatic obstruction with or without collateral channels may be the sole secondary evidence of nodal replacement. Confirmation by complementary procedures, notably venography, ultrasound, and computed tomography, is of value to demonstrate the presence of an enlarged replaced node or tumor mass (Figs. 9.54 B and C).

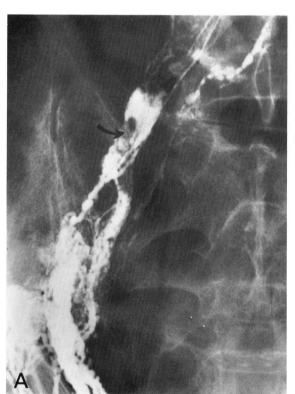
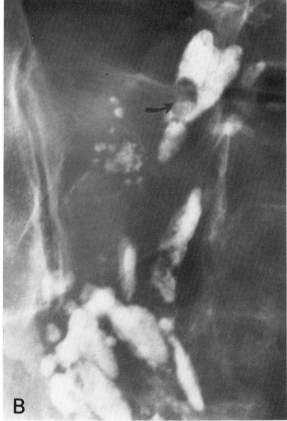

FIG. 9.52. CARCINOMA OF THE BLADDER

A: Metastases to a common iliac node (*arrow*), lymphatic phase. B: Nodal phase (*arrow*).

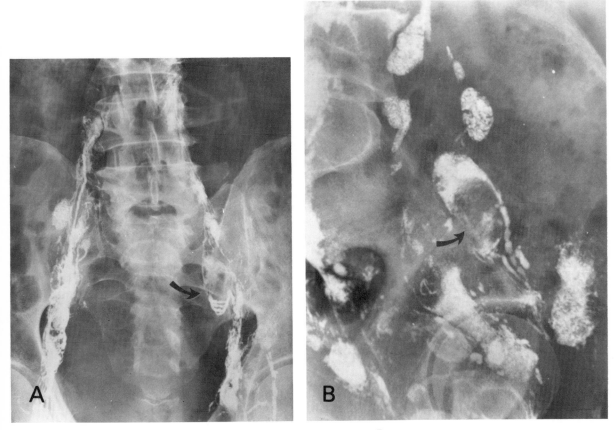

FIG. 9.53. CARCINOMA OF THE BLADDER

A: Metastasis to the left iliac node (*arrow*), lymphatic phase. *B:* Nodal phase (*arrow*).

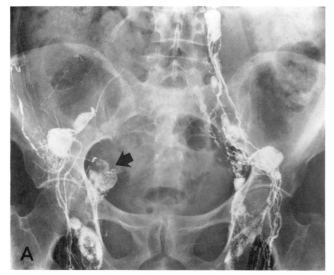

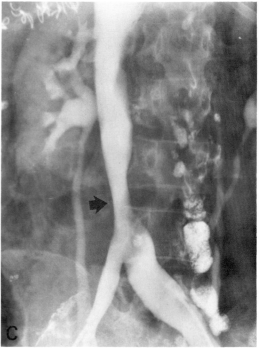

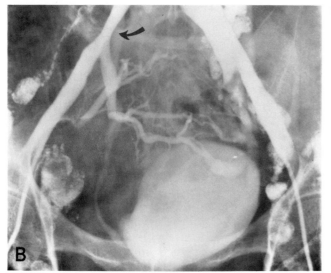

FIG. 9.54. CARCINOMA OF THE BLADDER

A: Primary evidence of metastasis is seen in a right external iliac lymph node, medial chain (*arrow*). Obstruction of lymphatics and collateral pathways are opacified. *B and C:* Venography yields complementary information by external compression of the right common iliac vein and inferior vena cava (*arrows*).

Results

From December 1966 to December 1974, 91 patients with carcinoma of the bladder had bilateral pedal lymphangiograms as a part of the assessment of metastatic disease. Surgical findings were correlated within 3 months of lymphangiographic interpretation in 49 patients. However, 56 of these 91 patients received preoperative irradiation (5000 rads tumor dose in 5 weeks through 10 × 10 cm fields) 6 weeks prior to surgical exploration. In all cases, surgical exploration included careful palpatory scrutiny of the pelvic and para-aortic lymph nodes and suspicious or enlarged lymph nodes were removed for histologic examination. Three pa-

tients underwent formal bilateral pelvic lymphadenectomy. The results of lymphangiographic and surgical correlation are shown in Table 9.10. No false positive lymphangiographic readings were encountered. In the 9 patients with

TABLE 9.10
LYMPHANGIOGRAPHIC-SURGICAL CORRELATION
(60 SURGICAL CASES)

Positive	9
False positive	0
Negative	46
False negative	5
Total	60

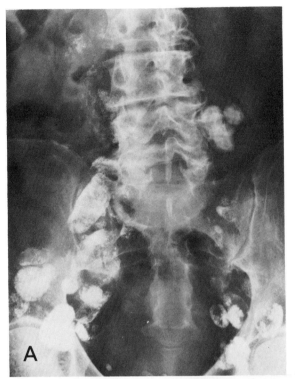

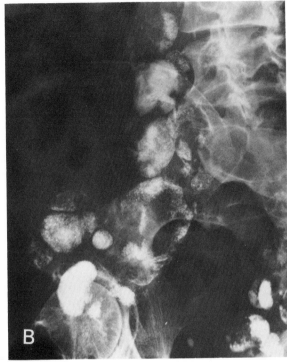

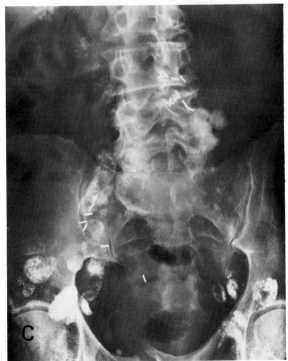

FIG. 9.55. CARCINOMA OF BLADDER AND LYMPHOMA

A: Diffuse nodal involvement is due to nodular lymphoma. Metastatic carcinoma from the bladder is seen in a right external iliac node, medial chain, anteroposterior view. *B:* Oblique view. *C:* Following therapy. The clips are at the sites of biopsy. The patient was treated by radiotherapy and chemotherapy.

TABLE 9.11
LYMPHANGIOGRAPHIC-SURGICAL CORRELATION
ACCORDING TO CLINICAL STAGE OF DISEASE

Interpretation	Clinical Stage				Total No. Patients
	B1	B2	C	D	
Positive	1	1	3	4	9
False positive	0	0	0	0	0
Negative[a]	14	12	16	4	46
False negative	1	0	2	2	5

[a] For the purpose of correlation and patient management, all equivocal or suspicious readings were considered negative.

proven nodal metastases diagnosed by lymphangiogram, an accuracy of 100%, the specific sites of the nodal involvement were the common iliac chain in 4 patients with a concomitant involvement of the para-aortic node in 1; the external chain was exclusively involved in 2 patients and in 2 others both the common and external chains were involved. The remaining 1 patient had both lymphomatous and carcinomatous disease in the same lymph nodes with extensive involvement of the pelvic and para-aortic nodes (Fig. 9.55). As might be expected, lymphangiograms positive for metastatic disease were encountered more frequently with the more advanced clinical stages as shown in Table 9.11. False negative interpretations were encountered in only 5 cases (9.8%). The sites of tumor involvement not diagnosed by lymphangiograms included the external iliac chains in 2 cases of metastasis, one of these 2 patients with microscopic foci, and another patient having lymphatic obstruction with incomplete filling of the external iliac nodes. An unexpected metastatic disease was encountered in the obturator nodes near the obturator foramen in 3 cases.

Our findings of positive lymphangiograms in 7% of patients with Stages B1 and B2 disease, 14% in patients with Stage C disease, and 40% in patients with fixation of the tumor to the pelvis or abdominal wall (Stage D1) underscores the value of this procedure in reducing the number of patients subjected to unnecessary and futile surgical exploration. Surgical treatment for patients with Stage D1 lesions has proven

highly unsatisfactory. Laplante and Brice treated 97 consecutive patients with pathologically demonstrated Stage D vesical carcinoma with only 5 patients free of neoplasm 5 years after radical cystectomy (1973). Only 6 of 35 patients with Stage D1 lesions (17%) undergoing radical cystectomy by Dretler and associates survived 5 years without evidence of recurrent disease. Our experience would suggest that equal or better results can be achieved with the use of radiotherapy alone and obviates the unnecessary risks and morbidity associated with radical surgery.

It is axiomatic that staging is the single most important factor in deciding upon therapy and determining the prognosis for carcinoma of the bladder. The accuracy of the commonly employed clinical methods for staging ranges from 50–81%. These methods are unable to accurately assess lymph node metastases in patients with clinically localized bladder carcinoma. When strict criteria are used for interpretation of the roentgenographic findings, lymphangiography becomes a simple direct highly reliable method of demonstrating clinically unsuspected metastases in the lymph nodes. It is the policy of this institution for all patients presenting with carcinoma of the bladder to have a complete routine examination for staging. Biopsies are taken to estimate the extent of the disease histologically, and if there is an invasive bladder carcinoma present (Stage B1-D) the patient is examined by a bilateral pedal lymphangiogram. If the lymphangiogram is negative for nodal metastasis and the patient has an invasive bladder carcinoma, he is then treated with preoperative external irradiation, 5000 rads with a four-field box technique, followed 6 weeks after completion of radiotherapy by a total cystectomy, prostatectomy, and ileal conduit urinary diversion procedure. If the lymphangiogram is positive for metastatic disease in the pelvic lymph nodes, the patient is randomized with half the patients receiving banjo or extended field radiotherapy and the other half of the group receiving pelvis irradiation. If the para-aortic nodes are involved, then the patient is treated with chemotherapy.

THE PROSTATE

Carcinoma of the prostate is the most prevalent neoplasm of the male genital organs. This tumor has become of increasing clinical importance because of the increasing number of men who are reaching later decades of life. Metastasis is predominantly through hematogenous routes, although lymphatic metastasis is common even in the early stage of the disease. The incidence of lymph node metastases is related to the size of the primary neoplasm as well as the presence of extraprostatic invasion (Tables 9.12–9.14).

TABLE 9.12
CARCINOMA OF PROSTATE

Stage A Two or less microscopic foci of cancer in a specimen obtained in the course of treatment of benign disease.

Stage B Palpable tumor confined within the capsule of the prostate.

Stage C Locally invasive (pelvic wall, base of bladder, etc.).

Stage D Distant metastases.

TABLE 9.13
RELATIONSHIP OF RECTAL SIZE OF PROSTATIC CANCER TO INCIDENCE OF LYMPH NODE METASTASES[a]

Size of Local Lesion	No. of Cases	No. with Positive Nodes	% with Positive Nodes
Nodule	29	2	7
<35 gm	132	26	20
35–80 gm	185	81	44
80–150 gm	55	28	51
>150 gm	12	11	92
Total	413	148	36

[a] From Flocks, R. H., Culp, D. and Porto, R.: Lymphatic spread from prostatic cancer. J. Urol., 81: 194, 1959.

The Lymphatic Drainage of the Prostate

The lymphatic networks of the prostate (Fig. 9.56) are drained by four collecting trunks:

1. The External Iliac Pedicle. It is formed by a single trunk of the lymphatics which arises from the superior surface and upper part of the posterior surface of the prostate. This trunk ascends along the medial border of the seminal vesicle and passes above the terminal segment of the ureter to terminate in one of the nodes of the middle group of the external iliac chain.

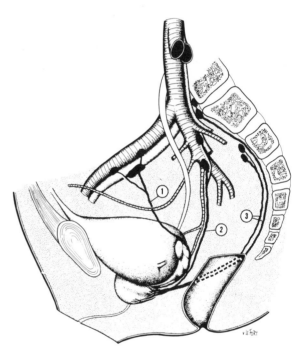

FIG. 9.56. LYMPHATICS OF THE PROSTATE

1, External iliac pedicle; *2,* hypogastric pedicle; and *3,* posterior pedicle.

TABLE 9.14
INCIDENCE OF LYMPH NODE METASTASES IN PATIENTS WITH DISEASE LIMITED TO PROSTATE AND WITH EXTRAPROSTATIC INVASION

	Disease Limited to Prostate	Lymph Nodes Positive	Extraprostatic Invasion	Lymph Nodes Positive
Whitmore (1963)[a]	2	0	18	9
Arduino and Glucksman (1962)[b]	54	5	17	14
Flocks et al. (1959)[c]	29	2	384	146
Total	85	7	419	169

[a] Whitmore, W. F., Jr.: The rationale and results of ablative surgery for prostatic cancer. Cancer, *16:* 1119, 1963.

[b] Arduino, L. J. and Glucksman, M. A.: Lymph node metastases in early carcinoma of the prostate. J. Urol., *88:* 91, 1962.

[c] Flocks, R. H., Culp, D. and Porto, R.: Lymphatic spread from prostatic cancer. J. Urol., *81:* 194, 1959.

2. The Hypogastric Pedicle. It is formed by a single trunk and arises from the inferior part of the prostate. It ascends on its posterior surface toward the superior surface of the gland, and then turns outward along the prostatic artery to terminate in one of the hypogastric nodes.

3. The Posterior Pedicle. It is composed of two or three trunks and arises from the posterior surface of the prostate. It is directed posteriorly in the medial aspect of the rectovesical fascia toward the sacrum and then terminates in lymph nodes located on the medial side of the second sacral foramen or in the nodes in the region of the promontory of the sacrum.

4. The Inferior Pedicle. It is usually formed by a single trunk and descends from the anterior border of the prostate to the floor of the perineum. There it follows the internal pudendal artery around the ischial spine into the pelvis and terminates in one of the hypogastric nodes near the origin of the internal iliac artery.

In summary, the first lymphoid echelon for the lymphatics of the prostate is represented by the entire lymphoid girdle at the superior strait of the pelvis, via the external iliac, the hypogastric and the promontory nodes. The lymphatics of the prostate are in communication with those of the bladder, the seminal vesicle and the rectum.

Lymphangiography in Carcinoma of the Prostate

Of the regional lymph nodes, only the external iliac nodes can be demonstrated on the lymphangiogram. Occasionally, the hypogastric nodes near the origin of the internal iliac artery may be visualized. The opacification of the promontory node is usually uncertain. The indications for lymphangiography in carcinoma of the prostate are suspicion of nodal metastasis and uncertainty about operability or further therapeutic measures.

The lymphangiographic findings in nodal metastases from carcinoma of the prostate are varied and show different architectural patterns. The lymph node may be enlarged with marginal filling defects or with partial replacement having crescentic appearance similar to that seen in classical carcinoma of epithelial origin (Figs. 9.57-9.59). The involved node may appear moderately enlarged, with irregular internal architecture and fairly well circumscribed filling defects simulating malignant lymphoma (Fig. 9.59). Fragmented nodes with multiple filling defects may also be seen. Lymphatic obstruction with or without collateral lymph channels is often associated with these abnormal nodes (Fig. 9.60). When the lymph node is completely replaced by tumor tissue with collateral lymphatic pathways, the presence of mass may be confirmed by venography.

Results and Summary

From August 1967 through February 1975, 59 patients with carcinoma of the prostate had pedal lymphangiograms. Fourteen of these patients had nodal metastases with positive lymphangiograms, 1 in Stage B, 7 in Stage C, and 6 in Stage D. The sites of nodal involvement were the common iliac and para-aortic nodes in 1 patient of Stage B, the external iliac nodes in 7 patients of Stage C, and both iliac and para-

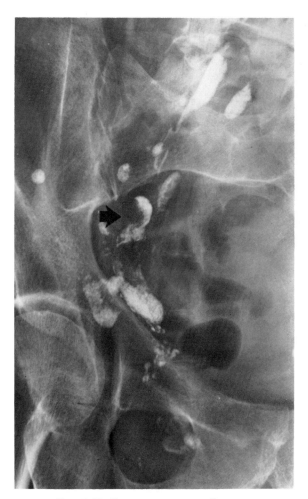

FIG. 9.57. CARCINOMA OF THE PROSTATE

Nodal phase demonstrates the crescentic configuration denoting metastatic carcinoma (*arrow*). Lymphatics failed to traverse this defect.

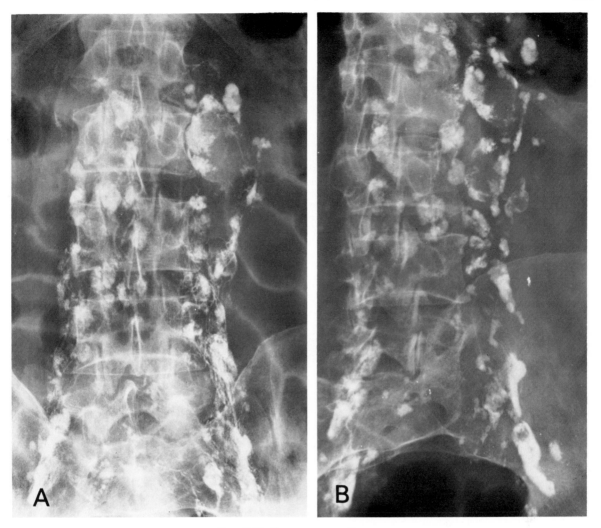

FIG. 9.58. CARCINOMA OF PROSTATE

Involvement of common iliac and para-aortic nodes on the left. *A:* Lymphatic phase; *B:* nodal phase.

aortic nodes in 5 patients of Stage D. One patient of Stage D had metastasis in the inguinal and external iliac nodes with lymphatic obstruction in the pelvic region and showed poor opacification of para-aortic nodes which was inadequate for proper interpretation. Two patients with pelvic and para-aortic metastases had supraclavicular nodal involvement. It should be emphasized that in one patient of Stage B the lymphangiogram showed a positive finding in common iliac and para-aortic nodes. It can probably be explained by the fact that the lymphatic spread in this patient was most likely through the hypogastric pedicle of the lymphatic drainage of the prostate. Generally speaking, as the

clinical stage increases from A to D, there is a progressive increase in the incidence of positive para-aortic lymph node involvement so that in Stage D patients almost all show positive para-aortic lymph node involvement as well as positive pelvic nodes. None of the 14 patients with positive lymphangiograms had an exploratory laparotomy. With strict diagnostic criteria, the interpretation of the lymphangiograms in carcinoma of the testicle, bladder, and cervix generally have excellent surgical correlation. Therefore a positive lymphangiogram in a patient with carcinoma of the prostate was considered definite evidence of metastasis and treated accordingly.

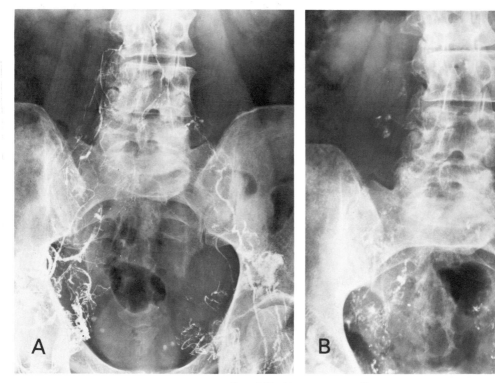

FIG. 9.59. CARCINOMA OF PROSTATE

Extensive involvement yields fragmented nodes at times simulating lymphoma. *A:* Lymphatic phase; *B:* nodal phase.

Lymph node metastases from carcinoma of the prostate have been demonstrated by lymphangiography in recent literature. Rummelhardt and Fussek (1970) performed lymphangiograms on 102 patients with carcinoma of the prostate and found 80.1% diagnostic accuracy of the abnormal lymphangiograms when correlated with nodes obtained at surgery or autopsy. Castellino et al. (1973) reported 89% accuracy in 9 patients with nodal metastases when correlated histologically with excised lymph nodes. Grossman et al. (1974) reported 58 patients with carcinoma of the prostate who had pedal lymphangiograms. Only 6 patients had a laparotomy and the correlation was excellent with all 6 patients having proven positive para-aortic nodes.

Depending primarily upon the stage of carcinoma of the prostate, various therapeutic modalities have been used for its treatment. The ability to accurately define the exact extent of the disease would be highly beneficial in the decision as to the choice of modality of treatment. Nodal metastases have been observed in early operable carcinoma of the prostate (Flocks et al., 1959). When the seminal vesicle is involved, there is a high incidence (at least 82.4%

or higher) of pelvic lymph nodes metastases (Arduino and Glucksman, 1962). The various clinical classifications are mainly based upon clinical methods and serum phosphatase levels and are often inaccurate. Lymphangiography is of great benefit in revealing lymph node metastases and in assessing the exact extent of disease, especially in patients with apparently localized disease. As to the management of carcinoma of the prostate at M. D. Anderson Hospital and Tumor Institute, lymphangiograms are routinely obtained in patients with Stage C, that is, locally invasive prostatic carcinoma involvement of the base of the bladder and/or seminal vesicle or fixation of the prostate to the pelvic wall. If the lymphangiogram is positive, then radiation therapy is not considered and the patient is treated with hormonal manipulation, usually orchiectomy and estrogens. If the lymphangiogram is negative, the patient either receives radiation therapy to the prostate or open surgical staging with lymphadenectomy and insertion of an infusion catheter and hypogastric artery infusion carried out over a protracted period of time.

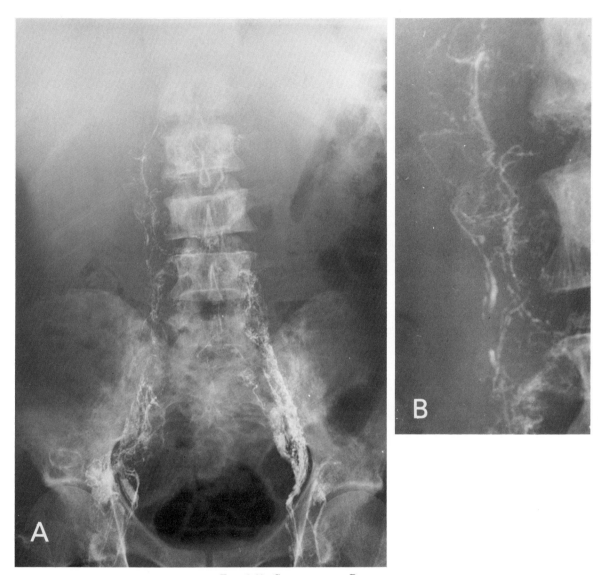

FIG. 9.60. CARCINOMA OF PROSTATE

A: Complete replacement of nodes by metastatic carcinoma produces distortion of the lymphatics which circumvent the totally replaced nodes. *B:* Magnified view (×2) of distorted para-aortic lymphatics. The bones are involved by osteoblastic metastases.

THE LARGE INTESTINE

Cancer of the lower intestinal tract is the second most common cause of death from cancer. Of all intestinal cancers, 75% arise in the colon, rectum, and anus. At the time of the initial surgical procedure, venous invasion and regional lymph node metastases are common. Blood vessel invasion has been reported in 36–41% dependent upon the site of the primary (Grinnell, 1942). This correlated with the presence or subsequent incidence of liver, lung, or other visceral involvement. When liver metastases were found, lymph node involvement was invariably present. Regional lymph node metastases noted during curative resection have been seen in one-half to two-thirds of the patients (Gilchrist, 1959; Keynes, 1961). Dukes and Bussey (1958) reported an overall 5-year survival rate with nodal metastases without venous invasion of 57.7% while with venous invasion it was 20%. Copeland et al. (1968) suggested that the survival rate varied inversely with the number of metastatic nodes: no nodes, 48%; one node, 26.8%; and 5 or more nodes, 9.1%. Crile et al. (1971) postulated that at one point in the growth of metastases in lymph nodes they begin to act as primary tumors and shed tumor cells into the blood. Such a period does not begin until the nodal metastasis is large and the tumor penetrates the capsule. Therefore lymph node involvement in carcinoma of the large intestine is a most important prognostic factor. The relative position and extent of lymph node metastasis determine the outcome far more than the size of the primary lesion or its penetration through the wall of the colon and rectum (Dukes, 1952).

Lymphatics of the Large Intestine

The lymphatics of the large intestine arise from the rich lymphatic plexuses of the wall and drain eventually to the central nodes of the superior mesenteric chain, the central nodes of the inferior mesenteric chain, or the latero- and preaortic nodes. Between the gut and terminal nodes are several sets of additional nodes, called the paracolic, the intermediate, and the principal nodes. The principal node is located near the root of the mesenteric vessels. The lymph vessels may pass through all of these sets of nodes in succession, or they may run directly to the principal nodes. There are important differences in the drainage of the right and left halves of the colon. The lymphatics of the ascending colon and proximal two-thirds of the transverse colon drain to the central nodes of the superior mesenteric chain. The remaining one-third of the distal transverse colon and the superior extremity of the descending colon are drained by the lymphatics that accompany the inferior mesenteric veins and terminate in the central nodes of the superior mesenteric chain. The greater part of the descending colon is drained to the nodes which accompany the left colic artery and then the nodes of the inferior mesenteric chain. The collecting trunks of the sigmoid colon are emptied into the central nodes of the inferior mesenteric chain. The central group of the inferior mesenteric chain is drained in turn by the left latero- and preaortic nodes, while the central group of the superior mesenteric chain is drained by the intestinal lymph trunk which usually anastomoses with one of the lumbar trunks above the renal artery, generally with the left or the initial part of the thoracic duct. Sometimes, as a normal variation, the efferent trunks from the central group of the superior mesenteric chain terminate in the left latero- and preaortic nodes immediately adjacent to the renal artery (Fig. 9.61A).

The lymphatics of the rectum and anal canal have numerous anastomoses with those of the prostate, seminal vesicle, vagina, and bladder. The collecting trunks are divided into three groups: inferior, middle, and superior. The inferior collecting trunks originate in the cutaneous part of the anus. They run forward and outward in the subcutaneous tissue of the perineum and the medial aspect of the thigh and drain into the superficial inguinal nodes. The middle collecting trunks, which arise from the anal canal and the inferior extremity of the rectum, usually follow the middle hemorrhoidal vessels and terminate in the hypogastric nodes. They may accompany the middle sacral and lateral sacral arteries and drain to the nodes of the promontory and to the lateral sacral nodes. The superior collecting trunks spring from the anal canal and extend through the entire length of the rectum and traverse one or several intercalating nodes along the course of the superior hemorrhoidal blood vessels. They finally terminate as follows: the short trunks, which come from every region of the rectum, terminate in the nodes situated at the level of the bifurcation of the superior hemorrhoidal artery. These are the most important lymph nodes draining the

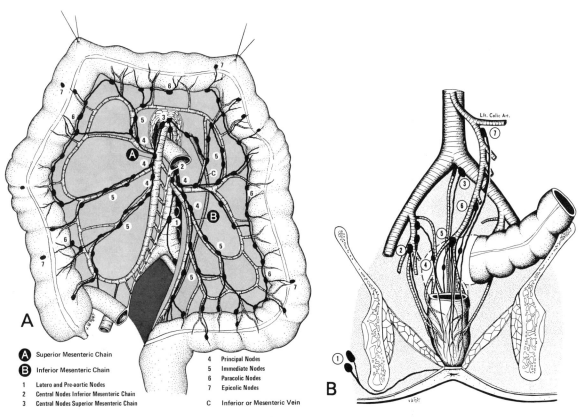

FIG. 9.61. LYMPHATICS OF THE COLON

A: Schematic drawing of the lymphatics of the colon and the sigmoid. *B:* Schematic drawing of the sigmoid and rectum. (Numbers *1–7* correspond to legend on Figure 9.61*A*.)

rectum. The middle trunks ascend, without stopping at the nodes of the bifurcation, to a node placed along the inferior mesenteric artery near the origin of its lowest sigmoid branch. The long trunks, which spring from the lower portion of the rectum, terminate in the nodes placed at the summit of the pelvic mesocolon near the origin of the left colic artery. By means of the efferent trunks of the inferior mesenteric chain, the rectal lymph is finally poured into the preaortic and left lateroaortic nodes (Fig. 9.61*B*).

Lymphangiography in Carcinoma of the Large Intestine

Despite the frequency of regional lymph node metastases at the time of the curative bowel resection, lymphangiography has not as yet been utilized routinely in carcinoma of the large intestine. By pedal lymphangiography the lymph nodes which can be demonstrated are the second echelon distribution of the nodes from the large intestine to the iliac and para-aortic regions. Nodal metastases from the right side of the colon are only rarely demonstrated. Metastasis from the left side of the colon and rectum can be visualized but occurs later in the course of the disease. Preliminary investigation of the value of this examination in patients with carcinoma of the colon and rectum was done at Thomas Jefferson University Hospital. Fifty-five patients who returned at varying intervals after the initial resection with complaints suggesting recurrence or metastases were studied by lymphangiography. Slightly more than 50% of these patients were found to have metastases as detected by this examination (Figs. 9.62–9.64).

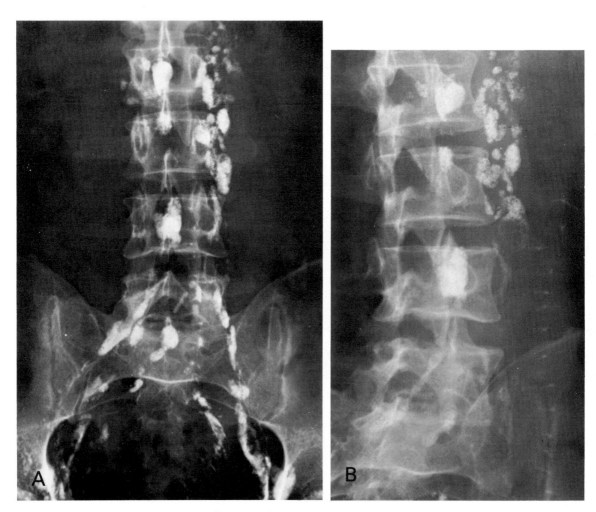

FIG. 9.62. CARCINOMA OF SIGMOID

A: Nodal phase of lymphangiogram performed just prior to resection of the sigmoid neoplasm. *B:* Five months after surgery a left para-aortic node was obviously involved by metastasis. *C:* Nodal phase of lymphangiogram performed just prior to resection of the sigmoid neoplasm in another patient. *D:* After 1½ years left para-aortic nodes were involved by metastases.

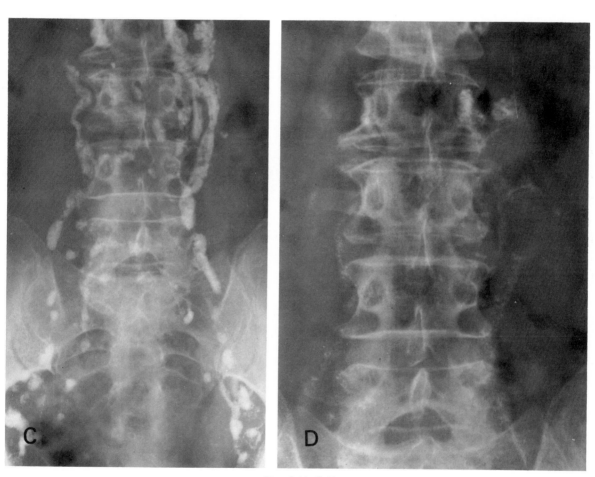

Fig. 9.62. C–D

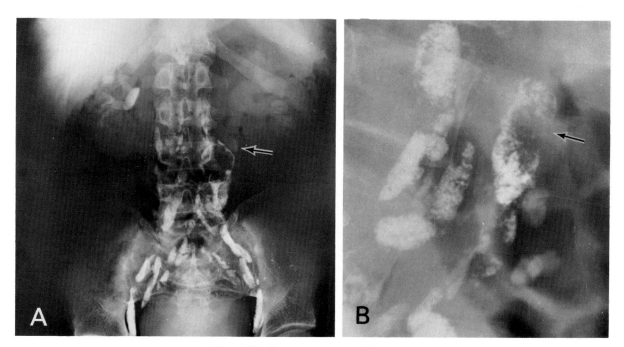

FIG. 9.63. CARCINOMA OF THE RECTUM

A: Metastasis to a lower para-aortic node (*arrow*) 6 months after resection of the primary neoplasm. *B:* Para-aortic metastases obstructing the left kidney (*arrow*) from a carcinoma of the rectum in another patient.

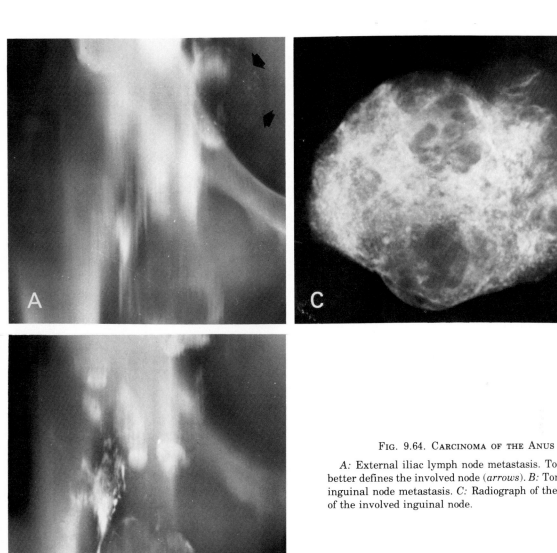

FIG. 9.64. CARCINOMA OF THE ANUS

A: External iliac lymph node metastasis. Tomography better defines the involved node (*arrows*). *B:* Tomogram of inguinal node metastasis. *C:* Radiograph of the specimen of the involved inguinal node.

THE BREAST

Carcinoma of the breast is the most common type of malignant neoplasm occurring in the female over 40 years of age. Prognosis depends upon the size of the primary carcinoma as well as the presence of lymph node metastasis. Despite all recent efforts in management, survival rates have not changed significantly. Earlier detection of the primary lesion will influence survival. The place of the lymphangiography of the upper extremity in the diagnosis and management of the patient with carcinoma of the breast has not as yet been established. Perhaps the more limited surgical approach of simple mastectomy or local excision of the breast mass plus radiotherapy may find new application for this procedure.

The Lymphatic Drainage of the Breast (Fig. 9.65)

Lymphatics of the Skin of the Breast. The lymphatics of the skin of the breast have a particular arrangement at the level of the nipple and of the areola. In this region, they form a dense areolar network with subareolar lymphatic plexuses (Fig. 9.65). To the outer side of the subareolar plexus, the lymphatic network has the same arrangement as the lymphatic network of the skin of the anterior chest wall and is continuous with the lymphatics of the skin of the surrounding region, forming an uninterrupted network over the entire surface of the chest, neck and abdomen. By this mechanism, the lymphatics of the skin of one breast communicate with those of the opposite breast. Collecting trunks of the skin of the breast may cross the midline and drain into the axillary nodes of the opposite side.

Lymphatics of the Breast Proper (Mammary Gland). The lymphatic network of the breast arises from the inter- or perilobular spaces. A few of the collecting trunks follow the lactiferous ducts and end in the subareolar plexuses of the lymphatics of the skin of the breast, but most of these trunks terminate in the axillary nodes. Some end in the internal mammary chain and rarely others empty into the supraclavicular nodes. The lymphatics of the breast may be grouped into the following pathways:

Principal Axillary Pathways. The axillary pathways are formed by the lateral and medial trunks. The lateral trunk receives a principal tributary from the superior part of the breast. The medial trunk passes below the areola and receives a principal tributary from the inferior part of the breast. After winding around the anterior border of the base of the axilla, the lateral and medial trunks traverse the axillary fascia of the base of the axilla and terminate in the nodes of the external mammary chain situated at the level of the second and third intercostal spaces. Some of the collecting trunks do not stop at the external mammary nodes but run directly into the nodes of the axillary vein group or to those of the central group. The efferent vessels of the axillary lymphatics unite to form the subclavian lymphatic trunks which may terminate in three ways: (a) they may empty directly into the jugulosubclavian confluence; (b) they may join the jugular and bronchomediastinal lymphatic trunks to form a common lymphatic duct and empty into the jugulosubclavian confluence; or (c) they may empty into the jugular lymphatic trunk.

Accessory Axillary Pathways. The accessory axillary pathways drain the upper medial region of the breast and are of two kinds. (a) Transpectoral lymph pathways consist of lymphatics which emerge from the periphery of the breast and pass across the pectoralis major.

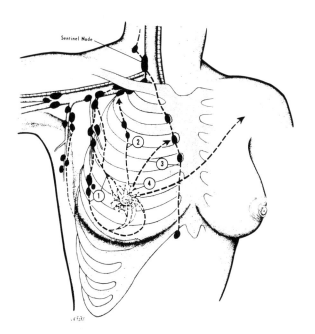

Fig. 9.65. Lymphatics of the Breast

1, Principal axillary pathways; *2*, accessory axillary pathways; *3*, internal mammary pathways; and *4*, subareolar lymphatic plexus.

Some of these traverse the pectoralis major with the pectoral branches of the superior thoracic and thoracoacromial arteries and terminate in subclavicular nodes. Others accompany the arterial rami which perforate the pectoralis major below the inferior border of the pectoralis minor and terminate in several axillary nodes. (b) Retropectoral lymph pathways consist of one or two lymph vessels which wind around the inferior border of the pectoralis major and ascend directly toward the subclavicular nodes by passing either behind the pectoralis minor, along the axillary vein, or between both pectoral muscles.

Internal Mammary Lymph Pathways. The internal mammary pathways drain the central and medial regions of the breast. The collecting trunks run along the perforating branches of the internal mammary blood vessels. They traverse the pectoralis major and the intercostal muscles and empty into the nodes of the internal mammary chain situated in the intercostal spaces at the sternal border—the internal mammary lymphatic duct (right), or the lowest lymph node (sentinel node) of the supraclavicular group—or directly into the jugulosubclavian vein confluence.

Supraclavicular Lymph Pathways. Although the lymphatic trunks coming from the superomedial part of the breast may terminate in some supraclavicular nodes as reported in 3 of 100 cases by Mornard, it is generally believed that the supraclavicular lymph nodes do not have direct connection with the breast but are rather involved by a retrograde permeation of the lymphatics which connect them with the deeply placed sentinel nodes. Sentinel nodes lie close to the confluence of the internal jugular and subclavian vein and are first to be involved by metastasis from the breast which reaches them by way of the subclavian or internal mammary lymphatic trunks.

Lymphangiography in Carcinoma of the Breast

In regional lymph node metastasis, the axillary nodes are often involved, probably because the upper outer quadrant of the breast is the common site of disease. In relatively few cases, the axillary nodes are by-passed and the first nodes involved are those of the subclavian supraclavicular groups. The internal mammary nodes are involved especially from the tumors of the inner quadrant of the breast. It is not rare for the nodes of the anterior mediastinum or even the opposite axilla to be involved.

Lymphangiographic demonstration of the lymph node metastasis from the breast is deficient in that upper limb lymphangiography does not opacify all the axillary nodes. In addition, the supraclavicular nodes are not constantly opacified and the internal mammary nodes are not demonstrated (Fig. 9.66).

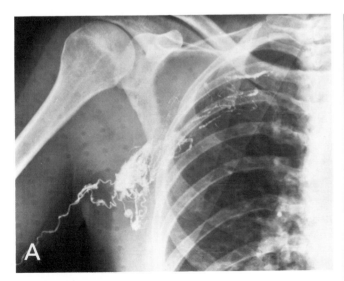
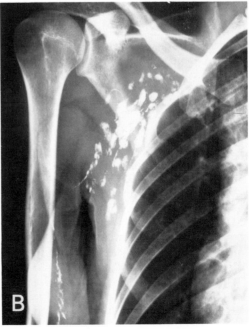

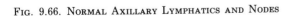

FIG. 9.66. NORMAL AXILLARY LYMPHATICS AND NODES

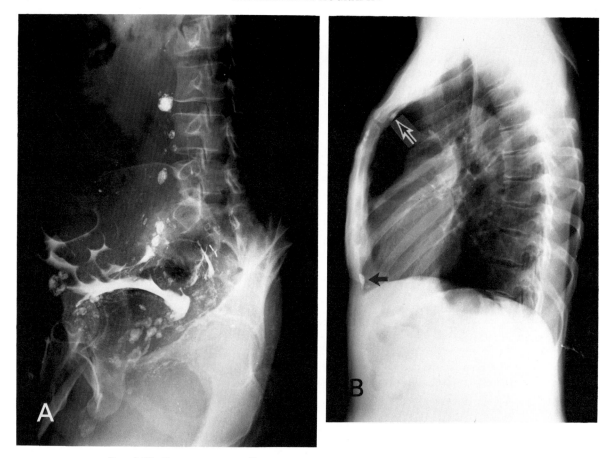

FIG. 9.67. OPACIFICATION OF INTERNAL MAMMARY NODES VIA PERITONEAL ROUTE

A: Fistulous tract into peritoneal cavity with contrast material outlining small bowel loops. *B:* Opacification of internal mammary nodes (*arrows*).

Currently, the indications for upper limb lymphangiography for carcinoma of the breast are detection of the axillary nodal metastasis and evaluation of postmastectomy and post irradiation edema of the upper extremity.

Opacification of the lymphatic drainage has been reported after the injection of contrast material directly into the breast. This is not consistent and has never received adequate clinical trial. Experimental opacification of internal mammary nodes has been accomplished by the intraperitoneal injection of contrast material. This same pathway has been appreciated in a patient with a carcinoma of the cervix staged by pelvic node biopsy. A lymphatic fistula into the peritoneal cavity was visualized during lower extremity lymphangiography. The contrast material outlined the small bowel. Eventually internal mammary lymph nodes were opacified (Fig. 9.67).

The diagnosis of metastatic carcinoma to the axillary lymph nodes can be established when the criteria previously described are employed (Fig. 9.68). This procedure has received adverse criticism because of the incomplete demonstration of all the axillary nodes (Kendall et al., 1963; Shibata et al., 1966; Kitt et al., 1972). However, when positive, the information has a high degree of pathologic correlation.

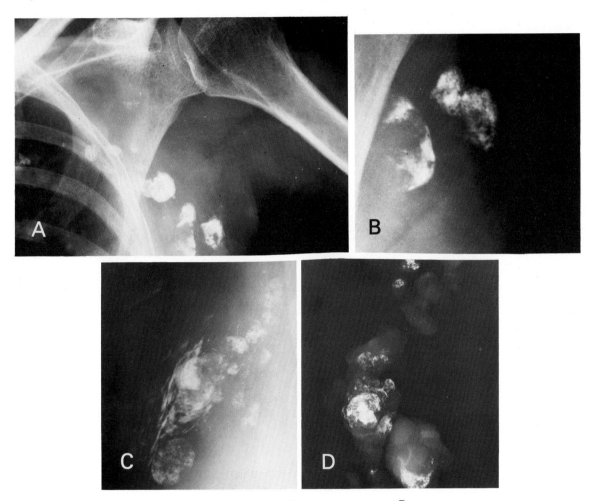

FIG. 9.68. METASTATIC CARCINOMA FROM THE BREAST

A: Metastases to the left axillary nodes from carcinoma of the breast. *B:* Magnification (×2) of nodes in *A*. *C:* Metastatic carcinoma to the right axillary nodes from carcinoma of the breast in another patient. *D:* Radiograph of specimen.

UPPER EXTREMITY EDEMA

In upper extremity edema (including post-mastectomy and postirradiation edema), lymphatic dynamics frequently depend on lymphatic-venous interplay. The etiology of many forms of secondary edema lies in the upset of balance which normally prevails between the two compartments. This is best presented by an analysis of the dynamics associated with the production of edema of an extremity. Differentiation of the mechanisms can be made by performing both lymphangiography and venography. Our findings can be classified as follows: (1) lymphatic obstruction; (2) venous occlusion—intrinsic and extrinsic; and (3) combined lymphatic and venous disease. These classifications are most dramatically illustrated in the variety of mechanisms seen in postmastectomy edema.

Radical mastectomy involves extensive dissection of the regional lymph nodes at the axilla which, in most instances, is beyond the regenerative power of the lymphatics to restore. The reestablishment of satisfactory lymphatic drainage is dependent upon the existence of the lymphatic vessels which are not resected at operation and the development of the collateral lymph channels with re-routing of lymph flow. Following radical mastectomy, obstruction of the lymph flow is usually seen in the axillary region. The collateral channels may be seen in the anterior chest wall to the internal mammary and mediastinal lymph nodes, and not infrequently to the opposite axillary nodes (Fig. 9.69). The cephalic (radial) lymphatic trunk is also a major pathway through which the collateral channels drain into the supraclavicular

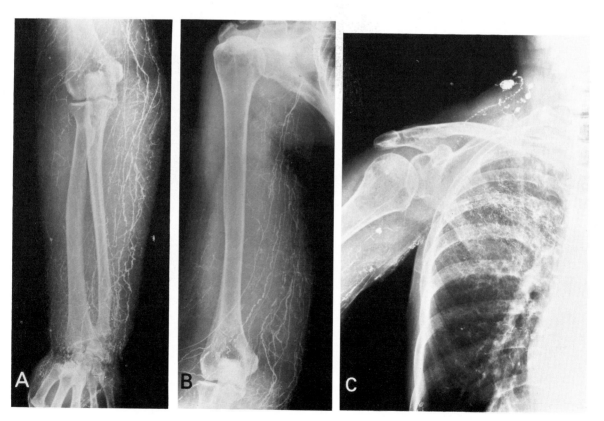

FIG. 9.69. LYMPHATIC OBSTRUCTION WITH COLLATERAL CIRCULATION POSTMASTECTOMY

A: Edematous forearm showing lymphatic obstruction. Opacification of multiple channels are a manifestation of obstruction. *B:* Edematous arm from obstruction in the axilla. Increase in the number of channels opacified. *C:* Collateral circulation of chest wall. *D:* Opacification of supraclavicular lymph nodes bilaterally, internal mammary nodes bilaterally, and left axillary lymph nodes due to collateral pathways. Anteroposterior projection. *E:* Lateral projection (*arrows,* opacified internal mammary nodes). *F:* Venogram. Patent axillary vein.

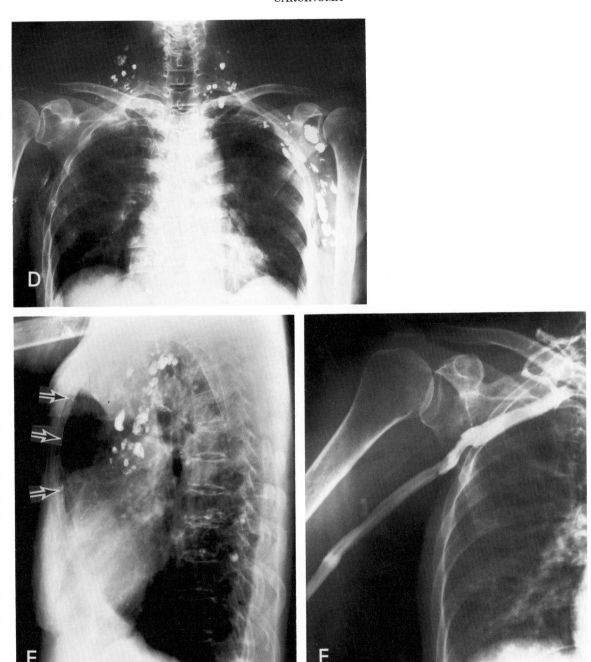

FIG. 9.69. D–F

nodes. Collateral channels through the lymphatics in the posterior chest wall to the paravertebral nodes and the opposite axillary nodes may be observed.

Lymphatic Obstruction. The sequelae of lymphatic obstruction have been described previously. Figure 9.70A shows a case of postmastectomy edema following radical mastectomy and axillary lymph node dissection; the lymphangiographic picture is that usually seen in cases with lymphatic obstruction. The site of the obstruction was in the axilla. Multiple collateral

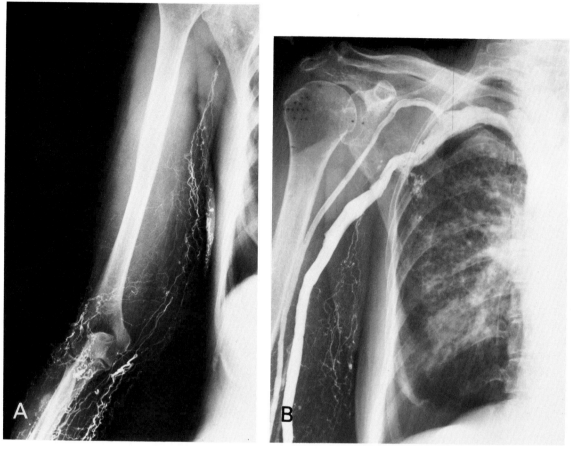

FIG. 9.70. POSTMASTECTOMY EDEMA

A: Lymphatic obstruction; and *B:* normal axillary vein.

channels are clearly seen attempting to circumvent the obstruction. The lymphatics are dilated and tortuous with associated dermal backflow. The venogram (Fig. 9.70*B*) was normal.

Venous Occlusion. Venous occlusion may be either intrinsic (thrombophlebitis) or extrinsic (vascular compression) in origin. The patient shown in Figure 9.71 had carcinoma of the breast which was treated by radical mastectomy and axillary dissection followed by radiation therapy. Postmastectomy edema gradually developed. The venogram revealed intrinsic disease, chronic thrombophlebitis. Lymphangiograms showed also a decrease in the caliber and number of the lymphatics opacified. It is believed by many that chronic thrombophlebitis is usually coupled with perivascular lymphangitis. In an attempt to explain our findings, it is

postulated that there is stasis in the lymphatics of the extremity, thereby making fewer channels available for active flow. On the other hand, perhaps the decrease in caliber is secondary to the increase in the interstitial tissue pressure, stasis, or spasm.

Extrinsic venous disease may be due to enlarged lymph nodes, inflammatory or neoplastic in origin, compressing the veins. It may also be produced by fibrotic or inflammatory changes in the perivascular tissues secondary to surgery or radiation therapy and may eventuate in an occlusion of the vein. Figure 9.72 shows extrinsic venous disease in a patient with a carcinoma of the breast. There was edema of the arm prior to any form of therapy. The lymph nodes compressing the vein proved to be inflammatory.

Combined Lymphatic and Venous Disease.

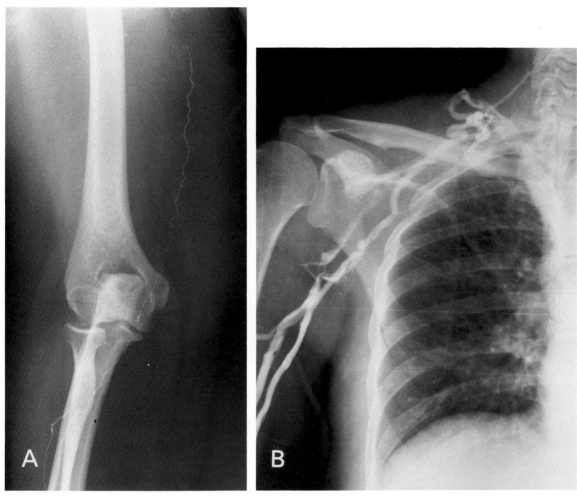

FIG. 9.71. POSTMASTECTOMY EDEMA – THROMBOPHLEBITIS

A: Normal lymphatics; and *B:* thrombophlebitis of axillary vein.

Most frequently encountered is a combination of these two entities. In such situations the vein is involved either by intrinsic or extrinsic disease. Lymphangiograms show lymphatic obstruction. There is usually an associated soft tissue suffusion of contrast material.

Obstruction of the superior vena cava and right subclavian vein by a carcinoma of the lung may also occlude lymphatic flow (Fig. 9.73). The increased venous pressure inhibits the normal flow of lymph into the subclavian vein at the venous angle. The lymphangiogram shows marked collateral lymphatic circulation in the axillary and supraclavicular areas and in the lateral chest wall. There are irregular supraclavicular lymph nodes demonstrated which are diagnostic of metastatic disease. Venograms demonstrate filling of accessory venous channels bypassing the occlusion.

Figure 9.74 shows a patient with Hodgkin's disease and extensive axillary lymph node involvement. The diagnosis was established by axillary lymph node biopsy and followed by radiation therapy to the axilla. There was progressive edema of the arm. The lymphangiogram shows an extensive collateral lymphatic

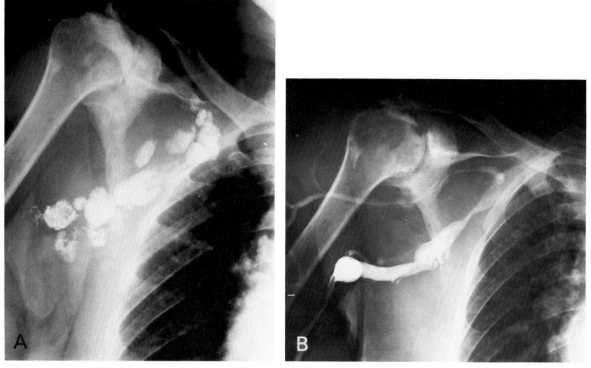

FIG. 9.72. EDEMA — EXTRINSIC VENOUS COMPRESSION

A: Enlarged nodes compressing the axillary vein. *B:* Venogram. Compression of axillary vein.

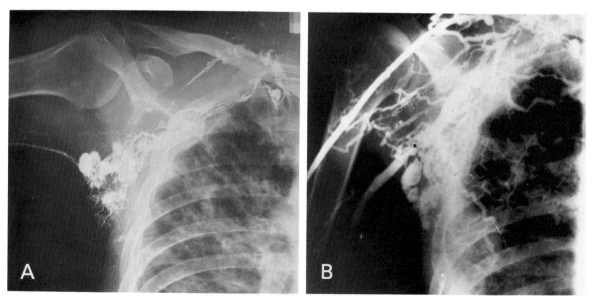

FIG. 9.73. EDEMA — LYMPHATICS AND VENOUS DISEASE IN CARCINOMA OF LUNG

A: Lymphatic obstruction with collateral circulation. *B:* Venous obstruction with collateral circulation.

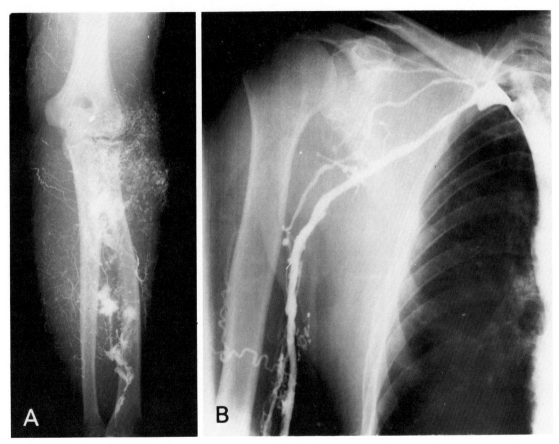

FIG. 9.74. EDEMA—LYMPHATIC AND VENOUS DISEASE IN HODGKIN'S DISEASE

After lymph node biopsy and radiation therapy. *A:* Lymphatic obstruction; and *B:* venous disease, thrombophlebitis.

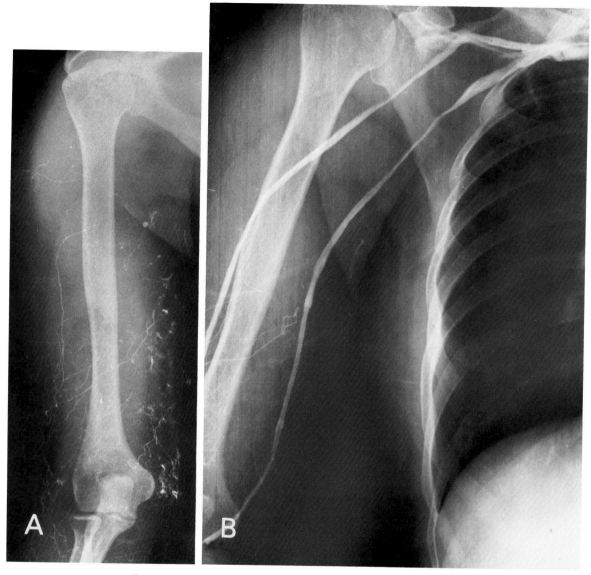

FIG. 9.75. EDEMA—POSTMASTECTOMY AND POSTRADIATION THERAPY

A: Lymphatic obstruction; and *B:* extrinsic compression of axillary and cephalic veins.

network; these vessels are, in general, fine in caliber and there is soft tissue suffusion of the radiopaque material. The venogram demonstrates an irregular axillary vein, suggesting thrombophlebitis.

Another patient with extrinsic venous disease in combination with lymphatic obstruction is shown in Figure 9.75. This patient developed edema of the arm following a radical mastec-tomy and radiation therapy. The axillary and cephalic veins are tapered in the axilla, suggesting extrinsic compression. The lymphangiogram reveals extensive collateral circulation through lymphatics of fine caliber and slight soft tissue suffusion of the contrast material. The lymphangiographic picture in such instances has been consistent.

SELECTED READINGS

Anatomy

Ackerman, L. V. and Del Regato, J. A.: *Cancer: Diagnosis, Treatment and Prognosis.* 4th ed. C. V. Mosby Co., St. Louis, 1970.

Bartels, P.: *Das Lymphgefaessystem.* Jena, 1909.

Plentl, A. and Friedman, E.: *Lymphatic System of the Female Genitals.* Vol II. W. B. Saunders Co., Philadelphia, 1971.

Reiffenstuhl, G.: *The Lymphatics of the Female Genital Organs.* J. B. Lippincott Co., Philadelphia, 1964.

Rouviere, H.: *Anatomy of the Human Lymphatic System.* trans. by J. M. Tobias, Edwards Co., Ann Arbor, 1938.

Cervix, Vulva and Uterus

Benninghoff, D. L., Herman, P. G. and Nelson, J. H., Jr.: Clinicopathologic correlation of lymphography and lymph node metastases in gynecological neoplasms. Cancer, *19:* 885, 1966.

Biggs, J. S.: Lymphography in carcinoma of the cervix. Aust. N. Z. J. Obstet. Gynaecol., *5:* 147, 1965.

Comas, M. R., Morris, C. H. and Averette, H. E.: Lymphography and vulvar carcinoma. Obstet. Gynecol., *33:* 177, 1969.

Conrad, J., Elkin, M. and Romney, S. L.: Pelvic angiography and lymphangiography in the evaluation of the patient with carcinoma of the cervix. Surg. Gynecol. Obstet., *122:* 983, 1966.

Davidson, J. W. and Van Lierop, M. J.: Lymphography and prognosis in carcinoma of the cervix. Am. J. Obstet. Gynecol., *112:* 669, 1972.

Delclos, L., Fletcher, G. H., Gutierrez, A. E. and Rutledge, F. N.: Adenocarcinoma of the uterus. Am. J. Roentgenol. Radium Ther. Nucl. Med., *105:* 603, 1969.

Dolan, P. A. and Hughes, R. R.: Lymphography in genital cancer. Surg. Gynecol. Obstet., *118:* 1286, 1964.

Doppman, J. L. and Chretien, P.: Visceral pelvic venography in carcinoma of the cervix. Radiology, *98:* 405, 1971.

Douglas, B., MacDonald, J. S. and Baker, J. W.: Lymphography in carcinoma of the uterus. Clin. Radiol., *23:* 286, 1972.

Fletcher, G. H. and Rutledge, F. N.: Carcinoma of uterine cervix. In *Modern Radiotherapy: Gynaecological Cancer*, edited by T. J. Deeley. Butterworths, London, 1971.

Fuchs, W. A. and Seiler-Rosenberg, G.: Lymphography in carcinoma of the uterine cervix. Acta Radiol. (Diagn.), *16:* 353, 1975.

Gerteis, W.: The frequency of metastases in carcinoma of the cervix and corpus. In *Progress in Lymphology*, edited by A. Ruttimann. Georg Thieme Verlag, Stuttgart, 1967.

Hagen, S. and Bjorn-Hansen, R.: Lymphography in the treatment of carcinoma of the vulva. Acta Radiol. (Diagn.), *11:* 609, 1971.

Hartgill, J. C.: Lymphogram control during pelvic lymphadenectomy. Proc. R. Soc. Med., *64:* 401, 1971.

Henriksen, E.: Distribution of metastases Stage I carcinoma of the cervix, study of 66 autopsied cases. Am. J. Obstet. Gynecol., *80:* 919, 1960.

Hliniak, I. and Vorbrodt, J.: The use of lymphangiography in cervical cancer. Radiol. Diagn. (Berl.), *13:* 655, 1972.

Hodari, A. A. and Hodgkinson, C. P.: Lymphography as a diagnostic aid in female genital malignancy. Obstet. Gynecol., *29:* 34, 1967.

Hreshchychyn, M. M. and Sheehan, R. R.: Collateral lymphatics in patients with gynecologic carcinoma. Am. J. Obstet. Gynecol., *91:* 118, 1965.

Jackson, R. J.: Lymphographic studies related to the problem of metastatic spread from carcinoma of the female genital tract. J. Obstet. Gynaec. Br. Commonw., *74:* 339, 1967.

Jackson, R. J.: Topography of the iliopelvic lymph nodes. Considerations relating to the treatment of carcinoma of the cervix. Am. J. Obstet. Gynecol., *104:* 1118, 1969.

Jing, B. S., McGraw, J. P. and Rutledge, F.: Gynecologic applications of lymphangiography. Surg. Gynecol. Obstet., *119:* 763, 1964.

Keating, G. M.: Lymphangioadenography in the study of malignant disease in gynecology. J. Med. Soc. N. J., *63:* 89, 1966.

Kittridge, R. D., Burger, R., Finby, N. and Draper, J.: An illustration of an approach to the diagnosis of pelvic disease. J. Urol., *89:* 607, 1963.

Kolbenstvedt, A.: Lymphography in the diagnosis of metastases from carcinoma of the uterine cervix stages I and II. Acta Radiol. (Diagn.), *16:* 81, 1975.

Lagrutta, J. and Grassi, G.: Lymphadenotomography in cancer of the cervix. Ann. Obstet. Gynecol., *87:* 497, 1965.

Lagrutta, J., Grassi, G. and Bonfante, M.: Radical vulvectomy and pelvilymphadenography. Panminerva Med., *9:* 94, 1967.

Lang, E. K., Simon, K. J., Cummings, D. H., et al.: Arteriography, pelvic pneumography and lymphangiography augmenting assessment and staging of carcinoma of the uterine cervix. South. Med. J., *63:* 1249, 1970.

Lecart, C. and Lenfant, P.: Critical appraisal of lymphangiography in cancer of the female genital tract. Lymphology, *4:* 100, 1971.

Lee, K. F., Greening, R., Kramer, S., Hahn, G. A., et al.: The value of pelvic venography and lymphography in the clinical staging of carcinoma of the uterine cervix. Am. J. Roentgenol. Radium Ther. Nucl. Med., *111:* 284, 1971.

Nair, M. K.: The diagnostic value of lymphangiography in the study of female genital cancer. Indian J. Cancer, *4:* 275, 1967.

Piver, M. S., Wallace, S. and Castro, J. R.: The accuracy of lymphangiography in carcinoma of the uterine cervix. Am. J. Roentgenol. Radium Ther. Nucl. Med., *111:* 278, 1971.

Reiffenstuhl, G.: The prognostic value of lymphography in carcinoma of the uterine cervix. In *Progress in Lymphology*, edited by A. Ruttimann. Georg Thieme Verlag, Stuttgart, 1967.

Tawil, E. and Belanger, R.: Prognostic value of the lymphangiogram in carcinoma of the uterine cervix. Radiology, *109:* 597, 1973.

Terry, L. N., Jr., Piver, M. S. and Hanks, G. E.: The value of lymphangiography in malignant disease of the uterine cervix. Radiology, *103:* 175, 1972.

Vincent, C. C.: Pelvic lymphangiography. The method, its diagnostic and therapeutic aid in female genital malignancies. J. Natl. Med. Assoc., *58:* 28, 1966.

Wallace, S. and Jackson, L.: Diagnostic criteria for lymphangiographic interpretation of malignant neoplasia. Cancer Chemother. Rep., *52:* 125, 1968.

Wallace, S. and Jing, B. S.: Lymphangiography in tumors of the female genital system. Radiol. Clin. North Am., *12:* 79, 1974.

Wallace, S., Jing, B. S. and Medellin, H.: Endometrial carcinoma: radiologic assistance in diagnosis, staging, and management. J. Gynecol. Oncol., *2:* 287, 1974.

Ovary

Athey, P. A., Wallace, S., Jing, B. S., Gallagher, H. S. and Smith, J. P.: Lymphangiography in ovarian cancer. Am. J. Roentgenol. Radium Ther. Nucl. Med., *123:* 106, 1975.

Douglas, B., MacDonald, J. S. and Baker, J. W.: Lymphography in carcinoma of the ovary. Proc. R. Soc. Med., *64:* 400, 1971.

Feldman, G. B., Knapp, R. C., Order, S. E. and Hellman, S.: Role of lymphatic obstruction in formation of ascites in murine ovarian carcinoma. Cancer Res., *32:* 2663, 1972.

Hanks, G. E., and Bagshaw, M. A.: Megavoltage radiation therapy and lymphangiography in ovarian cancer. Radiology, *93:* 649, 1969.

Hirabayashi, K. and Graham, J.: Genesis of ascites in ovarian cancer. Am. J. Obstet Gynecol., *106:* 492, 1970.

Jacobs, J. B.: Selective gonadal venography. Radiology, *92:* 855, 1960.

Marcille, M.: Lymphatiques et ganglions ilio-pelviens. Thèse de Paris, 1902, and **Tribune Mèdicale**, 1903, pp. 165–170.

Picard, J.: Lymphography in cancer of the ovary. Gynecol. Obstet., *63:* 585, 1964.

Wharton, J. T., Smith, J. P., Delclos, L. and Fletcher, G. H.: Tumors of ovary. In *Gynecology and Obstetrics.* F. A. Davis Co., Philadelphia, 1945.

Testicle

Busch, F. M., Sayegh, E. S. and Shenault, O. W., Jr.: Some uses of lymphangiography in the management of testicular tumors. J. Urol., *93:* 490, 1965.

Chiappa, S., Uslenghi, C. and Bonadonna, G.: Combined testicular and foot lymphangiography in testicular carcinomas. Surg. Gynecol. Obstet., *123:* 104, 1966a.

Chiappa, S., Uslenghi, C. and Galli, G.: Lymphangiography and endolymphatic radiotherapy in testicular tumors. Br. J. Radiol., *39:* 498, 1966b.

Cook, F. E., Lawrence, D. D., Smith, J. R. and Gritti, E. J.: Testicular carcinoma and lymphangiography. Radiology, *84:* 420, 1965.

Cuméo, B.: Note pur les lymphatiques du testicle. Bull. Mem. Soc. *46:* 574, 1959.

de Roo, T. and van Minden, S. H.: Lymphographic findings in a series of 258 patients with tumors of the testes. Lymphology, *6:* 97, 1973.

Fein, R. L. and Taber, D. O.: Foot lymphography in the testis tumor patients; a review of fifty cases. Cancer, *24:* 248, 1969.

Fuchs, W. A. and Girod, M.: Lymphography as a guide to prognosis in malignant testicular tumors. Acta Radiol. (Diagn.), *16:* 305, 1975.

Gagnon, J. H., Mount, B. M., Khonsari, H. and MacKinnon, K. J.: Lymphography in germinal tumors of the testis. Br. J. Urol., *44:* 136, 1972.

Johnson, D. E., ed., *Testicular Tumors.* Medical Examination Publishing Co., New York, 1972.

Jonsson, K., Ingemansson, S. and Ling, L.: Lymphography in patients with testicular tumors. Br. J. Urol., *45:* 548, 1973.

Maier, J. G. and Schamber, D. T.: The role of lymphography in the diagnosis and treatment of malignant testicular tumors. Am. J. Roentgenol. Radium Ther. Nucl. Med., *114:* 482, 1972.

van Minden, S. H.: The value of lymphography in tumors of the testes. Radiol. Clin. Biol., *40:* 274, 1971.

Wahlqvist, L., Hulten, L. and Rosencrantz, M.: Normal lymphatic drainage of the testis studied by funicular lymphography. Acta Chir. Scand., *132:* 454, 1966.

Wallace, N.: Lymphography in the management of testicular tumors. Clin Radiol., *20:* 453, 1969.

Wallace, S. and Jing, B. S.: Lymphography; diagnosis of nodal metastases from testicular malignancies. J.A.M.A., *213:* 94, 1970.

Kidney

Bell, R. D., Keyl, M. J. and Shrader, F. R.: Renal lymphatics: the internal distribution. Nephron, *5:* 454, 1968.

MacDonald, J. S.: Lymphography in renal tumors. Br. J. Radiol., *42:* 959, 1969.

Bladder and Prostate

Arduino, L. J. and Glucksman, M. A.: Lymphatic spread from prostatic cancer. J. Urol., *88:* 91, 1962.

Castellino, R. A.: The role of lymphography in "apparently localized" prostatic carcinoma. Lymphology, *8:* 16, 1975.

Castellino, R. A., Ray, G., Blank, N., Govan, D. and Bagshaw, M.: Lymphangiography in prostatic carcinoma; preliminary observations. J.A.M.A., *223:* 877, 1973.

Flocks, R. H., Culp, D. and Porto, R.: Lymphatic spread from prostatic cancer. J. Urol., *81:* 194, 1959.

Galesanu, M. R. and Rosenbaum, S.: Diagnosis of lymph node invasion of bladder and prostatic cancer by lympho- and pelvic phlebography. Int. Urol. Nephrol., *5:* 163, 1973.

Grossman, I., von Phul, R., Fitzgerald, J. P., Masih, S., Tuner, A. F., Kurohara, S. S. and George, F., III: The early lymphatic spread of manifest prostatic adenocarcinoma. Radiology, *120:* 673, 1974.

Higgs, B. and MacDonald, J. S.: Lymphography in the management of urinary tract tumors. Br. J. Urol., *40:* 727, 1968.

Hill, D. R., Quintous, E. C. and Walsh, P. C.: Prostate carcinoma; radiation treatment of the primary and regional lymphatics. Cancer, *34:* 156, 1974.

Jewett, H. J. and Strong, G. H.: Infiltrating carcinoma of the bladder: relation of depth of penetration of the bladder wall to incidence of local extension and metastases. J. Urol., *55:* 366, 1946.

Johnson, D. E., Kaesler, K. E., Kaminsky, S., Jing, B. S. and Wallace, S.: Lymphangiography as an aid in staging bladder carcinoma. South Med. J., *69:* 28, 1976.

Laplante, M. and Brice, M., II: The upper limits of hopeful application of radical cystectomy for visical carcinoma: does nodal metastasis always indicate incurability. J. Urol., *109:* 261, 1973.

MacDonald, J. S.: Lymphography in malignant disease of the urinary tract. Proc. R. Soc. Med., *63:* 1237, 1970.

Marshall, V. F.: Current clinical problems regarding bladder tumors. In *Bladder Tumors: A Symposium,* edited by V. F. Marshall, pp. 1–8. J. B. Lippincott, Philadelphia, 1956.

Miller, L. S. and Johnson, D. E.: Megavoltage irradiation for bladder cancer: alone, postoperative or preoperative? In *Proceedings of the Seventh National Cancer Congress.* J. B. Lippincott, New York, 1973.

Rummelhardt, S. and Fussek, H.: Lymphangioadenographie in der urologie. Erfahsungren and Ergebnisse Urologie, *9:* 933, 1970.

Wheeler, J. S.: Lymphography in early prostatic cancer. Urology, *3:* 444, 1974.

Whitmore, W. F., Jr.: The rationale and results of ablative surgery for prostatic cancer. Cancer, *16:* 1119, 1963.

Wirtanen, G. W. and Miller, R. C.: Bladder lymphatics and tumor dissemination. J. Urol., *109:* 58, 1973.

Penis

Janca, K., Popovic, L. and Dimkovic, D.: Lymphography in disease of the penis. Int. Urol. Nephrol., *4:* 59, 1972.

Riveros, M., Garcia, R. and Cabanas, R.: Lymphadenography of the dorsal lymphatics of the penis. Techniques and results. Cancer, *20:* 2026, 1967.

Large Intestine

Chiappa, S., Bonadonna, G., Uslenghi, C. and Veronesi, U.: Lymphangiography in the diagnosis of retroperitoneal node metastases in rectal cancer. Br. J. Radiol., *45:* 584, 1967.

Cohn, I.: Cause and prevention of recurrence following surgery for colon cancer. Cancer, *28:* 183, 1971.

Cole, W. H., Roberts, S. S., Webb, R. S., Strehl, F. W. and Oates, G. D.: Dissemination of cancer with special emphasis on vascular spread and implantation. Ann. Surg., *161:* 753, 1965.

Copeland, E. M., Miller, L. D. and Jones, R. S.: Prognostic factors in carcinoma of the colon and rectum. Am. J. Surg., *116:* 875, 1968.

Crile, G., Jr., Isbister, W. and Deodhar, S. D.: Demonstration that large metastases in lymph nodes disseminate cancer cells to blood and lungs. Cancer, *28:* 657, 1971.

Dukes, C. E. and Bussey, H. J. R.: The spread of rectal cancer and its effect on prognosis. Br. J. Cancer, *12:* 309, 1958.

Fisher, E. P. and Turnbull, R. B.: The cytologic demonstration and significance of tumor cells in the mesenteric venous blood in patients with colorectal carcinoma. Surg. Gynecol. Obstet., *100:* 102, 1955.

Fisher, E. P. and Fisher, B.: Experimental studies of factors influencing hepatic metastases: I. The effect of number of tumor cells injected and time of growth. Cancer, *12:* 926, 1959.

Fisher, B. and Fisher, E. P.: Experimental studies of factors influencing hepatic metastases: II. Effect of partial hepatectomy. Cancer, *12:* 929, 1959.

Fisher, B. and Fisher, E. P.: Experimental studies of factors influencing hepatic metastases: III. Effect of surgical trauma with special reference to liver injury. Ann. Surg., *150:* 731, 1959.

Fred, H. L., Eiband, J. M. and Collins, L. C.: Calcifications in intra-abdominal and retroperitoneal metastases. Am. J. Roentgenol. Radium Ther. Nucl. Med., *91:* 138, 1964.

Ghahremani, G. G. and Straua, F. H.: Calcification of distant lymph node metastases from cancer of the colon. Radiology, *99:* 65, 1971.

Gilchrist, R. K.: Lymphatic spread of carcinoma of the colon. Dis. Colon Rectum, *2:* 69, 1959.

Grinnell, R. S.: The lymphatic and venous spread of Ca of the rectum. Ann. Surg., *116:* 200, 1942.

Keynes, W. M.: Implantation from the bowel lumen in cancer of the large bowel. Ann. Surg., *153:* 357, 1961.

Marsili, E., Manfredi, L. and Borreani, B.: Lymphography in the study of cancer of the rectum. Panminerva Med., *9:* 62, 1967.

Messinger, N. H., Beneventano, T. C. and Siegelman, S. S.: Intra-flexural cancer of the colon: clinical-radiologic-pathologic correlations. Dis. Colon Rectum, *14:* 255, 1971.

Steidl, R. A.: Extensive calcified retroperitoneal lymph node metastases from a primary carcinoma of the cecum. Radiology, 89: 263, 1967.

Breast and Edema

Abbes, M.: Experience with lymphangiography in the surgical management of breast cancer. Int. Surg., 47: 243, 1967.

Askar, O. and Kassem, K. A.: The lymphatics of the leg in deep venous thrombosis. Br. J. Radiol., 42: 122, 1969.

Baltaxe, H. A., Meade, J. W. and Temes, G. D.: Lymphatic and venous examination of the postphlebitic extremity. Radiology, 91: 478, 1968.

Calnan, J. and Kountz, S. L.: Effect of venous obstruction on lymphatics. Br. J. Surg., 52: 800, 1965.

Danese, C. and Howard, J. M.: Postmastectomy lymphedema. Surg. Gynecol. Obstet., 120: 797, 1965.

Feldman, M. G., Kohan, P. and Edelman, S.: Lymphangiographic studies in obstructive lymphedema of the upper extremity. Surgery, 59: 935, 1966.

Hughes, J. H. and Patel, A. R.: Swelling of the arm following radical mastectomy. Br. J. Surg., 53: 4, 1966.

Hulten, L., Ahren, C. and Rosencrantz, M.: Lymphangio-adenography in carcinoma of the breast. Comparative clinical, roentgen, and histologic appraisal of the method for the demonstration of the lymph node metastases. Acta Chir. Scand., 132: 261, 1966.

Kendall, B. E., Arthur, J. F. and Patey, D. H.: Lymphangiography in carcinoma of the breast. Cancer, 16: 1233, 1963.

Kitchen, G.: Lymphangiographic studies in a case of postmastectomy lymphangiosarcoma. Br. J. Radiol., 45: 388, 1972.

Kitt, K., Lukacs, L. and Varga, G.: Diagnostic value of lymphography of the arm in the preoperative diagnosis of early metastases in breast cancer. Am. J. Surg., 123: 712, 1972.

Kreel, L. and George, P.: Postmastectomy lymphangiography detection of metastases and edema. Ann. Surg., 163: 470, 1964.

Pollard, W.: Lymphangiography in the surgical treatment of carcinoma of the cervix. Clin. Radiol., 20: 463, 1969.

Shibata, H. R., McLena, P., Vezina, J. L., Inglis, F. G. and Tabah, E. J.: Axillary lymphography in carcinoma of the breast. Surgery, 60: 329, 1966.

Smedal, M. I. and Evans, J. A.: Cause and treatment of edema of arm following radical mastectomy. Surg. Gynecol. Obstet., 111: 29, 1960.

Tsangaris, N. T. and Yutzy, C. V.: A lymphangiographic study of postmastectomy lymphedema. Surg. Gynecol. Obstet., 123: 1228, 1966.

Turner-Warwick, R. T.: The lymphatics of the breast. Br. J. Surg., 46: 574, 1957.

Miscellaneous

Ariel, I. M. and Resnick, M.: Altered lymphatic dynamics caused by cancer metastases. Arch. Surg., 94: 117, 1967.

Bellman, S. and Oden, B.: Regeneration of surgically divided lymph vessels. Acta Chir. Scand., 116: 99, 1959.

Berdon, W. E., Baker, D. H. and Poznanski, A.: Opacification of retrosternal lymph nodes following barium peritonitis. Report of two cases. Radiology, 106: 171, 1973.

Biggs, J. S. and Mackay, E. V.: Pelvic lymphocysts displayed by lymphography. J. Obstet. Gynaecol. Br. Commonw., 73: 264, 1966.

Bodie, J. F. and Linton, D. S., Jr.: Hepatic oil embolization as a complication of lymphangiography. Radiology, 99: 317, 1971.

Celis, A., Kuthy, J. and Del Castillo, E.: Importance of the thoracic duct in spread of malignant diseases. Acta Radiol., 45: 169, 1956.

Chavez, C. M.: The clinical significance of lymphatico-venous anastomosis. Its implications in lymphangiography. Vasc. Dis., 5: 35, 1968.

Chavez, C. M., Picard, J. D. and Davis, D.: Liver opacification following lymphangiography: pathogenesis and clinical significance. Surgery, 63: 564, 1968.

Edwards, J. M. and Kinmonth, J. B.: Lymphovenous shunts in man. Br. J. Surg., 56: 699, 1969.

Engeset, A.: An experimental study of the lymph node barrier. Injection of Walker carcinoma 256 in the lymph vessels. Extrait de Acta Union Internationale le Centre le Cancer, Vol. XV, 3-4, 1959.

Engeset, A.: Irradiation of lymph nodes and vessels. Acta Radiol., 1: (suppl. 229): 1, 1964.

Farrell, J.: Lymphangiographic demonstration of lymphovenous communication after radiotherapy in Hodgkin's disease. Radiology, 87: 630, 1966.

Gray, S. H. and Cohen, R. A.: Lymphaticovenous anastomoses involving the portal system: report of a case with metastatic carcinoma of vagina. Am. Surg., 32: 410, 1966.

Herman, P., Benninghoff, D. and Schwartz, J.: A physiologic approach to lymph flow in lymphography. Am. J. Roentgenol. Radium Ther. Nucl. Med., 91: 1207, 1964.

Job, T. T.: Lymphatico-venous communications in common rat and their significance. Am. J. Anat., 24: 467, 1918.

Koehler, P. R. and Schaffer, B.: Peripheral lymphatico-venous anastomoses. Report of two cases. Circulation, 35: 401, 1967.

Malek, P.: Some questions of the pathophysiology of the lymphatic system. Rev. Czech. Med., 5: 153, 1959.

Neyazaki, E., Kupic, E. A. and Marshall, W. H.: Collateral lymphatico-venous communications after experimental obstruction of the thoracic duct. Radiology, 85: 423, 1965.

Nielubowicz, J. and Olszewski, W.: Surgical lymphaticovenous shunts in patients with secondary lymphedema. Br. J. Surg., 55: 440, 1968.

Nielubowicz, J. and Olszewski, W.: Experimental lymphovenous anastomosis. Br. J. Surg., 55: 449, 1968.

Phillips, J. H.: The lymphatic system with particular reference to cardiac edema. Bull. Tulane Med. Fac., 14: 187, 1957.

Reichert, F. L.: The regeneration of the lymphatics. Arch. Surg., 13: 871, 1926.

Rivero, O. R., Calnan, J. S. and Reis, N. D.: Experimental peripheral lymphovenous communications. Br. J. Plast. Surg., 20: 124, 1967.

Roddenberry, H. and Allen, L.: Observations on the abdominal lymphaticovenous communications of the squirrel monkey (Saimiri sciures). Anat. Rec., 159: 147, 1967.

Roxin, T. and Bujar, H.: Lymphographic visualization of lymphaticovenous communications and their significance in malignant hemolymphopathies. Lymphology, 3: 127, 1970.

Rutledge, F., Dodd, G. D. and Kasilag, F. B.: Lymphocysts: a complication of radical pelvic surgery. Am. J. Obstet. Gynecol., 77: 1165, 1959.

Servelle, M.: Pathology of the thoracic duct. J. Cardiovasc. Surg. (Torino), 4: 702, 1963.

Steinberg, A. O., Madayag, M. A., Bosniak, M. A. and Morales, P. A.: Demonstration of two unusually large pelvic lymphocysts by lymphangiography. J. Urol, 109: 477, 1973.

Takashima, T. and Benninghoff, D. L.: Lymphatico-venous communications and lymph reflux after thoracic duct obstructions. An experimental study in the dog. Invest. Radiol., 1: 188, 1966.

Threefoot, S. A.: Gross and microscopic anatomy of the lymphatic vessels and lymphaticovenous communications. Cancer Chemother. Rep., 52: 1, 1968.

Threefoot, S. A. and Kossover, M. F.: Lymphaticovenous communications in man. Arch. Intern. Med., 117: 213, 1966.

Van Den Brenk, H. A. S.: Effects of ionizing radiations on regeneration and behavior of mammalian lymphatics; in vivo studies of Sandison Clark chambers. Am. J. Roentgenol. Radium Ther. Nucl. Med., 78: 837, 1957.

Wallace, S., Jackson, L. and Dodd, G. D.: Lymphangiographic interpretation. Radiol. Clin. North Am., 3: 467, 1965.

Wallace, S., Jackson, L. and Dodd, G. D.: Radiographic demonstration of lymphatic dynamics. Prog. Clin. Cancer, 3: 157, 1967.

Wolfel, D. A.: Lymphaticovenous communications, a clinical reality. Am. J. Roentgenol. Radium Ther. Nucl. Med., 95: 766, 1965.

Yune, H. Y. and Klatte, E. C.: Lymphography in lymphatic obstruction. Radiology, 92: 824, 1969.

10

Complications

MELVIN E. CLOUSE, M.D.

Lymphography, like all procedures which introduce a foreign substance into the body, is associated with complications. The major complications of lymphography are caused by the vital dyes and contrast materials rather than technique. The ideal contrast material — one that has no negative side effects and gives sharp delineation of lymph vessels and nodes for a period of time — is not yet available. Initially, water-soluble contrast media such as Cholegraphin were used (Tjernberg, 1956). Node detail was inadequate with these media, however, because they are diluted during passage through the lymphatic system. Ethiodol, a fat-soluble contrast agent, is the contemporary agent of choice: it offers sharp delineation and remains in the lymph nodes for several months (permitting follow-up of progressive lymph node changes). Ethiodol also has negative side effects, however.

Body Distribution of Ethiodol

Ethiodol passes from the lymph vessels into the venous system via the thoracic duct or by lymphaticovenous communications (usually caused by lymphatic obstruction peripheral to the thoracic duct). The lower the obstruction in the lymphatic system, the greater the chance of more oil entering the venous system and hence into the lungs, increasing the severity of pulmonary oil emboli.

Koehler et al. (1964) studied the body distribution of Ethiodol in dogs. After 3 days the highest concentration was in the lungs (50%), lymphatic system (25%), bone (4.2%), muscle (3.9%), brain (0.38%), and kidney (0.2%). The concentration in the lungs decreased to 9.8% after 17 days while that retained in lymph nodes remained almost constant at 20%. These figures are not directly applicable to humans because the number of iliac and retroperitoneal lymph nodes in the dog is considerably less than in humans.

On whole body scans performed after intraaortic injection of [131]I Ethiodol, Threefoot (1968) found the major portions in the liver, lungs, and

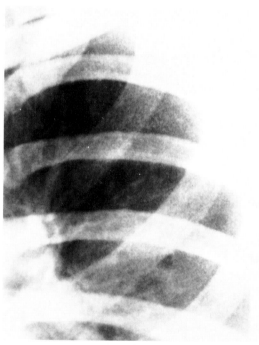

FIG. 10.1. ETHIODOL
Left upper lung field 24 hr after injection of 7 ml of Ethiodol into lymphatics of each lower extremity. Fine stippled densities indicate embolized Ethiodol. The patient was asymptomatic.

kidneys. This finding suggests that these organs have a more effective filter for oil than the other organs and peripheral regions. Further studies by Threefoot showed that 75–90% of the iodine in venous blood during the first 2 days was in the lipid form in the plasma. The iodine was redistributed in the plasma to lipid and aqueous states as well as being adhered to the red cells. After 9 days almost all of the plasma iodine was in the aqueous state. The iodine was excreted by the kidneys in this form with approximately 90% being recovered in 3 weeks. The fate of the lipid portion of the molecule is not completely known, but it is probably degraded by beta oxidation.

Pulmonary Oil Emboli

Because the lymphatics drain directly into the venous system, oil embolization occurs to a degree in every patient examined, but the amount of pulmonary oil embolization is difficult to determine. Even when constant amounts of contrast material are injected, variations occur in the amount retained in the nodes, the size and number of nodes, and the presence or absence of lymphaticovenous communications. Ethiodol can only be identified in 19–55% of routine postlymphography chest films (Bron et al., 1963; Clouse et al., 1966; MacDonald and Wallace, 1965) (Fig.10.1). Abrams et al.(1968) have shown considerable amounts of Ethiodol in small pulmonary arteries at postmortem in dogs that were not visible on the chest radiographs. Ethiodol can be differentiated from neutral fat in the tissues using brilliant cresyl blue and silver nitrate stain (Felton, 1952; Hallgrimsson and Clouse, 1965).

Pulmonary oil embolization usually does not produce clinical symptoms unless there is underlying cardiopulmonary pathology, excess amounts of contrast material are given (over 14–16 ml of Ethiodol), patent lymphaticovenous communications shunt more oil to the lungs, or the patient is hypersensitive to the oil. Fraimow et al. (1966) noted a decrease in diffusion capacity 2–24 hr after injection with a beginning of return to normal in 48 hr. Gold et al. (1965) also reported a decrease in diffusion capacity, pul-

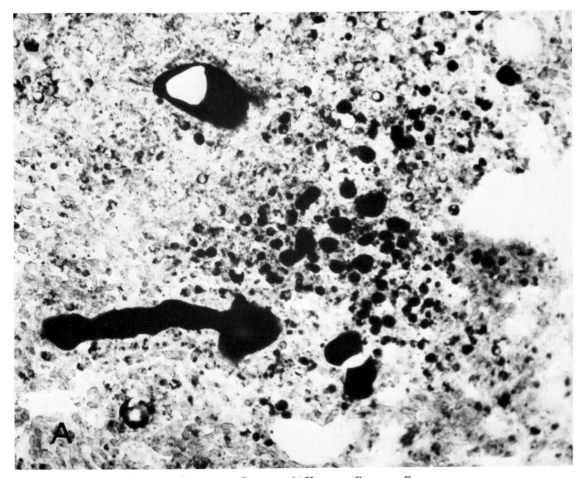

FIG. 10.2. PULMONARY REACTION 24 HR AFTER ETHIODOL EMBOLIZATION

A. Photomicrograph (×290) of guinea pig lung 24 hr after Ethiodol injection (fat stain). The oil is distributed in both small arterioles and alveoli.

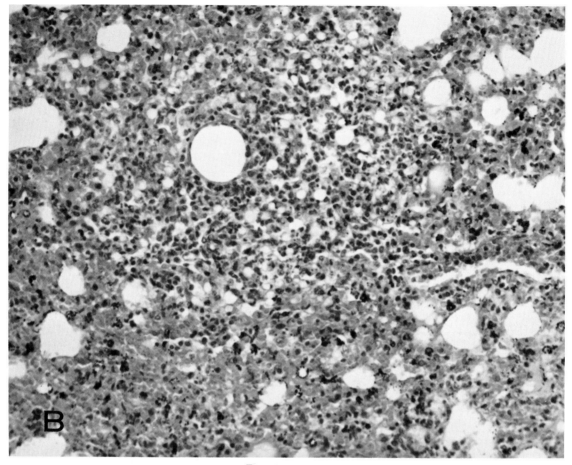

FIG. 10.2 (cont.)

B. Photomicrograph (×290) of guinea pig lung 24 hr after Ethiodol injection (H & E stain). Acute inflammatory infiltrate surrounding globules of oil (clear spaces).

monary capillary blood volume, and lung compliance without any clinical symptoms of pulmonary oil emboli. Gold et al. attributed the abnormality in diffusion capacity to a decrease in pulmonary capillary blood volume produced by oil emboli. Fraimow et al., however, believe it is caused by both a decrease in capillary blood volume and an inflammatory reaction in the alveolocapillary space. White et al. (1973) could not demonstrate an abnormality in the forced expiratory volume in 1 and 2 sec or vital capacity 1 month after lymphography. They concluded that only patients with severe lung disease would require careful assessment before lymphography.

To study the fate of Ethiodol in the lungs and the pulmonary reaction, 0.1 ml of Ethiodol was given intravenously to 0.4- and 0.5-kg guinea pigs. The animals were sacrificed 24 hr to 32 days after injection. Ethiodol was not visible roentgenographically after 12 days, but it was found microscopically in considerable amounts even after 32 days. The animal sacrificed at 24 hr showed Ethiodol in small pulmonary arteries as well as extravasation of serum and Ethiodol into the alveoli surrounded by large numbers of neutrophils and lymphocytes (Fig. 10.2). Histiocytes were present within 48 hr (Fig. 10.3), and after 8 days these predominated over the acute inflammatory response (Fig. 10.4).

The acute inflammatory response gradually regressed so that in 32 days there was clearing of most of the alveolar exudate and lipid material. Alveolar walls remained thickened by proliferation of capillary endothelium and alveolar lining cells. The remaining Ethiodol was scattered throughout the blood vessels of the lung with isolated oil granulomata (Fig. 10.5).

Ethiodol was demonstrated in pulmonary arteries and capillaries of 4 patients dying from causes unrelated to lymphography 1–33 days after lymphography. An endothelial reaction

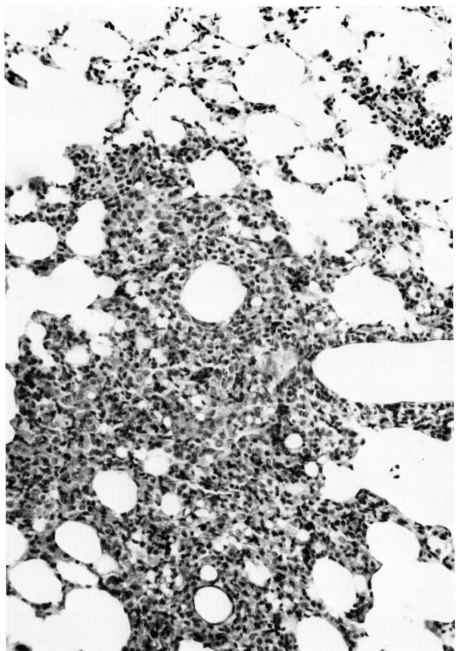

FIG. 10.3. PULMONARY REACTION 48 HR AFTER ETHIODOL EMBOLIZATION

Photomicrograph (×255) of guinea pig lung 48 hours after Ethiodol injection (H & E stain). Histiocytes now predominate over lymphocytes and neutrophiles. Oil is seen as clear spaces within infiltrate.

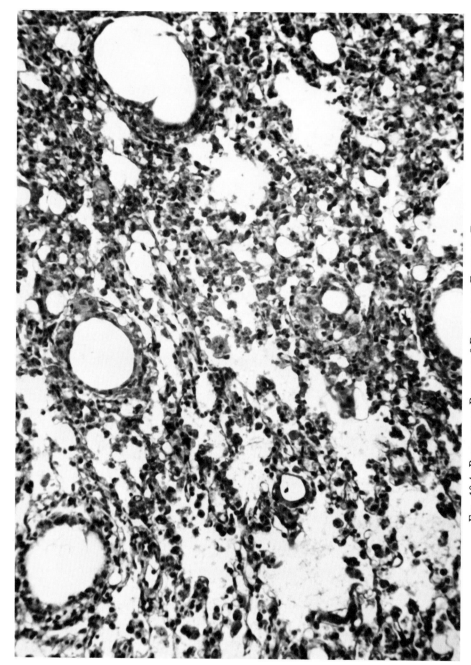

FIG. 10.4. PULMONARY REACTION 8 DAYS AFTER ETHIODOL EMBOLIZATION

Photomicrograph (×255) of guinea pig lung 8 days after Ethiodol injection. Oil granulomas are seen as clear spaces surrounded by giant cells and large histiocytes.

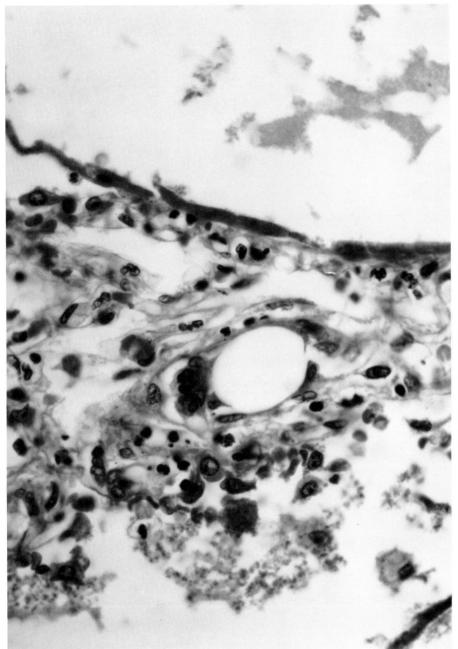

FIG. 10.5. HUMAN LUNG 11 DAYS AFTER LYMPHOGRAPHY

Photomicrograph (×725) of human lung 11 days after lymphography. Oil granuloma represented by a clear space with surrounding foreign body giant cells.

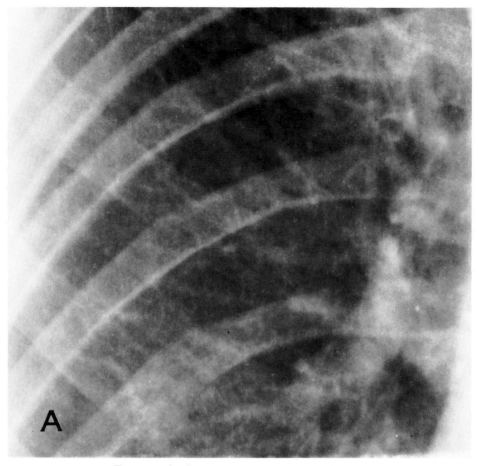

FIG. 10.6. OIL PNEUMONITIS AFTER LYMPHOGRAPHY

A. Chest normal on a 42-year-old female who had lymphography (7 ml of Ethiodol injected into each extremity) for carcinoma of the vulva.

consisting of histiocytic cells was identified within the lipid-containing vessels. These inflammatory changes presumably regressed without serious sequelae or the amount of oil reaching the lungs did not damage a significant number of alveolocapillary units. Schaffer et al. (1963) reported no Ethiodol in pulmonary capillaries in patients autopsied several months after lymphography. There have not been reports of significant long term effects of pulmonary oil embolization.

Pneumonia

The incidence of oil pneumonitis is probably more common than reported because it is not usually life-threatening. Patients with pneumonia usually spike a temperature of 101–104° within 6–12 hr after the injection. Roentgenograms of the chest in these patients show diffuse oil emboli as soft discrete nodular densities throughout both lungs (Fig. 10.6). Fever gradu-ally subsides within 4–5 days and the pulmonary infiltrate resolves within 5–7 days. Pneumonia has been reported in 5 of 108 consecutive examinations (4.6%) (Clouse et al., 1966) and 2.8% (Kutarna et al., 1972). In a survey of 32,000 examinations Koehler (1968) found an incidence of 1:2500 but believed it was much higher.

Pulmonary edema, infarction, and cardiovascular collapse associated with dyspnea, cyanosis, and pleuritic chest pain have been reported. These reactions are life-threatening and require oxygen, vasopressors, and digitalis (Bron et al., 1963; Fuchs, 1962; Schaffer et al., 1962).

Neurologic Complications

Cerebral complications after lymphography are rare. Twenty-two cases have been reported in the world literature (Boudin et al., 1967; Cardis, 1967; Colette, 1967; Collard et al., 1969; Davidson, 1969; Gerest et al., 1967; Gerhard and

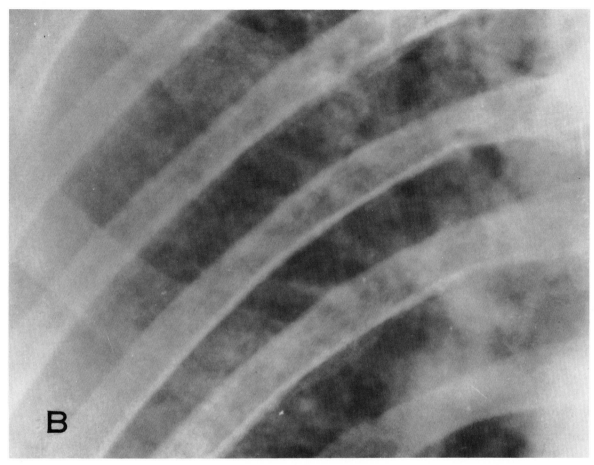

B. The patient's temperature was 102° 6 hr after injection. She was slightly dyspneic with no cough, chest pain or cyanosis. Chest roentgenogram 48 hr after injection revealed multiple small soft nodular densities in both lungs.

Brolsch, 1972; Gruwez, 1967; Koehler, 1968; Mikol et al., 1970; Moskowitz et al., 1972; Nelson et al., 1965; Okuda et al., 1971; Rasmussen, 1970; Sviridov, 1972; Veyssier et al., 1971). Three of these were fatal (Nelson et al., 1965; Gruwez, 1967; Gerhard and Brolsch, 1972). Nelson et al. reported the first fatality after injecting 20 ml of Ethiodol into each lower extremity. Gerhard and Brolsch reported a patient who received 15 ml of Lipiodol, but the patient had received irradiation for lymphoma. These patients experienced mental confusion, disorientation, motor weaknesses or paralysis, and coma. Rasmussen (1970) and Jay and Ludington (1973) reported temporary blindness in association with other cerebral symptoms of oil emboli in 2 patients. Both recovered completely within 6 weeks.

Ethiodol may short circuit the lung filter via intracardiac shunts, pulmonary arteriovenous fistulae, and possibly shunts within a lung tumor. Lymphaticovenous communications may also allow excess contrast material to reach the lung and overload its filter system. Animal experiments by Davidson (1969) suggest that radiation to the lung impairs the filter mechanism, presumably by capillary damage. This allows more oily contrast media to pass into the arterial circuit and become peripheral emboli.

Hypersensitivity

Patent Blue Dye. Hohenfellner and Ludvik (1964) reported the first patient having an allergic reaction to patent blue violet dye. Since then approximately 32 cases have been reported (Gruwez, 1967; Mortazavi and Burrows, 1971; Collard and Colette, 1967; Sieber, 1968). The true incidence is difficult to ascertain. Mortazavi and Burrows reported 3 cases in a series of 120 lymphograms. Two of their patients had negative skin tests to Xylocaine. Kropholler (1967), who does not mix patent blue with Xylocaine, reported 6 cases in 400 lymphograms. These and recent reports suggest that true inci-

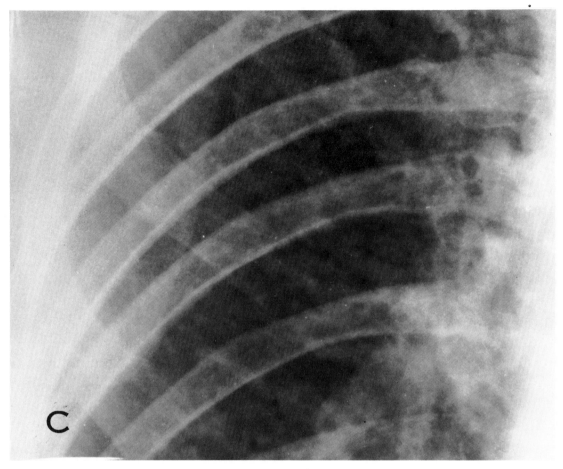

FIG. 10.6 (*cont.*)

C. The patient experienced daily temperature elevations gradually decreasing to normal over a 4-day period. Chest roentgenogram shows almost complete clearing after 9 days.

dence is much more common than originally reported, probably near 1%.

The allergic reaction usually manifests itself within minutes after injection by urticaria and blue wheals stained by blue serum from the dye. The reaction may require only subcutaneous epinephrine or intravenous antihistamines. More severe reactions may lead to bronchospasm; periorbital, glossal, and laryngeal edema; and hypotension. In such patients epinephrine, intravenous hydrocortisone, vasopressors, or tracheal intubation with respiratory assistance may be necessary. Death has not been reported.

Sokolowski and Engeset (1974) have recently reported marked cellular death and lymphocyte depletion in lymph nodes of dogs whose efferent vessels were ligated prior to the injection of patent blue violet dye. Similar but less severe changes were noted in nodes, the efferent ves-

sels of which were not ligated. These changes have not been reported in humans and probably are not clinically significant. The lymph nodes observed in humans almost always have superimposed inflammatory changes secondary to Ethiodol, however.

Ethiodol. Allergic reactions to the oily contrast media are sometimes difficult to evaluate because of the normal reaction of the lung to oil and superimposed pneumonia (which is probably always present even though it is not detected roentgenographically). Koehler (1968) reported an incidence of 1 in 800 lymphographies. Bray et al. (1970) reported two cases of Loeffler's syndrome in a series of 88 lymphograms. Symptoms began at 2 and 6 days after lymphography and were characterized by chills, fever, slight cyanosis, and blood-streaked sputum with eosinophiles. The white blood cell count demonstrated 22% and 6% eosinophilia. The syndrome slowly cleared spontaneously.

Wiertz et al. (1971) reported a case of intra-pulmonary hemorrhage and anemia occurring 5 days after lymphography. Dyspnea and hemoptysis were combined with a drop in the hematocrit from 43% to 28% over a 3-day period. The reaction did not impair pulmonary functions seriously and the lungs cleared spontaneously after 1 week. Kohler et al. (1969) reported 9 cases in a series of 1,000 lymphangiograms using 7-8 ml of ultrafluid Lipiodol for the lower extremities and 3-4 ml for the arm. This large series suggests that allergy to the contrast material approaches 1%.

Cardiac

No cardiac fatalities have been reported, but Leitsmann and Dietzsch (1972) reported abnormal electrocardiogram changes in 12 of 25 patients undergoing lymphography. The abnormalities were S-T segment depression and T-wave flattening.

Minor Complications

Fever may occur as an isolated complication. The patient may experience one transient temperature elevation 6–18 hr after lymphography. This may be caused by pyrogens entering the lymphatics or more likely, Ethiodol. This complication is missed when lymphograms are done as an outpatient procedure, but it is not significant.

Patients may also experience a low grade temperature (99-101°) with gradual return to normal after 3-4 days. Although it cannot be documented radiographically, this probably is a low grade oil pneumonitis or generalized low grade inflammatory reaction to the contrast material. Only symptomatic treatment is required.

Delayed wound healing which can be treated with warm saline soaks occurs in a few patients. Lymphangitis and wound infection rarely develop but do respond to antibiotics and warm saline soaks.

REFERENCES

Abrams, H. L., Takahashi, M. and Adams, D. F.: Clinical and experimental studies of pulmonary oil embolism. Cancer Chemother. Rep., *52:* 81, 1968.

Boudin, G., Pepin, B. and Vernant, J-C.: Manifestations neuropsychiatriques au decors d'une lymphographie. Bull. Soc. Med. Hop. Paris, *118:* 1027, 1967.

Bray, D. A., Brown, C. H., Herdt, J. R. and DeVita, V. T.: Loeffler's syndrome as a complication of bipedal lymphangiography. J.A.M.A., *214:* 369, 1970.

Bron, K. M., Baum, S. and Abrams, H. L.: Oil embolism in lymphangiography. Incidence, manifestations, and mechanisms. Radiology, *80:* 194, 1963.

Cardis, R.: Lymphography, panel discussion. II. A. Complications and accidents. In *Progress in Lymphology: Proceedings of the International Symposium on Lymphology, Zurich, Switzerland, July 19–23, 1966,* p. 323, Georg Thieme Verlag, Stuttgart, 1967.

Clouse, M. E., Hallgrimsson, J. and Wenlund, P. E.: Complications following lymphography with particular reference to pulmonary oil embolization. Am. J. Roentgenol. Radium Ther. Nucl. Med., *96:* 972, 1966.

Colette, J. M.: Lymphography, panel discussion. II. A. Complications and accidents. In *Progress in Lymphology: Proceedings of the International Symposium on Lymphology, Zurich, Switzerland, July 19–23, 1966,* p. 323, Georg Thieme Verlag, Stuttgart, 1967.

Collard, M. and Colette, J. M.: Les modalities cliniques de l'allergie au bleu patente violet. J. Belge Radiol., *50:* 407, 1967.

Collard, M., Leroux, G., Noel, G. and Declercq, A.: L'embolie cerebrale graisseuse diffuse: complication de la lymphographie lipiodolee. J. Radiol. Electrol. Med. Nucl., *50:* 793, 1969.

Collard, M. and Noel, G.: Embolies cerebrales graisseuses, complication de l'exame l'esamen lymphographique au lipiodol. Acta Neurol. Belg., *69:* 419, 1969.

Davidson, J. W.: Lipid embolism to the brain following lymphography. Case report and experimental study. Am. J. Roentgenol. Radium Ther. Nucl. Med., *105:* 763, 1969.

Felton, E. L., II: A method for the identification of Lipiodol in tissue sections. Lab. Invest., *1:* 3, 1952.

Fraimow, W., Wallace, S., Lewis, P., Greening, R. R. and Cathcart, R. T.: Changes in pulmonary function due to lymphography. Radiology, *85:* 231, 1966.

Fuchs, W. A.: Complications in lymphography with oily contrast media. Acta Radiol., *57:* 427, 1962.

Gerest, F., Rouves, L., Maleysson, M. and Saint-Paul, J.: Encephalopathie a semeiologie psychiatrique consecutive a une lymphographie. Lyon Med., *218:* 1435, 1967.

Gerhard, L. and Brolsch, C.: Morphology of the central nervous system with lipiodol following lymphography. Verh. Dtsch. Ges. Sch. Path., *56:* 401, 1972.

Gold, W. M., Youker, J., Anderson, S. and Nadel, J. A.: Pulmonary function abnormalities after lymphangiography. N. Engl. J. Med., *273:* 519, 1965.

Gruwez, J.: Lymphography, panel discussion. II. A. Complications and accidents. In *Progress in Lymphology: Proceedings of the International Symposium on Lymphology, Zurich, Switzerland, July 19–23, 1966,* p. 322, Georg Thieme Verlag, Stuttgart, 1967.

Hallgrimsson, J. and Clouse, M. E.: Pulmonary oil emboli after lymphography. Arch. Pathol., *80:* 426, 1965.

Hohenfellner, R. and Ludvik, W.: Die Lymphographie in der Urologischn diagnostik. Urologe [A], *3:* 87, 1964.

Jay, J. C. and Ludington, L. G.: Neurologic complications following lymphangiography. Possible mechanism and a case of blindness. Arch. Surg., *106:* 863, 1973.

Koehler, P. R.: Complications of lymphography. Lymphology, *1:* 116, 1968.

Koehler, P., Meyers, W. A., Skelley, J. F. and Schaffer, B.: Body distribution of Ethiodol following lymphography. Radiology, *82:* 866, 1964.

Kohler, I., Platzbecker, H. and Fritz, H.: Komplikationen bei de oligen Lymphographie – ein bericht uber 1000 lymphographische Untersuchungen. Cesk. Radiol., *23:* 48, 1969.

Kropholler, R. W.: Lymphography, panel discussion. II. A. Complications and accidents. In *Progress in Lymphology: Proceedings of the International Symposium on Lymphology, Zurich, Switzerland, July 19–23, 1966*, p.306, Georg Thieme Verlag, Stuttgart, 1967.

Kutarna, A., Hanecka, M., Saskova, B. and Javorkova, J.: Lung complications following lymphographies with iodinated poppyseed oil. Bratisl. Lek. Listy, *58:* 581, 1972.

Leitsmann, H. and Dietzsch, J.: Electrocardiographic changes following lymphography. Zentralbl. Gynaekol., *14:* 1392, 1972.

MacDonald, J. S. and Wallace, E.: Lymphangiography in tumors of the kidney, bladder and testicle. Br. J. Radiol., *38:* 93, 1965.

Mikol, J., Bousser, M. G., Grellet, F., Chomette, G., Sors, C. and Garcin, R.: Paraplegie au cours d'une lymphographie chez un malade atteinte d'un reticulosarcome glanglionnaire cervical: etude anatomo-clinique. Ann. Med. Interne (Paris), *121:* 355, 1970.

Mortazavi, S. H. and Burrows, B. D.: Allergic reaction to patent blue dye in lymphography. Clin. Radiol., *22:* 389, 1971.

Moskowitz, G., Chen, P. and Adams, D. F.: Lipid embolization to the kidney and brain after lymphography. Radiology, *102:* 327, 1972.

Nelson, B., Rush, E. A., Takasugi, M. and Wittenberg, J.: Lipid embolism to the brain after lymphography. N. Engl. J. Med., *273:* 1132, 1965.

Okuda, K., Matsuo, H. and Adachi, M.: Side effect of lymphography with special reference to pulmonary and cerebral embolism. Rinsho Hoshasen, *16:* 979, 1971.

Rasmussen, K. E.: Retinal and cerebral fat emboli following lymphography with oily contrast media. Acta Radiol. (Diagn.), *10:* 199, 1970.

Schaffer, B., Gould, R. J., Wallace, S., Jackson, L., Iuker, M., Leherman, P. R. and Felten, T. R.: Urological application of lymphangiography. J. Urol., *87:* 91, 1962.

Schaffer, B., Koehler, P. R., Daniel, R. C., Wohl, G. T., Rivera, E., Meyers, W. A. and Skelley, J. F.: A critical evaluation of lymphangiography. Radiology, *80:* 917, 1963.

Sieber, F.: Incidents after the subcutaneous instillation of patent blue (Patent blau) for lymphography. Med. Bild., *11:* 102, 1968.

Sokolowski, J. and Engeset, A.: The toxic effect of patent blue violet on rat lymph node lymphocytes. Lymphology, *7:* 28, 1974.

Sviridov, N. K.: Embolia mozga posle limfografii. Khirurgiia (Mosk.), *48:* 145, 1972.

Threefoot, S. A.: Pulmonary hazards of lymphography. Cancer Chemother. Rep., *52:* 107, 1968.

Tjernberg, B.: Lymphography as an aid to examination of lymph nodes. Acta Soc. Med. Upsalien, *61:* 207, 1956.

Veyssier, P., et al.: Embolie grasseuse cerebrale and lymphographie. Ann. Med. Interne (Paris), *122:* 1127, 1971.

White, R. J., Webb, J. A. W., Tucker, A. K. and Foster, K. M.: Pulmonary function after lymphography. Br. Med. J., *4:* 775, 1973.

Wiertz, L. M., Gagnon, J. H. and Anthonisen, N. R.: Intrapulmonary hemorrhage with anemia after lymphography. N. Engl. J. Med., *285:* 1364, 1971.

11

Radionuclide Lymphography

MAJIC S. POTSAID, M.D., AND KENNETH A. McKUSICK, M.D.

Of all the tissues in the body, the lymphatic system is the most prone to contain malignant neoplasms. These tumors may originate within the lymphoid tissue itself (e.g., lymphoma), but more often they are metastatic deposits from cancers arising elsewhere (e.g., carcinomas of breast, cervix, colon, etc.) (Abrams et al., 1950). The clinical problems associated with the common occurrence of malignant neoplasms in lymph nodes provided the impetus for the development of radionuclide lymphography.

Today, we view the modality as a diagnostic procedure, but the initial efforts centered around the idea of using beta ray-emitting radionuclides that could deliver therapeutic doses of radiation to lymph nodes containing cancer. Shortly after World War II, several investigators showed that radiocolloids (e.g., gold-198) concentrated in normally functioning reticuloendothelial cells following parenteral administration of the radiopharmaceutical, especially the accumulation of radioactivity in regional lymph nodes after a subcutaneous injection (Hahn and Sheppard, 1946; Sheppard et al., 1947; Walker, 1950). Colloidal gold-198 was investigated as a possible radiotherapeutic agent (Hahn and Carothers, 1951 and 1953; Sherman et al., 1950 and 1951; Sherman and Ter-Pogossian, 1953), but this approach was abandoned because the concentration of radionuclide was too often the highest in normal nodes and the lowest in nodes most heavily involved with tumor (Seaman and Powers, 1955).

As radiogold was being investigated for therapy, it became obvious that diagnostic information was being derived from knowledge about the distribution patterns of radioactivity in normal versus abnormal lymph nodes. It was fortuitous that gold-198 also emits a 412 keV peak photon that can be detected easily by external probes, and it was a relatively simple matter to obtain useful images of the distribution of radio-

activity in lymph nodes. During this same period, diagnostic radionuclide lymphography was advanced along with other nuclear medicine procedures by major technologic improvements in imaging instrumentation, which made organ and tissue scanning practical (Sage and Gozun, 1958b) (Figs. 11.1 and 11.2).

Colloidal gold-198, as a therapeutic agent, was found useful for the control of pleural and peritoneal effusions resulting from malignant tumors. Following intraperitoneal administration of the agent for the treatment of malignant ascites, accumulations of radiogold were noted in the mediastinum of some patients, indicating passage of colloid from the abdominal cavity to the lymph nodes in the chest (Muller, 1956). This finding indicated another manner in which radiocolloid could be used diagnostically.

When compared to roentgen lymphangiography, diagnostic radionuclide lymphography using colloidal gold-198 is a relatively simple procedure to perform. However, it has significant limitations and some of the disadvantages stem from the use of gold-198, a radionuclide that has to be restricted in amount because of the high radiation dose that can result from beta radiation. As a consequence, the low photon flux and poor statistics make the production of quality images difficult. In order to overcome these limitations, other agents have been tried, including technetium-99m as a colloid (Hauser et al., 1969). Because it is often desirable to obtain an image 1 or 2 days after administration of the agent and because technetium-99m has only a 6-hr physical half-life, that radionuclide has definite limitations as a lymphographic agent. More recently, colloidal indium-111, with a physical half-life of 2.8 days and no beta ray emissions, has shown considerable promise for the study of lymph nodes. Since millicurie amounts of indium-111 can be administered, imaging statistics can be improved markedly

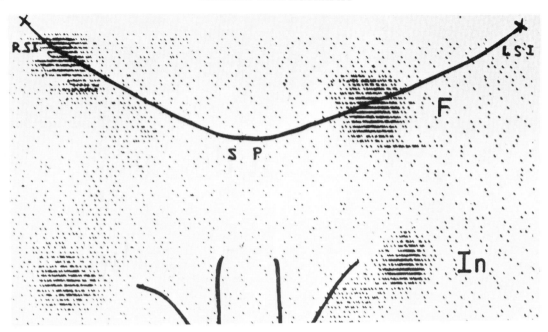

FIG. 11.1. NORMAL ANTERIOR SCAN

Scan shows radiogold in inguinal (*In*) and femoral (*F*) lymph nodes bilaterally after injection of colloidal gold-198 into the dorsum of each foot. (From Sage, H. H., Kizilay, D., Miyazaki, M., Shapiro, G. and Sinha, B.: Lymph node scintigrams. Am. J. Roentgenol. Radium Ther. Nucl. Med., *84:* 666–669, 1960.)

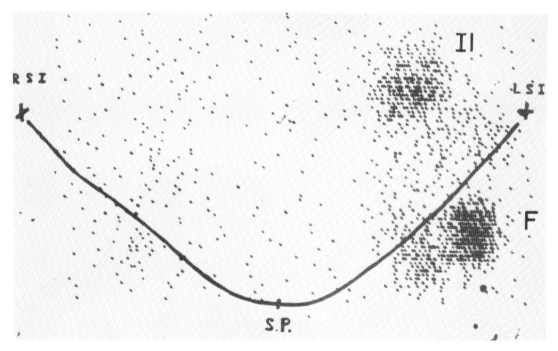

FIG. 11.2. ABNORMAL ANTERIOR SCAN

Scan shows little or no radioactivity in the lymph nodes on the right while the iliac (*Il*) and femoral (*F*) nodes on the left are well delineated in a woman who had external beam pelvic radiation on the right for uterine cancer. Absence of radioactivity was the result of tumor involvement of nodes and/or extensive radiation. (From Sage, H. H., Kizilay, D., Miyazaki, M., Shapiro, G. and Sinha, B.: Lymph node scintigrams. Am. J. Roentgenol. Radium Ther. Nucl. Med., *84:* 666–669, 1960.)

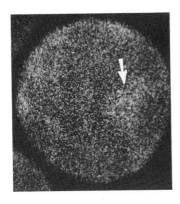 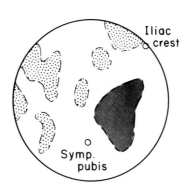 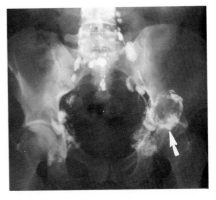

FIG. 11.3. ANTERIOR VIEW OF PELVIS

Through use of a gamma camera (*left*), abnormal selenium-75 activity (*arrow*) shown in left iliac lymph node region is illustrated further with a schematic drawing (*center*). Corresponding abnormal roentgen lymphangiogram (*right*) in this patient who has reticulum cell sarcoma (*arrow*). (From Ferrucci, J. T., Berke, R. A. and Potsaid, M. S.: Se-75 selenomethionine isotope lymphography in lymphoma: correlation with lymphangiography. Am. J. Roentgenol. Radium Ther. Nucl. Med., *109:* 793–802, 1970.)

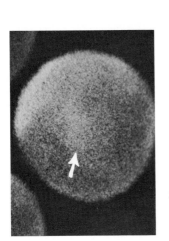 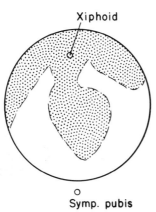 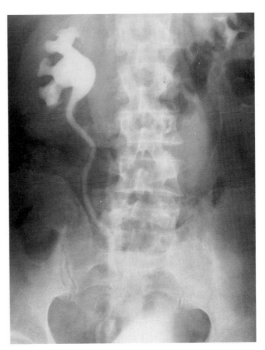

FIG. 11.4. ANTERIOR VIEW OF ABDOMEN

Gamma camera (*left*) shows abnormal selenium-75 activity in midabdominal lymph nodes (*arrow*) as detailed with schematic drawing (*center*). Normal activity in the liver and spleen are noted. An excretory urogram (*right*) in this same patient shows displacement and obstruction of the right ureter by lymphocytic lymphoma. (From Ferrucci, J. T., Berke, R. A. and Potsaid, M. S.: Se-75 selenomethionine isotope lymphography in lymphoma: correlation with lymphangiography. Am. J. Roentgenol. Radium Ther. Nucl. Med., *109:* 793–802, 1970.)

(Goodwin et al., 1969 and 1970). Even with the advent of indium-111, there may be little clinical application of colloids now that noncolloidal radiopharmaceuticals are available for the detection of tumor deposits in lymph nodes.

A practical noncolloidal method of radionuclide lymphography was discovered in the course of performing pancreas scans with intravenously administered ^{75}Se-L-selenomethionine, when it was observed that lymphomatous nodes concentrated that amino acid in sufficient quantities for the production of images (Herrera et al., 1965). This new method compared favorably with roentgen lymphangiography (Spencer et al., 1967; Ferrucci et al., 1970) (Figs. 11.3 and 11.4).

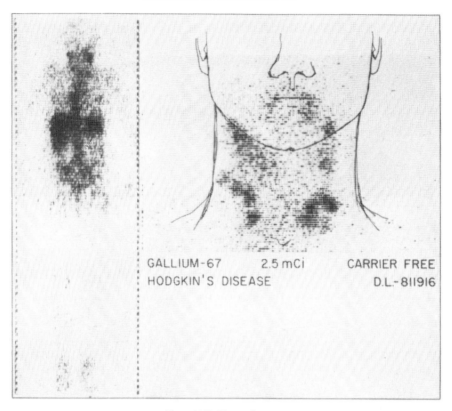

GALLIUM-67   2.5 mCi   CARRIER FREE
HODGKIN'S DISEASE   D.L.-811916

FIG. 11.5. NECK SCAN

Gallium-67 activity in cervical lymph nodes containing tumor is shown on the *right*. Posterior whole body scan on *left* shows normal activity in liver, spleen, and skeleton in the same patient with abnormal activity again noted in the neck region. (From Edwards, C. L. and Hayes, R. L.: Tumor scanning with ^{67}Ga citrate. J. Nucl. Med., *10:* 103–105, 1969.)

Lymphography with selenium-75 as seleno-methionine has a definite statistical advantage over the radiocolloid method in that the abnormal tissues show an increase of radioactivity, the opposite of the radiocolloid method which shows a decrease of activity when neoplasms are present. Simple intravenous administration of ^{75}Se-L-selenomethionine is a marked improvement over the more complex injection of the colloid. However, the total statistics are still relatively low because only a few hundred microcuries of selenium-75 can be administered to a patient.

During a study of the skeletal distribution of intravenously administered, carrier-free radio-gallium, a dramatic advance in radionuclide lymphography occurred when it was noted that gallium-67 concentrated in cervical lymph nodes containing Hodgkin's lymphoma (Edwards and Hayes, 1969) (Figs. 11.5 and 11.6). Not only is gallium-67 activity often increased in certain tumors, but the millicuries' dose of the administered nuclide results in higher quality images. This chapter will emphasize the use of tumor-localizing agents for lymphography, especially gallium-67 citrate, which is currently the most widely used radiopharmaceutical for direct detection of neoplasms.

RADIOCOLLOIDS

Radionuclides

Any radionuclide with photons having energy suitable for image formation and with chemical properties allowing the particular element to be prepared in colloidal form can be used for lymphography. Colloidal radionuclides that have been applied clinically are gold-198, technetium-99m, and indium-111 (Table 11.1).

Chemical Form

Elemental gold and indium assume the colloidal state readily and need little chemical ma-

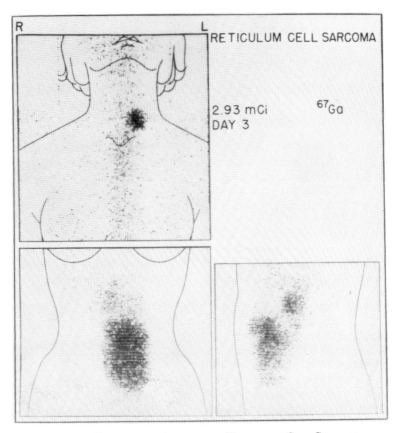

FIG. 11.6. THORAX AND ABDOMEN IN RETICULUM CELL SARCOMA

Anterior views of the thorax and abdomen and lateral view of abdomen showing abnormal concentrations of gallium-67 in the left supraclavicular and abdominal lymph nodes of a 45-year-old woman with reticulum cell sarcoma. (From Edwards, C. L. and Hayes, R. L.: Scanning malignant neoplasms with gallium-67. JAMA, *212:* 1182–1190, 1970.)

TABLE 11.1
RADIONUCLIDES USED CLINICALLY AS COLLOIDS FOR LYMPHOGRAPHY

Nuclide	T½ Physical	Photon Peak	Adult Dose
Gold-198	2.7 days	412 keV	0.10–0.20 mCi
Technetium-99m	0.25 days	140 keV	2.00–5.00 mCi
Indium-111	2.8 days	173 keV 247 keV	1.00–2.00 mCi

nipulation for the production of a suitable radio-pharmaceutical. Technetium-99m as a radiocolloid can also be obtained easily because the same agent that is used for routine liver-spleen scanning can be utilized for lymphography provided the colloid size is kept as small as possible. The colloidal properties of several agents were studied and radiogold was found best for lymphography because of its small size (Anghileri, 1967). In its biologic behavior as a colloid, indium may be comparable to gold because of size similarities.

Physiologic Principles

Localization of radiocolloids is through the mechanism of phagocytosis by reticuloendothelial cells within the lymph nodes. The particular group of lymph nodes to be studied determines the specific site of colloid injection. For the inguinal, pelvic, and abdominal nodes, the cutaneous tissues of the foot have been utilized (Sage et al., 1960 and 1964; Pearlman, 1970; Fairbanks et al., 1972; Hauser et al., 1969; Kazem et al., 1968; Drewett, 1973; Gates and Dore, 1971; Dunson et al., 1973). The axillary nodes have been examined by using the hand or the breast (Seaman and Powers, 1955; Sage et al., 1960 and 1964). Regional nodes for the breast, including the substernal nodes, have been evaluated after administration of the radiocolloid into the breast or adjacent to a breast carcinoma (Seaman and Powers, 1955; Vendrell-Torne et al., 1972). Substernal and other thoracic nodes have been studied by placing the radiopharmaceutical subcutaneously at the xiphoid as well as intraperitoneal placement (Schenk, 1966; Schenk et al., 1966; Atkins et al., 1970; Coates et al., 1973). Radiocolloid has been administered into the tongue and pharynx tissues for head and neck nodes (Sage et al., 1960) and into paracervical tissues of the uterus for pelvic node evaluation (Lang, 1960).

In order to enhance the movement of the colloid from the injection site into the lymphatic system, some investigators have administered hyaluronidase with the radiopharmaceutical (Lang, 1960; Sage and Gozun, 1958a; Pearlman, 1970; Fairbanks et al., 1972; Hauser et al., 1969). Most individuals using the method have preferred not to use a spreading agent.

In the course of studying the lymphatic system with radiocolloids, the liver and spleen may be visualized (Fig. 11.7). This is not surprising when one realizes that the terminal lymphatic channel, the thoracic duct, drains into the venous system at the junction of the internal jugular and subclavian veins. When a radiocolloid is allowed to pass through unobstructive lymphatics and is allowed to enter the venous system, it behaves in the same manner as a radiocolloid that is injected directly into a vein for a routine liver-spleen scan. The degree of visualization of the liver and spleen will depend on the amount of radiocolloid that has found its way into the venous system.

Imaging Procedure

Radionuclide images of the regions of interest are obtained from a few hours to several days after administration of the colloid. The usual protocol calls for the first scan to be performed at 4–6 hr after injection of a gold-198 or indium-111 colloid with additional views at 24 and 48 hr. Colloids of technetium-99m are scanned 2–3 hr after administration. Rectilinear scanners and gamma cameras can be used as the imaging devices. When the radionuclide has higher energy photons such as gold-198 (412 keV), the scanner is preferred because it is more efficient in the detection of such gamma rays than the gamma camera. There are no special rules for positioning the patient, although markers identifying key anatomic parts on the images are important as they permit a more precise localization of concentrations of activity as well as aid in identifying a decrease or absence of activity in nodal areas.

Clinical Applications

The first clinical applications of diagnostic radiocolloid lymphography were aimed at finding a simple method for the detection of breast carcinoma metastases. In addition to studying the lymph drainage from the breast to axillary and para-sternal nodes (Hultborn et al., 1955a; Leborgne et al., 1955), the procedure was used in the detection of lymph nodes following radical mastectomy (Hultborn and Jonsson, 1955). Microscopic distribution of colloidal gold-198 within regional lymph nodes containing cancer was determined by autoradiography in patients who underwent radical mastectomies. It was shown that occasionally nodes without tumor may fail to concentrate the radiocolloid as well as demonstrating significant radionuclide in nodes partially invaded by cancer (Seaman and Powers, 1955).

A more comprehensive investigation of normal mammary lymphatic drainage was carried out in 250 patients, with each group of 50 having an administration of the radiocolloid in a different site within the breast (i.e., each of the quadrants and the areola) (Vendrell-Torne et al.,

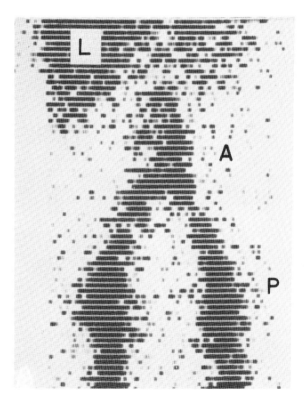

FIG. 11.7. LYMPH NODES AND LIVER FOLLOWING GOLD-198 COLLOID ADMINISTRATION

Normal pattern of pelvic (P) and abdominal (A) lymph nodes and liver (L) activity after the administration of gold-198 colloid into the tissues of both lower extremities. (From Kazem, I., Antoniades, J., Brady, L. W., Faust, D. S., Cross, M. N. and Lightfood, D.: Clinical evaluation of lymph node scanning utilizing colloidal gold-198. Radiology, 90: 905–911, 1968.)

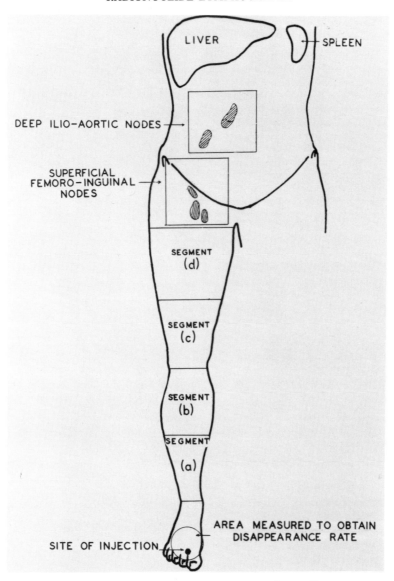

FIG. 11.8. RADIOCOLLOID MEASUREMENTS OF LYMPH FLOW

(From Sage, H. H., Sinha, B. K., Kizilay, D., et al.: Radioactive colloidal gold measurements of lymph flow and functional patterns of lymphatics and lymph nodes in the extremities. J. Nucl. Med., 5: 626–642, 1964.)

1972). This work emphasized the involvement of the internal mammary nodes in lymphatic drainage from all parts of the breast. Radioactivity was found in the internal mammary chain of nodes in 64% of patients who had the colloid injected in the lower outer quadrant of the breast, 36% after administration in the upper outer quadrant, and 20% from a subareolar injection. As expected, administrations into the inner quadrants generally produced the highest concentrations in the internal mammary nodes with 62% showing from the lower quadrant and 84% from the upper quadrant.

Assessment of inguinal lymph nodes following injection of radiocolloid was reported early

(Hultborn et al., 1955b). These initial studies were of limited clinical value since they produced crude numerical data (count rates) in the nodal areas following administration of colloidal gold-198 in the tissues of the calf. However, the feasibility of the technique as a diagnostic procedure was demonstrated, and with such improvements as foot injections, the lower extremity approach to studying the inguinal, pelvic, and abdominal lymph nodes became the most commonly applied radiocolloid lymphographic study. With the introduction of practical imaging equipment, pictorial displays of radiocolloid distribution were preferred, although there were attempts at deriving quantitative mea-

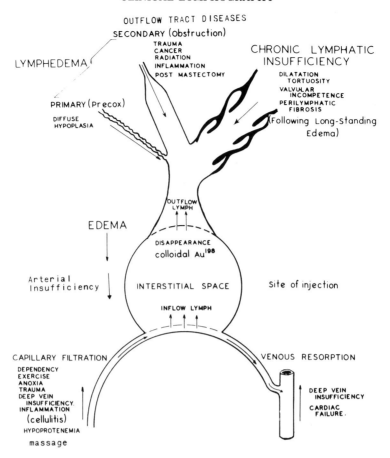

FIG. 11.9. PARAMETERS AFFECTING RADIOCOLLOID DISTRIBUTION
Physiologic and pathologic parameters that may influence radiocolloid distribution and measurements, which in turn reflect lymph flow. (From Sage, H. H., Sinha, B. K., Kizilay, D., et al.: Radioactive colloidal gold measurements of lymph flow and functional patterns of lymphatics and lymph nodes in the extremities. J. Nucl. Med., 5: 626–642, 1964.)

surements of lymph flow through the upper as well as lower extremities under normal conditions and in the presence of edema (Sage et al., 1964) (Figs. 11.8 and 11.9).

In one series of several hundred cases, radiogold lymphography was found to be clinically useful not only in the initial evaluation of patients, but also in their follow-up when it was deemed essential to determine the exact status of pelvic and aortic lymph nodes in individuals with cancer (zum Winkel and Scheer, 1965). In another series (Kazem et al., 1968), 75 cancer patients were evaluated with roentgen lymphangiography and gold-198 colloid lymphography; the correlation of the two modalities indicated a false positive rate of 5% for the radiocolloid procedure, using the x-ray study as the reference standard. This level of accuracy was based on the following scan features of abnormalities: (a) more than 24-hr delay in the transport of activity from the feet to the pelvic nodes,

unless there are obvious reasons to account for the delay, such as edema of the extremity; (b) absence or interruption of the chain of activity at one or more sites (Fig. 11.10); (c) marked assymmetry in the size and/or density of the activity within the lymph node areas; (d) mottled or patchy appearance of the activity accumulation within the nodal regions; (e) presence of abnormal collateral lymphatic pathways as evidenced by abnormal sites of activity on the scan; (f) undue enlargement of the activity in the next group; and (g) absence of activity accumulation in the liver area.

Tumors primary to the lymphatic system (e.g., lymphoma) have probably been studied by radionuclide lymphography more frequently than other neoplasms. A good correlation between the lymph node radiocolloid scan and the roentgen lymphangiograph was found in 40 patients with metastatic carcinoma and malignant lymphoma (Voutilainen and Wiljasalo,

1965). One hundred patients with histologically verified lymphoma had their pelvic and abdominal lymph nodes assessed for the presence of tumor by radiocolloid and roentgen methods, specifically to define the role of each modality (Pearlman, 1970). The criteria for abnormality were similar to the scan findings mentioned above. The major conclusions drawn from the latter investigation can be stated as follows: (1) the radiocolloid method is primarily a simple, rapid screening or evaluation procedure that is a supplement to x-ray lymphangiography; (2) in certain instances, radiocolloid lymphography alone may be sufficient to stage patients, to plan treatment and to follow the course of disease; and (3) a high incidence of unsuspected disease in abdominal nodes was found in asymptomatic patients with lymphosarcoma and reticulum cell sarcoma.

In an attempt to increase the number of photons available for image formation at less radiation exposure to the patients, colloids of Tc-99m were introduced with the hope of improving the quality of the studies (Fairbanks et al., 1972; Hauser et al., 1969; Coates et al., 1973; Dunson et al., 1973; Brunner et al., 1969; Marty, 1971; Thrall et al., 1973). It was soon learned that imaging of technetium-99m colloids in the abdominal nodes should be carried out within 3 hr after a foot injection, because the rate of accumulation of the radionuclide in those nodes was about equal to the rate of physical decay of technetium-99m at that time period (Hauser et al., 1969). With some colloids of technetium-99m, it was found necessary to scan at 2 hr because of apparent concentrations of radionuclide in the intestinal and urinary tracts that could be confused with lymph node activity, findings that indicate probable free pertechnetate (Fairbanks et al., 1972). The 2- to 3-hr limit with technetium-99m colloids compromised the study markedly as it did not allow time for the colloid to move into the superior nodes in the abdomen in sufficient amounts for satisfactory

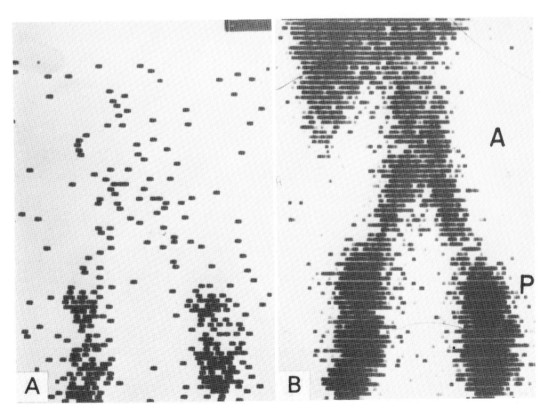

FIG. 11.10. RETICULUM CELL SARCOMA

Case of a 56-year-old woman with reticulum cell sarcoma involving the periaortic lymph nodes confirmed by laparotomy. Scan A, done at time of surgery, shows poor visualization of abdominal lymph nodes. Scan B, performed 3 months later and after combined chemotherapy and radiotherapy, shows an essentially normal pattern. A, Abdominal; P, pelvic. (From Kazem, I., Antoniades, J., Brady, L. W., Faust, D. S., Cross, M. N. and Lightfood, D.: Clinical evaluation of lymph node scanning utilizing colloidal gold-198. Radiology, 90: 905–911, 1968.)

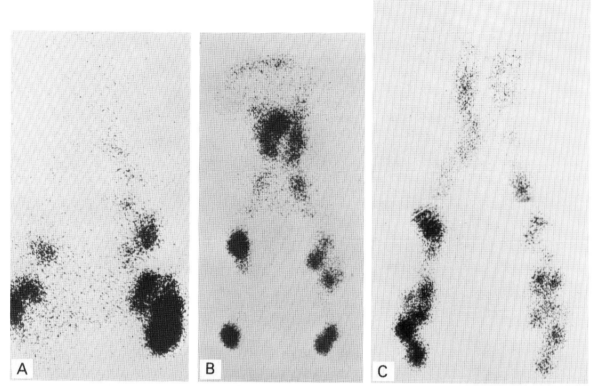

FIG. 11.11. ABNORMAL LYMPHOGRAPHIC PATTERNS PRODUCED WITH TECHNETIUM-99M COLLOID
A: A marked difference in the activity between the two sides. *B:* A prominent, broad pattern of activity in the para-aortic area. *C:* Linear confluence of nodes without clear delineation of individual nodes. (From Fairbanks, V. F., Tauxe, W. N., Kiely, J. M. and Miller, W. E.: Scintigraphic visualization of abdominal lymph nodes with ^{99m}Tc-pertechnetate labeled sulfur colloid. J. Nucl. Med., *13:* 185–190, 1972.)

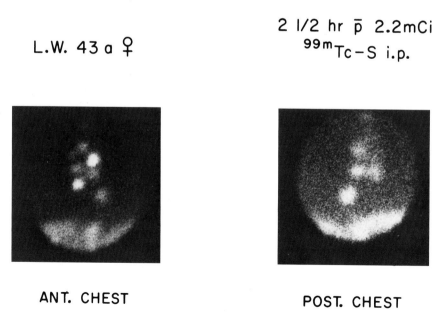

FIG. 11.12. DEMONSTRATION OF MEDIASTINAL LYMPH NODES AFTER INTRAPERITONEAL ADMINISTRATION OF TECHNETIUM-99M COLLOID
(From Atkins, H. L., Hauser, W. and Richards, P.: Visualization of mediastinal lymph nodes after intraperitoneal administration of ^{99m}Tc-sulfur colloid. Nucl. Med. (Stuttg.), *9:* 275–278, 1970.)

R.B. 65 M C.L.L

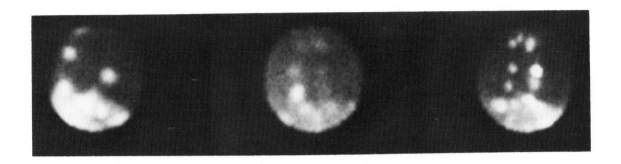

L. Lateral   Posterior   Anterior

FIG. 11.13. MEDIASTINAL LYMPH NODES

Demonstration of mediastinal lymph nodes after intraperitoneal administration of technetium-99m colloid in a patient with chronic lymphatic leukemia and a left pleural effusion. (Courtesy H. L. Atkins, M. D., Brookhaven National Laboratory, Upton, New York.)

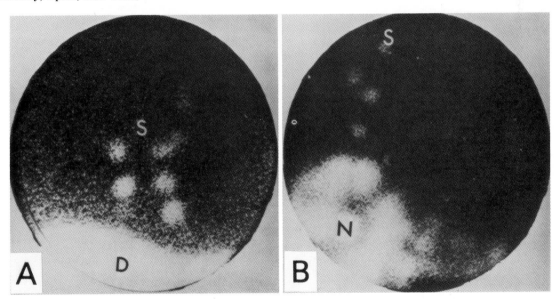

FIG. 11.14. MEDIASTINAL LYMPH NODES

A: Normal anterior gamma camera image of the distribution of radioactivity in the mediastinal lymph nodes 2 hr after intraperitoneal injection of 4 mCi of ^{99m}Tc-sulfur colloid. *S*, Sternal notch; *D*, activity in the peritoneal cavity and at the diaphragm. *B:* Anterior gamma camera image shows activity in the diaphragmatic lymph nodes (*N*) 2 hr after injection. (From Coates, G., Bush, R. S. and Aspin, N.: A study of ascites using lymphoscintigraphy with ^{99m}Tc sulfur colloid. Radiology, *107:* 577–583, 1973.)

image formation. An investigation of the effects of particle size on tissue distribution suggested that more favorable imaging statistics were achieved with technetium-99m "minicolloid" because a higher percentage of the administered dose passed through successive node levels (Dunson et al., 1973).

Thirty-one patients, 26 of whom had malignant lymphoma with and without abdominal pelvic node involvement, were studied with sulfur-sulfide colloid of technetium-99m (Fairbanks et al., 1972). The radionuclide lymphographs were correlated with findings on roentgen lymphangiography and/or at laparotomy.

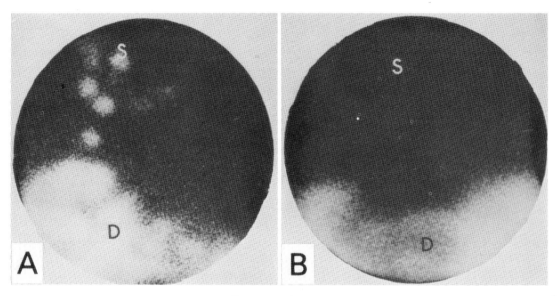

FIG. 11.15. ASCITES

A: Normal gamma camera image of a patient without ascites. *B:* Gamma camera image taken 5 months later shows no activity in the mediastinal nodes. Ascites is present. (From Coates, G., Bush, R. S. and Aspin, N.: A study of ascites using lymphoscintigraphy with ^{99m}Tc sulfur colloid. Radiology, *107:* 577–583, 1973.)

Abnormal patterns were characterized as illustrated in Figure 11.11. The investigators often found unsatisfactory visualization of uninvolved lymph nodes above the iliac level. However, they concluded that the method has value in given patients because of its low morbidity and of the ease with which it can be performed. Their conclusion of usefulness was influenced by the substantial errors, false positive and false negative, that occurred with roentgen lymphangiography as well as with radionuclide lymphography.

Technetium-99m colloid has been administered intraperitoneally to study mediastinal lymph nodes (Atkins et al., 1970). After appropriate animal research had shown good passage of technetium-99m-labeled sulfur-sulfide colloid from the abdomen into the mediastinal nodes, the procedure was applied clinically (Figs. 11.12 and 11.13). The authors made the point that the mediastinal nodes are not readily accessible for roentgen lymphangiographic contrast studies and that the method could prove to be useful in the study of Hodgkin's disease and carcinoma of the breast metastases, as well as in the evaluation of other neoplasms.

After an intraperitoneal injection radiocolloid distribution in the chest was analyzed in a group of 52 patients, most of whom had ascites, due to tumor (e.g., ovarian carcinoma) in 38 patients and due to liver cirrhosis in 6 instances (Coates et al., 1973). Figure 11.14 illustrates one

of their normal studies, the kind obtained in 5 of 6 cases of ascites due to liver cirrhosis. Patients with ascites due to tumor invariably showed no thoracic node activity. Of 23 patients with ascites due to ovarian carcinoma, 21 had no activity in thoracic nodes, 1 had "partial" concentration, and 1 had a normal distribution. In 2 cases of ovarian carcinoma without ascites, the thoracic distribution was within normal limits. Figure 11.15 is an example of a patient with ovarian carcinoma who initially had no ascites and a normal thoracic distribution of radiocolloid but 5 months later had ascites and no thoracic activity. Three patients with chylous ascites had normal thoracic radiocolloid lymphographs. Parasternal scintigraphy can be performed using technetium-99m colloid administered intraperitoneally or injected into the soft tissues about the xiphoid process (Goranson and Jonsson, 1974).

A radiocolloid scan superimposed upon a corresponding roentgenogram of a patient with a neonatal chylothorax is shown in Figure 11.16 (Gates et al., 1972). It shows leakage of radioactivity from the thoracic duct into the left pleural space, which was documented to have chyle by aspiration and chest roentgenograms. Fifteen microcuries of gold-198 colloid was injected subcutaneously into the first web space of each foot.

In primary congenital lymphedema of the leg, radiocolloid lymphography can show an absence of radioactivity in the inguinal and femoral lymph nodes on the affected side (Gates and Dore, 1971) (Fig. 11.17), whereas acquired lymphedema may allow the accumulation of radiocolloid in the inguinal nodes if the obstruction is above that level (Fig. 11.18). In an experiment with monkeys infected with microfilaria,

it was concluded that radiocolloids could be used to study lymphatic dynamics in that condition and that the method would probably diagnose subclinical (no external signs of lymphedema) phases of the disease (Thrall et al., 1973).

DIRECT TUMOR LOCALIZATION

The preceding section described techniques which are infrequently performed in most nuclear medicine departments because of the complexity, unfavorable radiation dose, and unacceptable incidence of false negative and false positive studies. Radiopharmaceuticals are usually given systemically by an intravenous route, not mechanically directed into an organ or system as in the case in intralymphatic or intra-arterial injection.

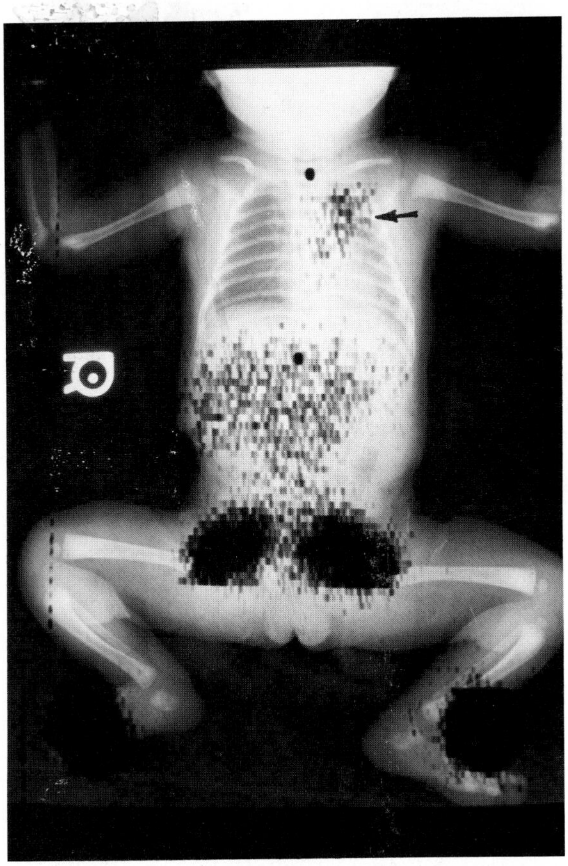

The most frequently performed in vivo radionuclide studies for tumor detection are studies of the brain, bones, and liver. The studies are safe, noninvasive, painless, relatively inexpensive, with a high sensitivity but with significant nonspecificity. For example, many skeletal metastases may be detected by bone scanning; however, the radiopharmaceuticals used show focal sites of increased radioactivity in regions of osteoblastic activity in benign as well as malignant processes. In spite of these limitations, nuclear medicine imaging studies have proven to be useful in clinical oncology, but there has been a continued interest in the development of more specific tumor-localizing radiopharmaceuticals. In fact, the use of radiopharmaceuticals that concentrate within the tumor itself has become the preferred radionuclide method for evaluating the lymphatic system of patients with cancer.

Radionuclide imaging of tumors depends mainly on four factors: (1) capabilities of imaging equipment, (2) physical characteristics of the radionuclide, (3) biological kinetics of the radiopharmaceutical, and (4) factors which determine the accumulation of the radionuclide.

Gallium-67 as citrate is the most widely used radionuclide for this purpose and will be the one emphasized in this presentation (Fig. 11.19). It accumulates most frequently in neoplasms arising in the liver, lung, and lymphatic system (Langhammer et al., 1972; Higasi and Nakayama, 1972; Littenberg et al., 1973a). It has been advocated for initial detection of occult tumor, as a complementary method for tumor staging, for noninvasive reassessment of patients during the course of their disease, and for measurements of the response of the tumor to therapy (Andrews and Edwards, 1975) (Fig. 11.20). The basic principles exhibited by gallium-67 citrate also apply to other tumor-seeking agents that may be employed in the search for neoplastic involvement of the lymphatic system (Fig. 11.21).

FIG. 11.16. RADIOCOLLOID LYMPHOGRAM WITH THE CORRESPONDING ROENTGENOGRAM

Patient has a left chylothorax showing leakage of gold-198 from the thoracic duct. Patency of the thoracic duct is evidenced by radioactivity in the liver. (From Gates, G. F., Dore, E. K. and Kanchanapoom, V.: Thoracic duct leakage in neonatal chylothorax visualized by ^{198}Au lymphangiography. Radiology, 105: 619–620, 1972.)

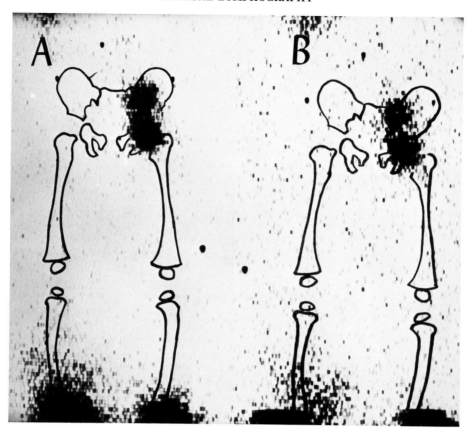

FIG. 11.17. PRIMARY CONGENITAL LYMPHEDEMA

Colloidal gold-198 scan shows no concentration of radioactivity in the right inguinal or femoral nodes over 96 hr. Left side is visualized normally as is liver (tip of which is noted above letters *A* and *B*). (From Gates, G. F. and Dore, E. K. Primary congenital lymphedema in infancy evaluated by isotope lymphangiography. J. Nucl. Med., *12:* 315–317, 1971.)

Clinical experience using gallium-67 since 1969 indicates this type of radiopharmaceutical has a role in the management of lymphoma patients (Edwards and Hayes, 1969; Kay and McCready, 1972; Turner et al., 1973; Bakshi and Bender, 1973; Silberstein et al., 1974). Concurrently, there has been a steady improvement in the prognosis of lymphomas, an improvement which may be attributed to both improved diagnosis and therapy. In part, this may be related to the more prevalent use of diagnostic laparotomy and bone marrow biopsy, which have led to an increased appreciation of the mode of spread of the disease and to more meaningful histologic classifications (Lukes, 1972).

The prognosis of lymphoma depends, in part, upon the extent of the disease upon its first presentation and upon the histologic classification of the tumor (Jones et al., 1973; Hellman, 1974; Smithers, 1972). Hodgkin's lymphoma commonly presents as a painless peripheral node, although any organ can be involved (Ro-

senberg and Kaplan, 1966). A modification of the Rye Conference Classification (Carbone, 1971) (Table 11.2) has supplanted the classification of Jackson and Parker and reflects the predominant histologic feature of the tumor at the time of diagnosis (Lukes et al., 1966). The cell type may reflect the immunologic state of the host, and is usually characterized by an inverse relationship between the number of lymphocytes and Reed-Sternberg cells (Lukes, 1972). The disease is usually chronic when the Reed-Sternberg cells are infrequent and is more virulent when there is a paucity of lymphocytes (Lukes, 1972). Prognosis is also related to the cellular characteristics of the non-Hodgkin's lymphomas as classified by Rappaport (Table 11.3) (Jones et al., 1973). The nodular non-Hodgkin's lymphomas have a more favorable prognosis than the diffuse lymphomas with a similar cell type.

It is probable that both the Hodgkin's and non-Hodgkin's lymphomas spread in a nonran-

E.S.

99m CA BREAST
TcS COLLOID

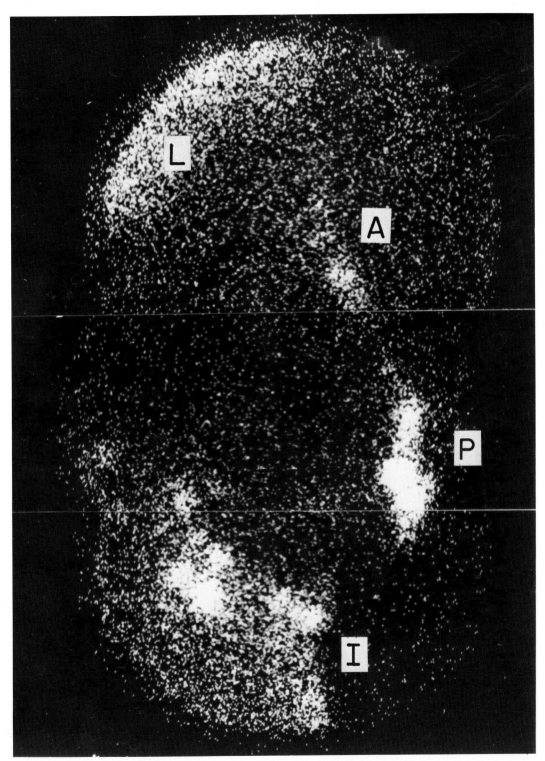

FIG. 11.18. ACQUIRED LYMPHEDEMA RIGHT LOWER EXTREMITY IN A PATIENT WITH METASTATIC BREAST CARCINOMA
Composite of gamma camera views of technetium-99m colloid distribution after subcutaneous injection in the right foot.
Study shows right inguinal node activity (*I*) with a cross-over of the radiocolloid to the left pelvic (*P*) and abdominal (*A*)
nodes due to right iliac node involvement and obstruction. Note radiocolloid in the liver (*L*). (Courtesy H. L. Atkins, M. D.,
Brookhaven National Laboratory, Upton, New York.)

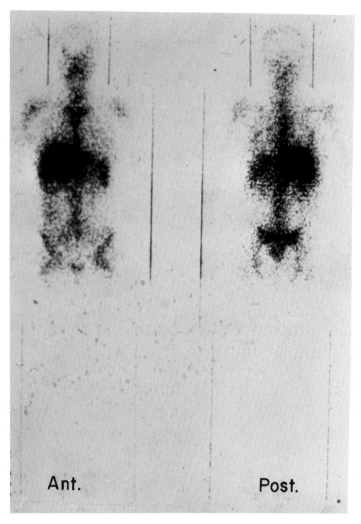

FIG. 11.19. NORMAL ^{67}GA-CITRATE SCAN

dom contiguous manner (Rosenberg and Kaplan, 1966). Extension occurs along lymphatic channels. The thoracic duct provides a pathway between the left lower cervical and supraclavicular nodes and the upper para-aortic nodes, and is also a mode of entry for tumor into the blood stream. Bone marrow and gastrointestinal tract involvement are more frequently observed in the non-Hodgkin's lymphomas, and are more likely to be widespread on initial presentation than the Hodgkin's lymphomas. The extent of the disease is a major determinant in the plan of therapy. The most widely used staging classification is the Ann Arbor Clinical Staging Classification (Table 11.4). In establishing the stage of the disease, the intra-abdominal region is relatively inaccessible to clinical examination (Figs. 11.22 and 11.23). Manual palpation may detect lymphadenopathy or organomegaly, but the mere presence of splenomegaly or hepatomegaly is of varying clinical significance. Hellman (1974) noted that the preoperative assessment of the spleen by radionuclide colloid scanning was unreliable with a false positive rate of 20% and a false negative of 23%. The most reliable finding on spleen scanning is that of splenomegaly greater than 15 cm on the posterior view, or the presence of focal splenic defects (Milder et al., 1973). Even then, the scan was only 43% sensitive in detecting intrasplenic tumor. The nonoperative clinical assessment of the liver in Hodgkin's disease is unreliable (Rosenberg, 1972; Milder et al., 1973). The presence of hepatic lymphomatous involvement is exceedingly rare without concomitant splenic involvement (Ferguson et al., 1973; Rosenberg,

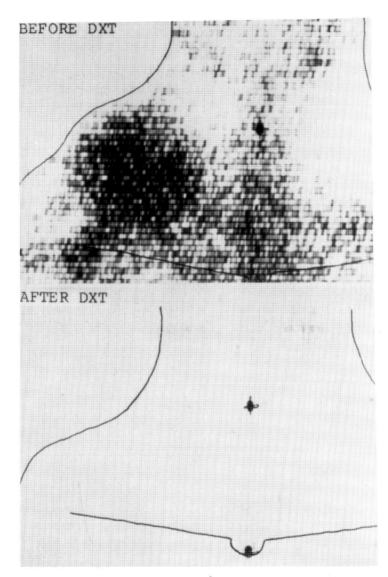

FIG. 11.20. SCAN OF THE RIGHT NECK REGION OF A MALE PATIENT AGED 23

Huge right cervical nodes are clearly seen prior to deep x-ray therapy. A repeat scan after treatment showed no specific concentration of ^{67}Ga in the neck region. (From Kay, D. N. and McCready, R. V.: Clinical isotope scanning using ^{67}Ga citrate in the management of Hodgkin's disease. Br. J. Radiol., *45:* 437–443, 1972.)

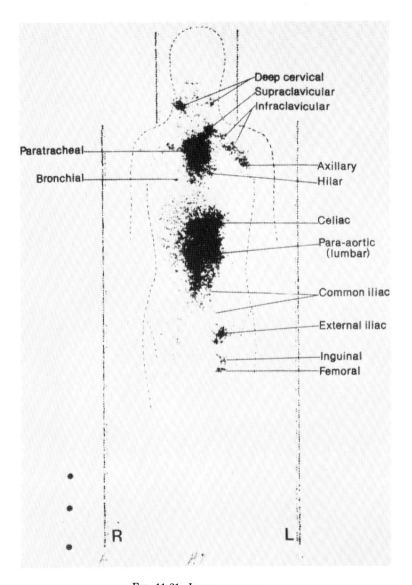

FIG. 11.21. LYMPHOSARCOMA
Commonly visualized lymph node groups are shown on anterior ⁶⁷Ga scan of a woman with widespread lymphosarcoma. (From Milder, M. S.: Interpretation of the ⁶⁷Ga photoscan. J. Nucl. Med., *14:* 1973.)

1972). When lymphoma does extend below the diaphragm, the spleen is involved in greater than 80% of the cases (Rosenberg, 1972).

Extralymphatic abdominal disease may be detected by endoscopy, gastrointestinal contrast studies, and roentgen arteriography, venography, and urography. Intra-abdominal lymph node tumor may be detected by bipedal lymph-

TABLE 11.2
CLASSIFICATION OF HODGKIN'S DISEASE

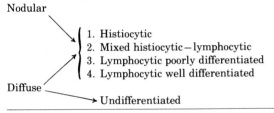

Jackson and Parker, 1947	Lukes et al., 1966
Paragranuloma	Lymphocyte predominant
Granuloma	Nodular sclerosis
Sarcoma	Lymphocyte depleted

TABLE 11.3
HISTOLOGIC CLASSIFICATION OF NON-HODGKIN'S LYMPHOMA*

Nodular

1. Histiocytic
2. Mixed histiocytic—lymphocytic
3. Lymphocytic poorly differentiated
4. Lymphocytic well differentiated

Diffuse → Undifferentiated

* Classified according to criteria of Rappaport et al. (1956) and Jones et al. (1973).

TABLE 11.4
ANN ARBOR MODIFICATION OF RYE STAGING SYSTEM*

Stage	Classification
I	Disease limited to one anatomic region (1) or a localized extralymphatic organ or site (1E).
II	Disease in two or more anatomic regions on same side of diaphragm (11), or solitary involvement of an extralymphatic organ or site of one or more lymph node regions on same side of diaphragm (11E). Spleen may be involved in case of localization below diaphragm.
III	Disease in anatomic regions on both sides of diaphragm (111); may be accompanied by involvement of spleen (111S), or by localized involvement of an extralymphatic organ or site (111E), or both (111SE).
IV	Diffuse or disseminated involvement of one or more extralymphatic organs or tissues with or without associated lymph node involvement.

* From Carbone, 1971.

angiography, but it entails some risk of reaction of the contrast agent and is only 74% sensitive (Takahashi and Abrams, 1967) with a false positive incidence of 33% (Hellman, 1974).

Because of the need for diagnostic accuracy, many lymphoma patients undergo an exploratory laparotomy. The operation is not performed unless the patient's medical condition will allow it or unless it will affect the plan of therapy. Some modification of treatment was made in 40 of 114 patients in one series (Hellman, 1974). In addition, splenectomy permits a reduction in the size of the radiation field reducing radiation damage to the base of the left lung and the kidney, and in some patients may allow more aggressive chemotherapy by increasing the total white cell and platelet count (Pannettiere and Coltman, 1973). There is some concern about serious post-operative infections in splenectomized children (Eraklis et al., 1967).

There would clearly be a role for a noninvasive test which would reliably detect the extent

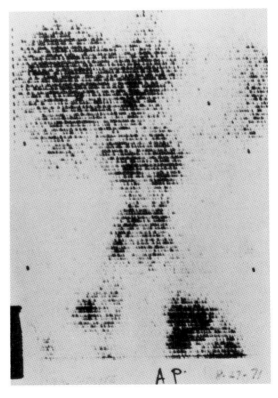

FIG. 11.22. HODGKIN'S LYMPHOMA
Anterior scintigram with ^{67}Ga citrate in a patient with Hodgkin's lymphoma involving abdominal and pelvic lymph nodes. (From Bakshi, S. and Bender, M. A.: Use of gallium-67 scanning in the management of lymphoma. J. Surg. Oncol., 5: 539–549, 1973.)

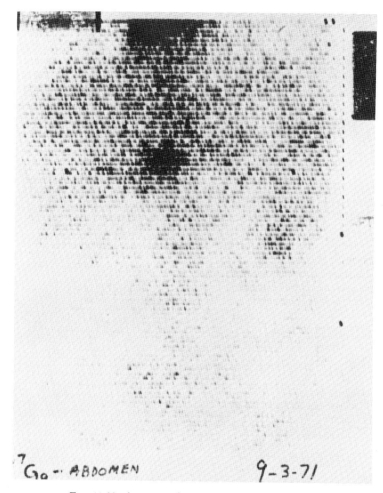

FIG. 11.23. ANTERIOR SCINTIGRAM OF THE ABDOMEN

Scintigram demonstrates one solitary lymph node 2 cm in diameter in the epigastric region proven to be diseased at laparotomy. (From Bakshi, S. and Bender, M. A.: Use of gallium-67 scanning in the management of lymphoma. J. Surg. Oncol., 5: 539–549, 1973.)

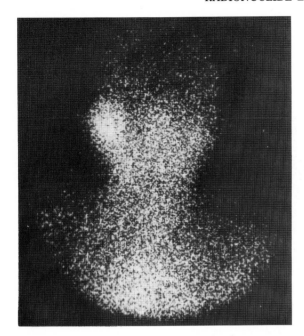

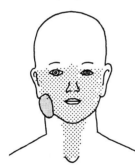

FIG. 11.24. HODGKIN'S DISEASE

Anteroposterior view head and upper thorax. Increased uptake can be seen in the upper cervical lymph nodes on the right. Note the normal uptake pattern of the face and mediastinum. (From Berelowitz, M. and Blake, K. C. H.: ^{67}Gallium in the detection and localization of tumours. S. Afr. Med. J., 45: 1351–1359, 1971.)

of lymphoma, especially if the test could be performed repeatedly. Numerous investigations, therefore, have ensued following the initial report of Edwards and Hayes (1969) of the accumulation of gallium-67 citrate in cervical lymph nodes in a patient with Hodgkin's disease (Figs. 11.24 and 11.25). Langhammer et al. (1972) observed positive gallium-67 scans in 17 of 50 patients with non-Hodgkin's lymphoma and 14 of 17 patients with Hodgkin's disease. Abnormal gallium scans were reported in 14 of 24 non-Hodgkin's lymphoma patients and 19 of 27 Hodgkin's patients, in a follow-up study by Edwards and Hayes (1971). Kay and McCready

(1972) reported that in 50 Hodgkin's lymphoma patients, 76 of 96 "active" sites of tumor were gallium-positive. Turner et al. (1972) were able to identify 23 of 29 Hodgkin's sites using gallium-67 citrate. To date, the largest combined group of patients studied was that of the Cooperative Group Study for Localization of Radiopharmaceuticals (Johnston et al., 1974; Greenlaw et al., 1974). Their observations on 151 untreated Hodgkin's and 168 non-Hodgkin's lymphoma patients (Table 11.5) indicate that gallium-67 scanning may be sensitive in the detection of patients with lymphoma, but it is insensitive in the detection of all individually histologically proven sites of disease.

The incidence of false positive gallium-67 foci is 5% (Greenlaw et al., 1974; Johnston et al., 1974; Alder et al., 1975). Other than retained fecal activity (Fig. 11.26), the most common reason for false positive results is the presence of an unsuspected infection (Fig. 11.27). Numerous inflammations and infections have been noted to accumulate gallium (Lavender et al., 1971), and in fact, gallium-67 citrate scanning is advocated for the assessment of patients with sepsis or fevers of undetermined origin (Littenberg et al., 1973b; Silva and Harvey, 1974; Teates and Hunter, 1975) (Fig. 11.28). Unusual pulmonary gallium-67 activity may occur in patients who have undergone previous roentgen lymphangiography. Abnormal ^{67}gallium lung activity was noted in 14 of 28 patients who had undergone contrast lymphangiography within 1 month prior to the radionuclide study (Lentle et al., 1975). The unexpected pulmonary collection of gallium-67 may be a reflection of a pulmonary response to contrast oil embolization.

Gallium-67 scanning appears to be most sensitive in the detection of lymphoma in the region of the neck and chest (Figs. 11.29 and 11.30), and least sensitive in the abdomen and inguinal-femoral region (Greenlaw et al., 1974; Johnston et al., 1974; Alder et al., 1975; McCready, 1972). Furthermore, gallium-67 scanning is more likely to detect the disease within lymph nodes than within intralymphatic tumors. In one series of 59 untreated Hodgkin's patients who underwent laparotomy, 38 had splenic tumor present, but only 14 (37%) had a significant splenic gallium activity (Johnston et al., 1974). Gallium-67 accumulates in the normal spleen as well as in the normal liver so that it may be difficult to determine what constitutes an abnormal accumulation. ^{67}Gallium accumulation in a focal defect seen on a radionuclide liver scan should be considered indicative of

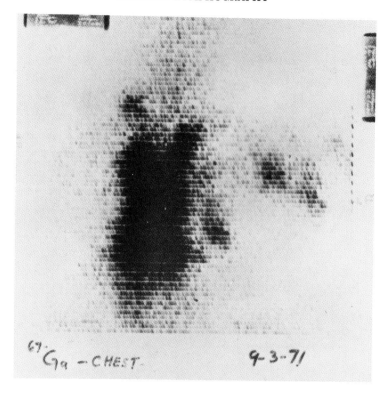

FIG. 11.25. ABNORMAL ANTERIOR SCINTISCAN OF CHEST WITH ⁶⁷GA CITRATE
There is marked abnormal uptake in the diseased areas involving the mediastinum, left parahilar, right cervical, and left axillary regions in a patient with Hodgkin's disease. (From Bakshi, S. and Bender, M. A.: Use of gallium-67 scanning in the management of lymphoma. J. Surg. Oncol., 5: 539–549, 1973.)

TABLE 11.5
SCANNING RESULTS IN UNTREATED TUMOR*

	No.	Positive		Negative	
		No.	%	No.	%
Hodgkin's lymphoma					
Patients	151	137	91	14	9
Sites—all	596	416	70	180	30
Sites—histologically proven	249	161	65	88	35
Non-Hodgkin's lymphoma					
Patients	168	133	79	35	21
Sites—all	714	373	52	341	48
Sites—histologically proven	270	139	51	131	49

* Based on reports of Johnston et al. (1974) and Greenlaw et al. (1974).

pathology (Suzuki et al., 1971; Lomas et al., 1972). It is unlikely that the spleen will contain lymphoma, however, if the ⁶⁷Ga activity in the spleen is absent or considerably reduced (Alder et al., 1975; Turner, 1972; Greenlaw et al., 1974).

The concentration of gallium-67 in the tumor is, in part, related to the degree of differentiation of the cell and to the amount of the viable tissue as opposed to necrotic tumor (Edwards and Hayes, 1970). There is also a relationship to cell type. In the Cooperative Study, 70% of histiocytic lymphomas and only 31% of poorly differentiated lymphocytic lymphoma sites were gallium-positive. In Hodgkin's disease, the highest incidence of positive ⁶⁷gallium sites was in those patients with nodular sclerotic disease. The sites of lymphocyte-depleted Hodgkin's lymphoma were too small to be considered significant, but the overall incidence in the lymphocyte-predominant Hodgkin's was 64%.

Intralymphatic injection of gallium-67 citrate in the hopes that the radiopharmaceutical would accumulate in intralymphatic lymphoma has been disappointing (Edwards et al., 1971). The intralymphatically injected radiopharmaceutical shortly becomes distributed in a manner similar to the same radiopharmaceutical administered intravenously. It was concluded in that study that gallium was not transferred directly from lymph to lymph tissue.

The mechanisms by which gallium-67 citrate accumulates in tumor are not fully understood.

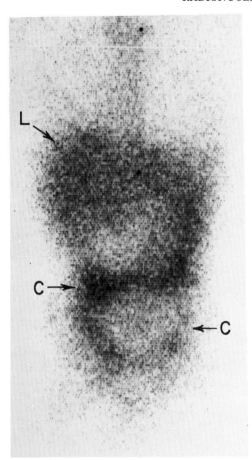

FIG. 11.26. PERSISTENT COLON RADIOACTIVITY

Anterior projection demonstrating colon radioactivity (C) persisting 48 hr after intravenous injection of ^{67}Ga citrate. This could obscure abnormal concentration of ^{67}Ga in intra-abdominal lymph nodes. There is normal accumulation in other sites in this patient, including the liver (L).

A subcellular localization of gallium-67 in association with lysosomes in both murine lymphoma and Buffalo rat hepatoma has been demonstrated (Swartzendruber et al., 1971; Hayes et al., 1971). There is a rapid association of gallium-67 on the plasma membrane of lymphocytes in culture, with an increase in uptake on the membranes when those lymphocytes are stimulated with phytohemagglutinin (Merz et al., 1974). A membrane association has also been observed in mice fetal membrane and decidua (Otten et al., 1973). They showed that ^{67}gallium accumulation is not necessarily related to cell proliferation as indicated by the lack of ^{67}gallium association with proliferating intestinal crypt cells, which do accumulate labelled thymidine. The effect of blood flow on gallium-67 concentration in tumors is uncer-

tain. No relationship of gallium accumulation of blood flow was noted in colon tumors, but was observed to be in the highest concentration in the leading edge of the tumors (Nash et al., 1972).

In the Periodic Table, gallium is an element of Group IIIA which also includes aluminum and indium. Most salts of gallium are hydrolized in aqueous media and are insoluble at a physiologic pH. Citrate produces a soluble salt of gallium and is, therefore, usually used as the radiopharmaceutical. Gallium-67 citrate is absorbed poorly from the intestine. It is, therefore, injected intravenously. Approximately one-third of the injected dose combines with plasma proteins initially, then to transferrin, and then

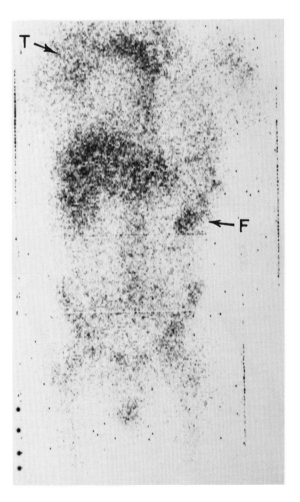

FIG. 11.27. TWO OTHER CAUSES FOR FALSE-POSITIVE GALLIUM-67 SCANS

This patient had a right subclavian-brachial thrombophlebitis (T) and a gastrocolic fistula (F) secondary to diverticulitis.

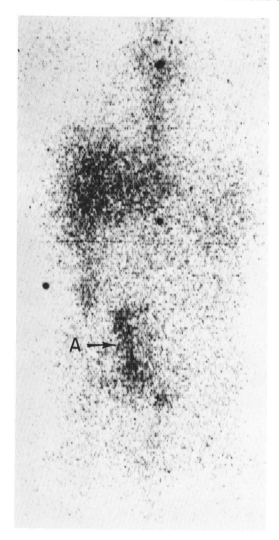

FIG. 11.28. PERIAPPENDICEAL ABSCESS

[67]Ga concentration in periappendiceal abscess (*A*). Sites of sepsis must be differentiated from tumor.

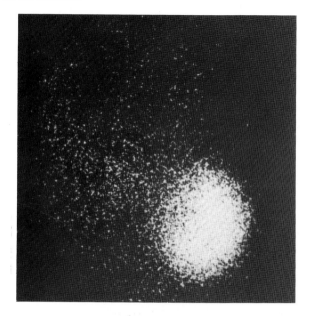

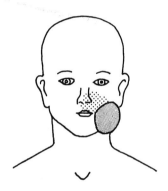

FIG. 11.29. LYMPHOSARCOMA

Anteroposterior view head and neck. A marked area of uptake is present in the upper cervical lymph nodes on the left. (From Berelowitz, M. and Blake, K. C. H.: [67]Gallium in the detection and localization of tumours. S. Afr. Med. J., *45:* 1351–1359, 1971.)

to haptoglobin and albumin (Hartman and Hayes, 1969; Gunasekera et al., 1972). The soluble remainder diffuses throughout the extracellular space or is excreted by the kidneys. Within the first 24 hr, 12% of the dose is excreted in the urine. Overall, 26% is excreted by this route in the first week as measured in one series of patients with neoplasia (Nelson et al., 1972). An additional 10% is excreted by the gastrointestinal tract (Edwards and Hayes, 1970). Plasma clearance is relatively slow because of protein binding. Tissue distribution does vary among normal individuals. The highest initial concentrations are considered to be in the liver and kidney (Table 11.6), and later shift to the liver

and spleen (Lavender, 1971). Spleen activity is distributed within phagocytic cells, while in the liver both the Kupffer cells and hepatocytes concentrate the radionuclide (Nelson et al., 1972). The large intestines, kidney, liver, and spleen receive the highest radiation dose (Table 11.7). Whole body radiation dose is 0.26 rads/mCi with the critical organ being the large intestine 0.9 rads/mCi (MIRD/Dose Estimate, 1973).

In order to maximize the target-to-nontarget ratio, imaging is usually performed 48–72 hr following an intravenous injection of 50–100 μCi/kg of gallium-67 citrate. Effective bowel cleansing is necessary to remove excreted radio-

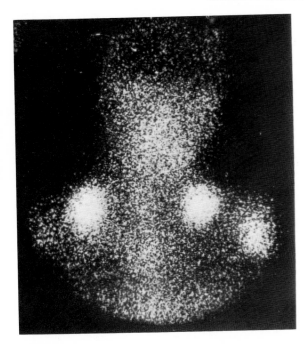

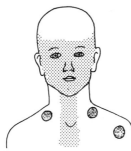

Fig. 11.30. Reticulum Cell Sarcoma
Anteroposterior view head, neck, and upper thorax. Obviously abnormal uptake of ^{67}Ga is demonstrated in the apical lymph nodes of the left axilla and in both supraclavicular regions. (From Berelowitz, M. and Blake, K. C. H.: ^{67}Gallium in the detection and localization of tumours. S. Afr. Med. J., *45:* 1351–1359, 1971.)

TABLE 11.6
CONCENTRATION OF Ga-67 IN VARIOUS TISSUES*†

Tissue	% Administered Activity/Kg Mean
Spleen	4.1
Kidney cortex	3.8
Adrenal	3.8
Marrow	3.6
Liver	2.8
Bone	2.6

* Data from MIRD/Dose Estimate, 1973.

† Radioassay of autopsy tissue corrected for radioactive decay and normalized to a body weight of 70 kg.

activity contained with the feces. If, however, fecal activity persists and interferes with the interpretation of a particular region, the patient may receive additional cathartics and return the following day for further studies for comparison. Over the several days following injection, there is minimal additional intestinal excretion.

The physical characteristics of gallium-67 are listed in Table 11.8. The 184 and 300 keV photo peaks may be utilized for imaging either with a rectilinear scanner or an Anger scintillation camera. The procedure requires 60–90 min to complete.

It is imperative that any physician, in interpreting a gallium-67 scan, become thoroughly familiar with the normal gallium scan and is

TABLE 11.7
SUMMARY OF ESTIMATED ABSORBED DOSE PER UNIT OF ADMINISTERED ACTIVITY FROM A SINGLE INTRAVENOUS ADMINISTRATION OF RADIOACTIVE Ga-67-CITRATE*

Tissue	Radioisotope of Gallium (rads/mCi injected)
	Ga-67
Gastrointestinal tract	
Upper large intestine	0.56
Lower large intestine	0.90
Gonads	
Ovaries	0.28
Testes	0.24
Kidneys	0.41
Liver	0.46
Marrow	0.58
Skeleton	0.44
Spleen	0.53
Total Body	0.26

* Data from MIRD/Dose Estimate, 1973.

TABLE 11.8
PHYSICAL CHARACTERISTICS OF Ga-67*

Radionuclide	^{67}Ga	
Physical half-life	78.0 hr	
Decay constant	0.00885 hr^{-1}	
Mode of decay	Electron capture	
Equilibrium dose constant for nonpenetrating radiation (gm-rad/μCi-hr)	0.0873	
Principal photons:	E_i (MeV)	n_i
E_i, energy	0.0933	0.380
	0.1845	0.239
n_i, mean number/dis	0.3002	0.161
	0.3936	0.043

* Data from MIRD/Dose Estimate, 1973.

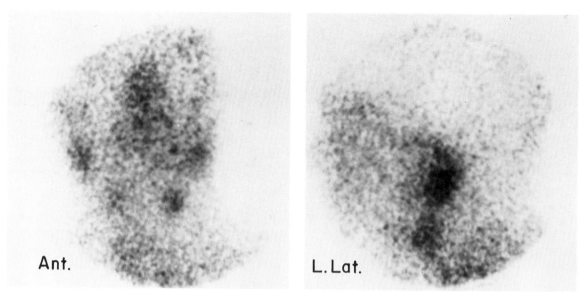

FIG. 11.31. SALIVARY GLAND ⁶⁷GA ACTIVITY
Anterior and lateral projections in patient with Hodgkin's lymphoma. This can occur following radiation therapy.

aware of the benign processes which may concentrate the radiopharmaceutical. Figure 11.19 is an illustration of a normal gallium study. There is usually some definition of the bony structures of the head, spine, and pelvis with the accentuation of activity in the region of the epiphyses, especially in children (Larson et al., 1973). Although long bones are not usually seen, regions of osteoblastic activity secondary to fracture, infection, or tumor and areas of very active bone marrow will concentrate the radiopharmaceutical. In the face, some gallium activity is seen in the region of the nose, the lacrimal glands, and the salivary glands. A normal parotid gland will show an increase in concentration following radiation therapy to the neck and may lead to misinterpretation (Kashima et al., 1974) (Fig. 11.31). Sternal activity can be pronounced but may be separated from abnormal mediastinal concentration by utilizing a lateral projection. Numerous benign processes within the lung may concentrate gallium including pneumoconiosis, pneumonia, sarcoidosis (Siemsen et al., 1974; Kinoshita et al., 1974; McKusick et al., 1973; Heshiki et al., 1974). Breast tissue under the stimulation of cyclic estrogen or progestational agents or during lactation or menarche may show a marked concentration (Larson and Schall, 1971; Fogh, 1971) (Fig. 11.32). The liver and spleen normally accumulate gallium in a pattern similar to that seen on a ⁹⁹ᵐTc sulfur colloid scan. During the first 24 hr, the kidneys may be visualized. Renal

activity at 48 hr or later is usually abnormal and suggests the presence of pathology such as pyelonephritis, urinary obstruction, or tumor (Fig. 11.33). Retained fecal radioactivity is often seen at 48 hr. Normally the fecal activity will decrease with time and change position within the abdomen where a fixed concentration in pathologic tissue will become more apparent with the passage of time. Re-examination of the patient for a period of as long as a week may be necessary.

What is the role of gallium-67 scanning in the management of patients with lymphomas? The variable sensitivity precludes its use for initial detection of patients or as a single test for the staging of lymphoma. It does have a complementary role; 43% of unsuspected sites of disease were first detected by gallium-67 scanning in one series (Johnston et al., 1974; Greenlaw et al., 1974). It may be used to detect potential sites for biopsy. It can be used as one measurement of response to therapy. Gallium-67-positive sites of tumor have been shown to revert to gallium-negative state following adequate treatment (Andrews and Edwards, 1975; Higasi and Nakayama, 1972; Bakshi and Bender, 1973; Henkin et al., 1974; Edwards and Hayes, 1970). In patients with known lymphoma who have undergone therapy, gallium scanning provides a relatively simple and noninvasive technique for assessing new symptoms that may arise in relatively inaccessible areas. Six cases were reported by Kay and McCready in 1972, in which

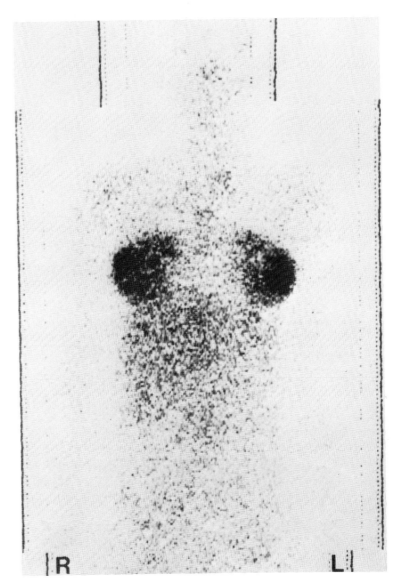

FIG. 11.32. ANTERIOR ⁶⁷GA SCAN OF 25-YEAR-OLD WOMAN PERFORMED AT 6 WEEKS POSTPARTUM
Intense ⁶⁷Ga uptake in both breasts was confirmed by finding of high activity in breast milk. (From Milder, M. S.: Interpretation of the ⁶⁷Ga photoscan. J. Nucl. Med., *14:* 1973.)

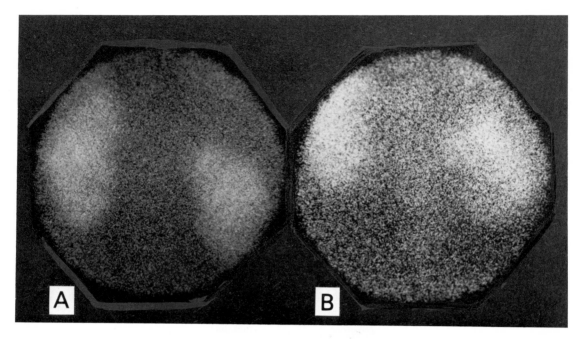

FIG. 11.33. PYELONEPHRITIS
Persistent renal gallium-67 activity (B) at 48 hr in a patient with pyelonephritis. For exact localization, ^{99m}Tc-DTPA (A) renal scan was performed.

gallium scanning detected active mediastinal disease in patients who were considered by chest x-ray to have changes only secondary to previous radiation therapy.

Over the past quarter of a century, a number of radiopharmaceuticals have been used in attempts to increase the specificity of tumor detection. These include the simple salts of P^{32}, ar-

senic-74, mercury-197, gallium-67, and a more complex structure such as radioiodinated fibrin. More recently, antineoplastic agents such as bleomycin have been labelled with CO^{57} or indium-111 with varying degrees of success for tumor localization (Poulose et al., 1975; Blum et al., 1973).

REFERENCES

Abrams, H. L., Spiro, R. and Goldstein, N.: Metastases in carcinoma – analysis of 1,000 autopsied cases. Cancer, 3: 74–85, 1950.

Alder, S., Parthasarathy, K. L., Bakshi, S. P., et al.: Gallium-67 citrate scanning for the localization and staging of lymphomas. J. Nucl. Med., 16: 225–260, 1975.

Andrews, G. A. and Edwards, C. L.: Tumor scanning with gallium-67. J.A.M.A., 233: 1100–1103, 1975.

Anghileri, L. J.: Lymph node distribution of several radiocolloids: migration ability through the tissues. J. Nucl. Biol. Med., 11: 180–184, 1967.

Atkins, H. L., Hauser, W. and Richards, P.: Visualization of mediastinal lymph nodes after intra-peritoneal administration of ^{99m}Tc-sulfur colloid. Nucl. Med. (Stuttg.), 9: 275–278, 1970.

Bakshi, S. and Bender, M. A.: Use of gallium-67 scanning in the management of lymphoma. J. Surg. Oncol., 5: 539–549, 1973.

Berelowitz, M. and Blake, K. C. H.: ^{67}Gallium in the detection and localization of tumors. S. Afr. Med. J., 45: 1351–1359, 1971.

Blum, R. H., Carter, S. K. and Agre, K.: A clinical review of bleomycin – a new antineoplastic agent. Cancer, 31: 903–914, 1973.

Brunner, P. N., Kann, D. E. and Peterson, R. E.: Comparison of lymphadenoscintigraphy using subcutaneous injections of ^{99m}Tc-sulfur colloids in aqueous media with similar colloids in emulsified media. J. Nucl. Med., 10: 390, 1969.

Carbone, P. P.: Report of the Committee on Hodgkin's Disease Staging Classification. Cancer Res., 31: 1860–1861, 1971.

Coates, G., Bush, R. S. and Aspin, N.: A study of ascites using lymphoscintigraphy with ^{99m}Tc sulfur colloid. Radiology, 107: 577–583, 1973.

Drewett, J.: Lymph node scanning and imaging using colloidal ^{198}Au. J. Nucl. Med., 14: 471, 1973.

Dunson, G. L., Thrall, J. H., Stevenson, J. S. and Pinsky, S. M.: ^{99m}Tc minicolloid for radionuclide lymphography. Radiology, 109: 387–392, 1973.

Edwards, C. L. and Hayes, R. L.: Tumor scanning with ^{67}Ga citrate. J. Nucl. Med., 10: 103–105, 1969.

Edwards, C. L. and Hayes, R. L.: Scanning malignant neoplasms with gallium-67. J.A.M.A., 212: 1182–1190, 1970.

Edwards, C. L. and Hayes, R. L.: Localization of tumors with radioisotopes. In Clinical Uses of Radionuclides; Critical Comparison with Other Techniques. Oak Ridge USAEC Conf-71101, 1971.

Edwards, C. L., Hayes, R. L., Ominsky, S. et al.: Intralymphatic injection of ^{67}Ga for visualizing intra-abdominal lymph nodes. J. Nucl. Med., 12: 431, 1971.

Eraklis, A. J., Kevy, S. V., Diamond, L. K. et al.: Hazard of overwhelming infection after splenectomy in childhood. N. Engl. J. Med., 276: 1225–1229, 1967.

Fairbanks, V. F., Tauxe, W. N., Kiely, J. M. and Miller, W. E.: Scintigraphic visualization of abdominal lymph nodes with ^{99m}Tc-pertechnetate labeled sulfur colloid. J. Nucl. Med., 13: 185–190, 1972.

Ferguson, D. J., Allen, L. W., Griem, M. L. et al.: Surgical experience with staging laparotomy in 125 patients with lymphoma. Arch. Int. Med., 131: 356–361, 1973.

Ferrucci, J. T., Berke, R. A. and Potsaid, M. S.: Se-75 selenomethionine isotope lymphography in lymphoma: correlation with lymphangiography. Am. J. Roentgenol. Radium Ther. Nucl. Med., 109: 793–802, 1970.

Fogh, J.: ^{67}Ga accumulation in malignant tumors and in prelactating or lactating breast. Prog. Soc. Exp. Biol. Med., 138: 1086–1090, 1971.

Gates, G. F. and Dore, E. K.: Primary congenital lymphedema in infancy evaluated by isotope lymphangiography. J. Nucl. Med., 12: 315–317, 1971.

Gates, G. F., Dore, E. K. and Kanchanapoom, V.: Thoracic duct leakage in neonatal chylothorax visualized by ^{198}Au lymphangiography. Radiology, 105: 619–620, 1972.

Goodwin, D. A., Finston, R. A., Colombetti, L. G., Beaver, J. E. and Hupf, H.: 2.8 day 198-Au colloid for lymphatic scintiphotography (abstr.). J. Nucl. Med., 10: 337, 1969.

Goodwin, D. A., Finston, R. A., Collombetti, L. G., Beaver, J. E. and Hupf, H.: ^{111}In for imaging: lymph node visualization. Radiology, 94: 175–178, 1970.

Goranson, L. R. and Jonsson, K.: Parasternal scintigraphy with technetium-99m sulfide colloid in human subjects. Acta Radiol. Diag., 15: 639–649, 1974.

Greenlaw, R. H., Weinstein, M. B., Brill, A., Bertrand, et al.: ^{67}Ga-citrate imagining in untreated lymphoma; preliminary report of cooperative group. J. Nucl. Med., 15: 404–407, 1974.

Gunasekera, S. W., King, L. J. and Lavender, P. H.: The behavior of tracer gallium-67 towards carrier proteins. Clin. Chim. Acta, 39: 401–406, 1972.

Hahn, P. F. and Carothers, E. L.: Radioactive metallic gold colloids coated with silver and their distribution in the lung and its lymphatics following intra-pulmonary administration: therapeutic implication in primary lung and bronchiogenic tumors. Br. J. Cancer, 5: 400–404, 1951.

Hahn, P. F. and Carothers, E. L.: Lymphatic draining following intrabronchial instillation of silver-coated radioactive gold colloids in therapeutic quantities. J. Thorac. Cardiovasc. Surg., 25: 265–279, 1953.

Hahn, P. F. and Sheppard, C. W.: Selective radiation obtained by the intravenous administration of colloidal radioactive isotopes in diseases of the lymphoid system. South. Med. J., 39: 559–562, 1946.

Hartman, R. E. and Hayes, R. L.: The binding of gallium by blood serum. J. Pharmacol. Exp. Ther., 168: 193–198, 1969.

Hauser, W., Atkins, H. L. and Richards, P.: Lymph node scanning with ^{99m}Tc sulfur colloid. Radiology, 92: 1369–1371, 1969.

Hayes, R. L., Nelson, B., Swartzendruber, D. C. et al.: Studies in the intracellular deposition of ^{67}gallium. J. Nucl. Med., 12: 364, 1971.

Hellman, S.: Current studies in Hodgkin's disease. N. Engl. J. Med., 290: 894–897, 1974.

Henkin, R. E., Polcyn, R. E. and Quinn, J. L., III: Scanning treated Hodgkin's disease with ^{67}Ga citrate. Radiology, 110: 151–154, 1974.

Herrera, N. E., Gonzalez, B. and Schwartz, R. D.: Se methionine as diagnostic agent in malignant lymphoma. J. Nucl. Med., 6: 792–804, 1965.

Heshiki, A., Schatz, S. L., McKusick, K. A. et al.: Gallium-67 citrate scanning in patients with pulmonary sarcoidosis. Am. J. Roentengol. Radium Ther. Nucl. Med., 122: 744–749, 1974.

Higasi, T. and Nakayama, Y.: Clinical evaluation of ^{67}gallium-citrate scanning. J. Nucl. Med., 13: 196–201, 1972.

Hultborn, K. A. and Jonsson, L. I.: Use of colloidal Au^{198} for detection of lymph nodes in radical excision of breast. Acta Radiol., 43: 132–138, 1955.

Hultborn, K. A., Larsson, L. G. and Ragnhult, I.: Lymph drainage from breast to axillary and parasternal lymph nodes studied with aid of colloidal Au-198. Acta Radiol., 43: 52–64, 1955a.

Hultborn, K. A., Larsson, L. G. and Ragnhult, I.: Study of lymph drainage of lower limb with use of colloidal radiogold (Au-198). Acta Radiol., 43: 139–144, 1955b.

Jackson, J., Jr. and Parker, J., Jr.: Hodgkin's Disease and Allied Disorder. New York, Oxford University Press, 1947.

Johnston, G., Benua R. S., Teates, C. D. et al.: ^{67}Ga-citrate imaging in untreated Hodgkin's disease. Preliminary report of Cooperative Group. J. Nucl. Med., 15: 399–403, 1974.

Jones, S. E., Fuks, Z., Bull, M. et al.: Non-Hodgkin's lymphomas IV: clinicopathological correlation in 405 cases. Cancer, 31: 806–823, 1973.

Kashima, H. K., McKusick, K. A., Malmud, L. S. et al.: Gallium-67 scanning in patients with head and neck cancer. Laryngoscope, 84: 1078–1089, 1974.

Kay, D. N. and McCready, V. R.: Clinical isotope scanning using ^{67}Ga citrate in the management of Hodgkin's disease. Br. J. Radiol., 45: 437–443, 1972.

Kazem, I., Antoniades, J., Brady, L. W., Faust, D. S., Cross, M. N. and Lightfood, D.: Clinical evaluation of lymph node scanning utilizing colloidal gold-198. Radiology, 90: 905–911, 1968.

Kinoshita, F., Ushio, T., Maekawa, A. et al.: Scintiscanning of pulmonary disease with ^{67}Ga citrate. J. Nucl. Med., 15: 227–233, 1974.

Lang, E. K.: Demonstration of blockage and involvement of the pelvic lymphatic system by tumor with lymphangiography and scintiscanograms. Radiology, 74: 71–73, 1960.

Langhammer, H., Glaubitt, G., Grebe, S. F. et al.: ^{67}Ga for tumor scanning. J. Nucl. Med., 13: 25–29, 1972.

Larson, S. M., Milder, M. S. and Johnston, G. S.: Interpretation of the ^{67}Ga photoscan. J. Nucl. Med., 14: 208–214, 1973.

Larson, S. M. and Schall, G. L.: Gallium-67 concentration in human breast milk. J.A.M.A., 218: 257, 1971.

Lavender, J. P., Lowe, J., Barker, J. R. et al.: Gallium-67 citrate scanning in neoplastic and inflammatory lesions. Br. J. Radiol., *44:* 361–366, 1971.

Leborgne, F. E., Leborgne, R., Schaffner, E. and Leborgne, F. E., Jr.: Study of lymphatics of mammary gland with radioactive gold. Thorax, *4:* 233–244, 1955.

Lentle, B. C., Castor, W. R., Khaliq, et al.: The effect of contrast lymphangiography on localization of ⁶⁷Ga-citrate. J. Nucl. Med., *15:* 374–376, 1975.

Littenberg, R. L., Alazraki, N. P., Taketa, R. M. et al.: A clinical evaluation of gallium-67 citrate scanning. Surg. Gynecol. Obstet., *137:* 424–430, 1973a.

Littenberg, R. L., Taketa, R. M., Alazraki, N. P. et al.: Gallium-67 for localization of septic lesions. Ann. Intern. Med., *79:* 403–406, 1973b.

Lomas, F., DiBos, P. and Wagner, H. N., Jr.: Increased specificity of liver scanning with the use of ⁶⁷Ga citrate. N. Engl. J. Med., *286:* 1323–1329, 1972.

Lukes, R. J.: Prognosis and relationship of histological features to clinical stage. J.A.M.A., *222:* 1294–1296, 1972.

Lukes, R. J., Carver, L. F., Hall, T. C. et al.: Report of the Nomenclature Committee. Cancer Res. *26:* 1311, 1966.

Marty, R.: Radioisotope lymphangiography using technetium-sulfur colloid. J. Nucl. Med., *12:* 382, 1971.

McCready, R. V., Dance, D. R., Hammersley, P. et al.: Clinical and experimental observation on 67-Ga citrate uptake in tumors and other lesions. In *Symposium on Medical Radioisotope Scintigraphy, Monte Carlo, Principality of Monaco, October 23–28, 1972.* I.A.E.A./SM - 164/42.

McKusick, K. A., Ghiladi, A. and Wagner, H. N., Jr.: Gallium-67 in pulmonary sarcoidosis. J.A.M.A., *223:* 688, 1973.

Merz, T., Malmud, L. S., McKusick, K. A. et al.: The mechanism of ⁶⁷Ga association with lymphocytes. Cancer Res. *34:* 2495–2499, 1974.

Milder, M. S., Larson, S. M., Bagley, C. M. et al.: Liver-spleen scan in Hodgkin's disease. Cancer, *31:* 826–834, 1973.

MIRD/Dose Estimate Report No. 2. J. Nucl. Med., *14:* 755–756, 1973.

Muller, J. H.: Intraperitoneal application of radioactive colloids. In *Therapeutic Use of Artificial Radioisotopes,* edited by P. F. Hahn, p. 269, New York, John Wiley & Sons, 1956.

Nash, A. G., Dance, D. R., McCready, V. R. et al.: Uptake of ⁶⁷gallium in colonic and rectal tumors. Br. Med. J., *3:* 508–510, 1972.

Nelson, B., Hayes, R. L., Edwards, C. L. et al.: Distribution of gallium in human tissues after intravenous administration. J. Nucl. Med., *13:* 92–100, 1972.

Otten, J., Johnston, G. S. and Pasten, I.: Cyclic AMP levels in fibroblasts: relationship to growth rate and contact inhibition of growth. Proc. Soc. Exp. Biol. Med., *142:* 92–95, 1973.

Pannettiere, F. and Coltman, C. A.: Splenectomy effects on chemotherapy in Hodgkin's disease. Arch. Int. Med., *131:* 362, 1973.

Pearlman, A. W.: Abdominal lymph node scintiscanning with radioactive gold (Au-193) for evaluation and treatment of patients with lymphoma. Am. J. Roentgenol. Radium Ther. Nucl. Med., *109:* 780–792, 1970.

Poulose, K. P., Watkins, A. E., Reba, R. C. et al.: Cobalt-labeled bleomycin—a new radiopharmaceutical for tumor localization. A comparative clinical evaluation with gallium citrate. J. Nucl. Med., *16:* 839–841, 1975.

Rappaport, H., Winter, W. J. and Hicks, E. B.: Follicular lymphoma. Cancer, *9:* 792–821, 1956.

Rosenberg, S. A.: Updated Hodgkin's disease; place of splenectomy in evaluation of management. J.A.M.A., *222:* 1296–1298, 1972.

Rosenberg, S. A. and Kaplan, H. S.: Evidence for an orderly progression in spread of Hodgkin's disease. Cancer Res. *26:* 1225–1231, 1966.

Sage, H. H. and Gozun, B. V.: Lymphatic scintigrams: method for studying function of lymphatics and lymph nodes. Cancer, *11:* 200–203, 1958a.

Sage, H. H. and Gozun, B. V.: Methods for studying lymphatic function in intact man utilizing Au-198. Proc. Soc. Exp. Biol. Med., *97:* 895–896, 1958b.

Sage, H. H., Kizilay, D., Miyazaki, M., Shapiro, G. and Sinha, B.: Lymph node scintigrams. Am. J. Roentgenol. Radium Ther. Nucl. Med., *84:* 666–669, 1960.

Sage, H. H., Sinha, B. K. Kizilay, D. et al.: Radioactive colloidal gold measurements of lymph flow and functional patterns of lymphatics and lymph nodes in the extremities. J. Nucl. Med., *5:* 626–642, 1964.

Schenk, P.: Szintigraphic Darstellung des Parasternalen Lymphsystems. Stahlentherapie, *130:* 504–510, 1966.

Schenk, P., zum Winkel, K. and Becker, J.: Die Szingraphie des Parasternalen Lymphsystem. Nucl. Med. (Stuttg.), *5:* 388–396, 1966.

Seaman, W. B. and Powers, W. E.: Studies on the distribution of radioactive colloidal gold in regional lymph nodes containing cancer. Cancer, *8:* 1044–1046, 1955.

Sheppard, C. W., Goodell, J. P. B. and Hahn, P. F.: Colloidal gold containing the radioactive isotope Au-198 in the selective internal radiation therapy of diseases of the lymphatic system. J. Lab. Clin. Med., *32:* 1437–1441, 1947.

Sherman, A. I., Bonebrake, M. and Allen, W. M.: The application of radioactive colloidal gold in the treatment of pelvic cancer. Am. J. Roentgenol. Radium Ther. Nucl. Med., *66:* 624–638, 1951.

Sherman, A. I., Nolan, J. F. and Allen, W. N.: The experimental application of radioactive colloidal gold in the treatment of pelvic cancer. Am. J. Roentgenol. Radium Ther. Nucl. Med., *64:* 75–85, 1950.

Sherman, A. I. and Ter-Pogossian, M.: Lymph node concentration of radioactive colloidal gold following interstitial injection. Cancer, *6:* 1238–1240, 1953.

Siemsen, J. K., Sargent, E. N., Grebe, S. F. et al.: Pulmonary concentration of Ga-67 in pneumoconiosis. Am. J. Roentgenol. Radium Ther. Nucl. Med., *120:* 815–820, 1974.

Silberstein, E. B., Kornblut, A., Shumrick, D. A. et al.: ⁶⁷Ga as a diagnostic agent for the detection of head and neck tumors and lymphoma. Radiology, *110:* 605–608, 1974.

Silva, J. Jr. and Harvey, W. C.: Detection of infections with gallium-67 and scintigraphic imaging. J. Infect. Dis., *130:* 125–131, 1974.

Smithers, D. W.: Updated Hodgkin's disease; patterns of spread. J.A.M.A., *222:* 1298–1299, 1972.

Spencer, R. P., Montana, G., Scanlon, G. T. and Evan, O. R.: Uptake of selenomethionine by mouse in human lymphomas with observations on selenite and selanate. J. Nucl. Med., *8:* 197–208, 1967.

Suzuki, T., Honjo, I., Hamamoto, K. et al.: Positive scintiphotography of cancer of the liver with ⁶⁷Ga citrate. Am. J. Roentgenol. Radium Ther. Nucl. Med., *113:* 90–103, 1971.

Swartzendruber, D. C., Nelson, B. and Hayes, R. L.: ⁶⁷Gallium localization in lysosomal-like granules of leukemic and non-leukemic murine tissues. J. Natl. Cancer Inst., *46:* 941–952, 1971.

Takahashi, M. and Abrams, H. L.: The accuracy of lymphoangiographic diagnosis in malignant lymphoma. Radiology, *89:* 448–460, 1967.

Teates, C. D. and Hunter, J. G.: Gallium scanning as a test for inflammatory lesions. Radiology, *116:* 383–387, 1975.

Thrall, J. H., Reddington, B., Johnson, M. C. and Pinsky, S. M.: Technique for radionuclide study of lymphatic dynamics. J. Nucl. Med., *14:* 640–641, 1973.

Turner, D. A., Pinsky, S. M., Gottschalk, A. et al.: The use of ^{67}Ga scanning in the staging of Hodgkin's disease. Radiology, *104:* 97–101, 1972.

Vendrell-Torne, E., Setoain-Quinquer, J. and Domenech-Torne, F. M.: Study of normal mammary lymphatic drainage using radioactive isotopes. J. Nucl. Med., *13:* 801–805, 1972.

Voutilainen, A. and Wiljasalo, M.: On the correlation of lymphography and lymphoscintigraphy in metastases of tumours of the pelvic region. Ann. Chir. Gynaecol. Fenn., *54:* 268–277, 1965.

Walker, L. A.: Localization of radioactive colloids in lymph nodes. J. Lab. Clin. Med., *36:* 440–449, 1950.

zum Winkel, K. and Scheer, K. E.: Scintigraphic and dynamic studies of the lymphatic system with radiocolloids. Minerva Nucl., *9*: 390–398, 1965.

12

Immunospecific Radionuclide Immunoglobulin Lymphography

STANLEY E. ORDER, M.D., F.A.C.R.

HISTORICAL PERSPECTIVE OF THE USE OF IMMUNOGLOBULIN

The development of passive immunotherapy began in 1890 in the same era in which radioactive substances were discovered. Emil von Behring and Paul Erlich collaborated to develop the first horse diphtheria antitoxin (von Behring, 1890). This clinical advance which was associated with success in the patients in whom it was used was soon supplanted by active immunization to prevent susceptibility to diphtheria toxin (von Behring, 1913). Other attempts to produce heterologous immunospecific antibodies were carried out with tetanus toxoid and pneumococcal antigens (Wainwright, 1926; Dochez and Gillespie, 1913). The identification of specific pneumococcal antigens led to the development of antiserum against each of the major antigenic types. The most successful use of a heterologous antiserum was in type 1 pneumococcal antiserum. Perhaps the classic study in the use of immunospecific heterologous antibody was the lead publication of Sutliff and Finland in the February issue of the *New England Journal of Medicine* in 1934. They stated that "the foregoing data and similar results obtained by other observers, leave no room to doubt that concentrated type 1 antipneumococcic serum exerts a striking symptomatic effect and reduces the death rate by one half in type I lobar pneumonia in adults." Carmichael Tilghman of Johns Hopkins reported with Finland in 1937 the marked improvement noted in the treatment of type VII pneumococcal pneumonia with concentrated type specific antibody. The

dosage used routinely was as much as 45 cc at 2-hr intervals with the antiserum being given intravenously. Serum was administered as late as 8–10 hr after a third dose if it seemed clinically indicated, especially in the type I pneumococcal treatment. This highly refined bacterial antigen was used to immunize both horses and rabbits. Horsefall et al. found that the antipneumococcal rabbit antiserum was more successful than horse antiserum in therapeutic trials in lobar pneumonia and reported their results in the *Journal of the American Medical Association* in 1937. The advent of antibiotics made further exploration of type specific heterologous antibody unnecessary. However, the retrospective 50% cure rate cannot be ignored, especially in light of a 10% survival in untreated controls.

In more recent times the clinical trials of antilymphocyte antiserum as well as antilymphocyte globulin reactivated interest in the use of heterologous antibodies. The specificity of such antisera had not been clearly defined as in the case of pneumococcal antisera and these agents have been of questionable benefit. Clinically, exploration of antibodies derived against human fibrin and ferritin has followed the tradition of immunologic specificity and represented attempts to utilize highly specific antigens to produce specific immunoglobulins for diagnostic purposes (Bale et al., 1962; Order et al., 1974).

316

TUMOR ANTIGENICITY

Tumor antigenicity was recognized first by Witebsky in 1929, and later Hirzfeld et al. (1929) confirmed these conclusions. Abelev (1971) isolated an alpha-globulin which he subsequently called alpha-fetoprotein and demonstrated that it was an oncofetal antigen in both rodents and human hepatomas.

Gold and Freedman reported in 1965 a carcinoembryonic antigen which was subsequently demonstrated in a variety of neoplastic and inflammatory disorders but more recently has had an isomer identified which seems to be more specific.

Several points of confusion still seem to surround the topic of tumor specific antigens. Experimental tumor antigens have been discovered which seem to be specific for the tumor and not for other tissues. However, the careful elimination of possible cross reactive proteins in all other organs and tissues has not been thoroughly reviewed in such models. The true and possibly unique specificity of these tumor antigens remains questionable. Tumor antigens, however, have been demonstrated to be increased in concentration and have been called tumor-associated antigens by some authors (Order, 1975). These antigens which are increased in concentration offer the possibility of specific targeting in tumor-bearing sites with an appropriate immunospecific immunoglobulin and are more central to the issue of lymphangiographic

visualization of microfoci of tumor.

Similarly, the technical restriction requiring the expression of unique antigenic specificity from tumors may not be a serious concern for lymphangiographic visualization. A unique protein may exist in a tumor which on immunization produces an antibody in a heterologous species. This antibody may cross react with other normal tissue proteins having a similar biochemical structure. For example, a human splenic ferritin which is used to immunize a rabbit produces an antiserum which recognizes human splenic ferritin and will precipitate with it and will similarly react and precipitate with other human ferritins (Eshhar et al., 1974) such as liver ferritin and diverse ferritins such as horse ferritin. All of these ferritins have a similar biochemical structure with some of the variable portions of the molecule defined by electrophoretic migration or by biochemical means rather than by the immunoglobulin which precipitates with the family of ferritin molecules.

At present the human tumor antigens which have been demonstrated have definitely been increased in concentration rather than specific. These increased concentrations of well characterized proteins present in tumor-bearing sites may be used for binding specific antibody in order to localize tumor masses and possibly for therapeutic purposes.

EXPERIMENTAL THERAPEUTIC TRIALS WITH HETEROLOGOUS ANTIBODY

Attempts were made to utilize various antitumor antisera with outbred strains of animals or with inbred strains when the antigen was cross reactive with circulating proteins (Reif, 1971; DeCarvalho and Rand, 1962; Ghose and Nigam, 1972). Linkage of immunospecific antibody with boron for subsequent irradiation with neutrons or with diphtheria toxin as a cytotoxic agent was attempted to deliver cytotoxic agents to tumors (Hawthorne et al., 1972; Moolten et al., 1972). In other models tumor was often not established for any duration in the host and the results were unconvincing. The antigens used for production of immunospecific immunoglobulin similarly often lacked discernible specificity.

Order et al.(1973) reported a successful therapeutic effect with a crude tumor antiserum derived against an antigen present on the cell surface of an ovarian cancer in a syngeneic strain of mice. This antiserum cured animals

even after several days of tumor implantation. Multiple doses of antiserum were toxic. However, by refining the antigen and producing a more specific antiserum, not cross reactive with normal tissue, multiple dose therapy without toxicity was achieved (Order et al., 1974). Treated animals have as high as a 90% survival in contrast to the 10% survival in the untreated group. Specific cytotoxicity against tumor-bearing cells in contrast to normal spleen cells also supported the hypothesis that production of a specific antigen and its purification was a more practical method for the development of highly immunospecific antibody than was sequential absorption of a crude antiserum. Certainly, if clinical use of similarly developed reagents is to be considered, absorption techniques would be unacceptable because of contamination of the antiserum with other human tissues, viruses, and possible pathogens.

IMMUNOSPECIFIC RADIONUCLIDE IMMUNOGLOBULIN FOR DIAGNOSIS

In 1959 an isolated antifibrin was radiolabelled and used for subsequent tumor localization, since fibrin was often present in tumors due to the inflammatory process associated with local tumor invasion (Day et al., 1959). Fibrin, however, was not a tumor-associated antigen since the fibrin was not related to the proliferation of the neoplastic cells. These findings did demonstrate that a protein in high concentration in tumor-bearing sites could be used for localization of tumors. A total of 179 scans were attempted in patients with rabbit immunospecific antifibrin antibody, and 113 positive tumor scans were visualized (Spar et al., 1967). The attractiveness of this approach was diminished by the lack of association of the fibrin directly with the neoplastic process and its lack of specificity for any given neoplasm.

Attempts to use rabbit antiglioma antibody by intracarotid infusion of radiolabelled immunoglobulin were associated with minimal success; however, the specificity of the antiserum was questionable (Mahaley et al., 1965). Similar localization as obtained with immunospecific globulin did not occur with nonspecific radioiodinated serum albumin.

More recent attempts at tumor scanning with anti-CEA antibody in experimental systems have been successful; however, the xenogenic host did not provide a normal tissue background competitive with the tumor proteins as would occur in patients (Hoffer et al., 1974; Goldenberg et al., 1974; Mach et al., 1974). Thus if an antigen was cross reactive with normal bowel and human colon cancer but would have been in higher concentration in the colon cancer, the opportunity for absorption or cross reactive binding was eliminated in these xenogenic experiments. The autoradiograph and gamma camera visualization of the ovarian tumor were carried out in a model system in which the normal tissue background and the tumor had the same genetic characteristics and were similar to the clinical situation.

PRINCIPLES FOR APPLICATION OF IMMUNOSPECIFIC REAGENTS BY THE LYMPHANGIOGRAPHIC ROUTE

Certain principles have become clear from the extensive investigation of immunospecific reagents and tumor-associated antigens.

1. A high concentration of the antigen of interest must be present in the tumor-bearing site.

2. Isolation and characterization of the antigen must be accomplished prior to the production of an immunospecific agent for possible clinical use.

3. The resultant highly specific immunoglobulin should not require absorption and after radiolabelling must be pyrogen-free.

4. It has yet to be determined whether immunoglobulin or Fab fragments (the papain derivative of the whole immunoglobulin molecule) will be more advantageous reagents.

5. If the Fab fragment is effective, then both the immunogeneticity of the foreign proteins as well as the potential increased binding in the tumor-bearing site could offer many advantages.

6. The potential cross reactivity of the immunospecific globulin and normal tissues, both in the lymphatic systems as well as in visceral organs, particularly the lung and kidneys, should be known prior to consideration of the use of immunospecific globulins.

7. The proposed agent to be used must be demonstrated to be pyrogen-free and nonallergenic in skin and conjunctival testing prior to its administration.

8. The lymphangiographic infusion of radiolabelled immunoglobulin offers the distinct advantage of presenting the immunoglobulin to potential tumor-bearing sites prior to its entering the general circulation where competitive cross reactive proteins might otherwise reduce its binding potential.

PRESENT RESULTS WITH LYMPHANGIOGRAPHIC INFUSION

Details concerning antigen isolation and purification, antiserum production, radiolabelling, and subsequent preclinical testing of the immunospecific radionuclide immunoglobulin have been reported (Order et al., 1975).

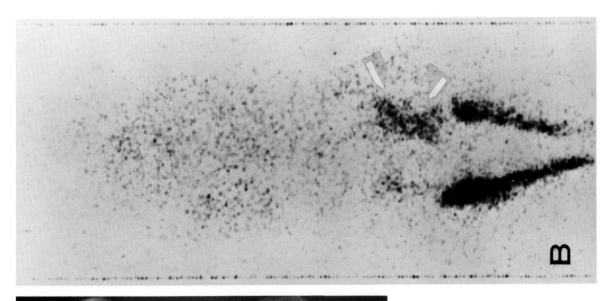

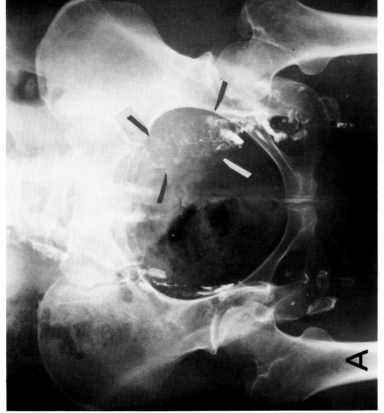

FIG. 12.1. LEFT PELVIC MASS IN A PATIENT WITH RECURRENT HODGKIN'S DISEASE
Lymphangiogram and radionuclide lymphangiographic 21-hr scan demonstrating the left pelvic mass. The scan views from the head to the feet.

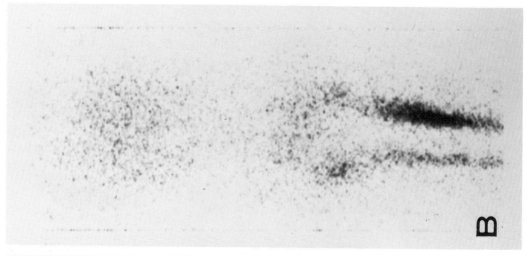

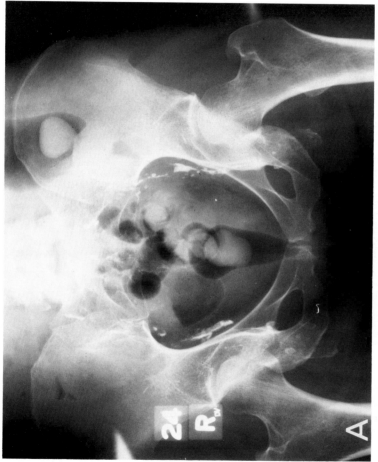

Fig. 12.2. Lymphangiogram of a Patient with Recurrent Hodgkin's Disease
Hodgkin's disease was seen in the epidural space with negative pelvic and para-aortic nodes. Scan obtained at 42 hr was consistent with the negative lymphangiographic x-ray.

LYMPHANGIOGRAPHIC TECHNIQUE

Using aseptic conditions, 5 mg gamma globulin, specific for F (ferritin) antigen of Hodgkin's disease, in 2 ml of 0.1 M phosphate buffer (pH 7.4) were combined with 50 μg lactoperoxidase (Calbiochem) and 1 mCi carrier-free NaI[131] (New England Nuclear). The reaction was initiated by the addition of 20 μl freshly prepared 0.5 M hydrogen peroxide and allowed to proceed for 30 min at room temperature with vigorous mixing. Unbound iodide was removed by successive cycles of buffer addition and vacuum dialysis until chromatographic determinations showed less than 3% unbound iodide. Specific activity of the iodinated gamma globulin was 0.47 Ci/gm. The entire sample was passed through a sterile 0.22 μm Millipore membrane filter. Pyrogen testing in three rabbits showed a total temperature rise of 0.5°C, well within the USP limits for pyrogenicity. Dermal and conjunctival tests for sensitivity to rabbit gamma globulin in the patient were negative.

The patient received Lugol's solution prior to the study. Standard technique was employed in cannulating the lower extremity lymphatics. Each lower extremity was infused with 2 ml Ethiodol at a flow rate of 0.13 ml/min to insure intralymphatic infusion prior to the introduction of 250 μCi antiserum. Total body scanning from the knees to the mandible was carried out with a dual probe rectilinear scanner (Ohio Nuclear) using a 3.5-inch focused medium energy collimator. Scanning was performed daily for 4 days and on the 7th day following infusion. Activity over the pelvis, right groin, and heart was monitored with a scintillation detector for the first 8 postinfusion days.

Similar techniques were applied to a second patient since the original publication. This patient within 15 min of the infusion had radioactive counts measurable over the thoracic duct representing a distinct difference between the 2 patients.

In the 2 patients receiving radionuclide immunoglobulin by intralymphatic administration, both infusions were preceded by 1–2 ml of Ethiodol. Intercomparison of both the lymphangiographic radiograph and the scan demonstrated clear correlation in both cases (Figs. 12.1 and 12.2). The first patient had clearly delineated left pelvic mass whereas the second patient did not have recurrent tumor in the axial lymphatics of either the pelvis or para-aortic regions. Both patients demonstrated some retention in one of the lower extremities and this could not be related to either pelvic masses or to technique. However, the preadministration of Ethiodol may cause sufficient resistance in the lymphatic system to cause the transudation of the immunoglobulin. In more recent studies this has proven to be true.

External monitoring during the radionuclide lymphangiogram revealed a remarkable difference in the two patients. The first patient having pelvic and para-aortic tumor did not have significant radioactive counts over the thoracic duct as late as 50 min whereas the second patient, lacking tumor, had high counts within 15 min. The background in the general circulation was also higher in the patients without tumor. The scan after 20 hr in both patients also showed a remarkable difference with retention of the isotope over the tumor-bearing region and in the pelvic nodes in the patient with known recurrence. An appropriate dissimilar circumstance was noted in the patient without pelvic recurrence.

Perhaps the two most critical questions remaining to be determined are the relationships between the radiolabelled antibody and the tumor infiltrate on a microscopic level and the technical question relating to the preinfusion use of Ethiodol.

It has been clear from the present experience that immunospecific radionuclide immunoglobulin lymphangiographic infusion has potential as both a diagnostic and therapeutic tool. Further investigation of tumor antigens, tumor antibodies, fragments of immunospecific antibody, and radiolabelling techniques and isotopes will be needed before the complete potential of these techniques for clinical use may be realized. The possibility of determining micrometastatic disease and the use of antibody-directed radiotherapy opens a new avenue for research in both diagnostic and therapeutic radiology and is the present state of these investigative efforts.

REFERENCES

Abelev, G. I.: Alpha fetoprotein in oncogenesis and its association with malignant tumors. Adv. Cancer Res., *14:* 295–358, 1971.

Bale, W. F., Spar, I. L. and Goodland, R. L.: Research directed toward the use of I[131] labeled fibrinogen in the localization and treatment of tumors. AEC Research and Development Report, UR-612: 1–16, 1962.

Day, E. O., Planisek, J. A. and Pressman, D.: Localization of radioiodinated rat fibrinogen in transplanted rat tumors. J. Natl. Cancer Inst., *23:* 799–812, 1959.

DeCarvalho, S. and Rand, H. J.: Effects of iso and heteroantibodies against specific antigens of the transplantable Novikoff hepatoma of the rat. Nature, *193:* 950–952, 1962.

Dochez, A. R. and Gillespie, L. J.: A biological classification of pneumococci by means of immunity reactions. J.A.M.A., *61:* 722–730, 1913.

Eshhar, Z., Order, S. E. and Katz, D.: Ferritin: a Hodgkin's disease associated antigen. Proc. Natl. Acad. Sci., *71:* 3956–3960, 1974.

Ghose, T. and Nigam, S. P.: Antibody as a carrier of chlorambucil. Cancer, *29:* 1398–1400, 1972.

Gold, P. and Freedman, S. O.: Demonstration of tumor specific antigen in human colonic carcinomata by immunologic tolerance and absorption techniques. J. Exp. Med., *121:* 439–462, 1965.

Goldenberg, D. M., Preston, D. F., Primus, F. J. and Hansen, H. J.: Photoscan localization of GW-39 tumors in hamsters using radiolabelled anticarcinoembryonic antigen immunoglobulin G. Cancer Res., *34:* 1–9, 1974.

Hawthorne, M. F., Wiersema, R. J. and Takasugi, M.: Preparation of tumor specific boron compounds. I. In vitro studies using boron labeled antibodies and elemental boron as neutron targets. J. Med. Chem., *15:* 449–452, 1972.

Hirzfeld, L., Halber, W. and Laskowski, J.: Unterschungen uber die serologischen eigenschaften der Gewebe 11. Ueber serologischen eigenschaften der neubildungen. Z. Immunitaetsforsch. *64:* 81–113, 1929.

Hoffer, P. B., Lathrop, K., Bekerman, C., Fang, V. S. and Refetoff, S.: Use of I[131]-CEA antibody as a tumor scanning agent. J. Nucl. Med., *15:* 323–327, 1974.

Horsefall, F. L., Goodner, K. and MacLeod, C. M.: Antipneumococcus rabbit serum as a therapeutic agent in lobar pneumonia. J.A.M.A., *108:* 1483–1490, 1937.

Mach, J. P., Carrel, S., Merenda, C., Sordat, B. and Cerottini, J. C.: In vitro localization of radiolabelled antibodies to carcinoembryonic antigen human colon carcinoma grafted into nude mice. Nature, *248:* 704–706, 1974.

Mahaley, M. S., Mahaley, J. and Day, E. D.: The localization of radioantibodies in human brain tumors. II. Radioautography. Cancer Res., *25:* 779–793, 1965.

Moolten, F. C., Copparell, N. J. and Cooperband, S. R.: Antitumor effects of antibody diphtheria toxin conjugates: use of hapten coated tumor cells as an antigenic target. J. Natl. Cancer Inst., *49:* 1057–1062, 1972.

Order, S. E.: Antigenic analysis of the lymphomas. Br. J. Cancer, *31:* 128–139, 1975.

Order, S. E., Bloomer, W. D., Jones, A. G., Kaplan, W. D., Davis, M. A., Adelstein, S. J. and Hellman, S.: Radionuclide immunoglobulin lymphangiography: a case report. Cancer, *35:* 1487–1492, 1975.

Order, S. E., Colgan, J. and Hellman, S.: Distribution of fast and slow migrating Hodgkin's tumor associated antigens. Cancer Res., *34:* 1182–1186, 1974.

Order, S. E., Donahue, V. and Knapp, R.: Immunotherapy of ovarian carcinoma, an experimental model. Cancer, *32:* 537–579, 1973.

Order, S. E., Kirkman, R. and Knapp, R.: Serologic immunotherapy: results and probable mechanism of action. Cancer, *34:* 163–171, 1974.

Reif, A. E.: Studies on the localization of radiolabelled antibodies to a mouse myeloma protein. Cancer, *27:* 1433–1439, 1971.

Spar, J. L., Bale, W. F., Marrock, D., Dewey, W. C., McCardle, R. J. and Harper, P. V.: I[131] labeled antibodies to human fibrinogen. Diagnostic studies and therapeutic trials. Cancer, *20:* 865–870, 1967.

Sutliff, W. D. and Finland, M.: Type I pneumococci infections with especial reference to specific serum treatment. J. Exp. Med., *210:* 237–245, 1934.

Tilghman, R. C. and Finland, M.: Clinical significance of bacteremia in pneumococci pneumonia. Arch. Int. Med., *59:* 602–619, 1937.

von Behring, E.: Unterschungen uber das zustandekommeh der diptherie – immuntat bei tehieren. Dtsch. Med. Wochenschr., *16:* 1145–1148, 1890.

von Behring, E.: Ueber ein neues diptherieschutzmittel. Dtsch. Med. Wochenschr., *39:* 873–876, 1913.

Wainwright, J. M.: Tetanus: its incidence and treatment. Arch. Surg., *12:* 1062–1079, 1926.

Witebsky, E.: Disponibilitat, und spezifitat alkoholloslicher struktturen von oraganen and bosartigen geschwulsten. Z. Immunitaetsforsch., *62:* 35–73, 1929.

Index

A

Abdominoaortic lymphatics, 38–49, 292–293
Abelev, G. I., 317
Abrams, H. L., 40, 44, 51, 166–167, 275
Ackerman, T., 105
Aging, effect of, 76
Akisada, M., 133
Albrecht, A., 133
Albumin disappearance curve, 97–99
Allen, E. V., 89
Allenby, F., 100
Alpha chain disease, 155
Angiosarcoma, 106–107
Ann Arbor clinical staging classification, 300
Antibody, heterologous, 317
Antigenicity, tumor, 317
Aortic lymphatics. *See* Abdominoaortic lymphatics *or specific nodal group*
Aortography, 128
Aplasia in lymphedema, 94–97
Arger, P. H., 128
Arnulf, G., 91
Arteriography, 303
Arthritis, 122–124
Arts, V., 67
Ascites, 103–104, 218, 222–223, 296
Asellius, G., 1–3
Atrial septal defect, 94
Axillary nodes
  in fibrolipomatosis, 131
  in lymphadenopathy, 133
  normal, 54–55, 260–261
  obstructed, 111

B

B cells, 142–145, 148–149, 151–152
Basca, S., 133
Bagshaw, M. A., 222
Bartels, P., 59, 191
Bartholin, T., 1, 3, 4
Bassani, G., 138
Baum, H., 110
Beales, J. S., 68
Bennett, M. H., 155
Biligrafin, 6, 11
Biopsy, 68–70, 163–164, 211
Bizzozero, G., 59
Bladder, urinary, 84, 243–248
Blalock, A., 105, 108
Blaudow, K., 133
Boerhaave, H., 4
Bollman, J. L., 59
Bottcher, J., 136
Bray, D. A., 282
Breast
  carcinoma, 260–262
  consequences of surgery, 90–91, 97, 100, 265–266
  lymphography, 68
  radionuclide studies, 290–292
Brice, M., II, 248
Broder, S., 143, 146, 152
Brolsch, C., 281

Bron, K. M., 110
Brucellosis, 134–136
Bruun, S., 64
Burke, J. F., 4, 11
Burkitt lymphoma, 149, 155
Burn, J. I., 90
Burrows, B. D., 62, 281
Bursa of Fabricius, 142
Busch, F. M., 225
Bussey, H. J. R., 254
Butler, J. J., 125

C

Calnan, J., 90
Camiel, M. R., 108
Carcinoma, 185–273. *See also specific organ or type*
Carvalho, R., 5
Casley-Smith, J. R., 4, 59
Castellino, R. A., 168–169, 170, 252
Catovsky, D., 153
Cavography, 74, 128, 160, 187, 236
Cellulitis, 97
Cervical nodes, 55, 68
Cervix, carcinoma of, 116, 187, 208–212
Charles, H., 102
Charles procedure, 102
Chemotherapy, changes due to, 189
Chest roentgenograms, 133
Chiappa, S., 36, 225
Child, C. G., 59
Cholegraphin, 274
Chylothorax, 104
Chylous syndromes, 103–106
Chyluria, 104–106
Cirrhosis, 59
Cisterna chyli, 1–4, 14, 51
Clark, E. L., 58
Clark, E. R., 58
Clementz, B., 67
Cloquet, node of, 22
Collagen disease, 84
Collargol, 6
Collateral lymphatic vessels
  after irradiation, 138
  in carcinoma, 186, 199
  in lymphedema, 91, 264–265
  in lymphoma, 167
  in obstruction, 108–109
  in retroperitoneal fibrosis, 128
Collins, R. D., 141
Compana, F. P., 68
Concanavalin, A., 143
Contrast media
  complications due to, 274–283
  current use, 64–67
  early applications, 5–11
Cook, F. E., 225
Cook, P. L., 108
Copeland, E. M., 254
Crampton, A. R., 91, 102
Craven, C. E., 108
Crile, G., Jr., 254
Cruikshank, W., 1, 3–4, 9
Cunningham, J. B., 108
Cusick, H., 67

D

Damascelli, B., 63
Davidson, J. D., 118
Davidson, J. W., 160, 163, 281
Davis, H. K., 50–51
Day, T., 58
DeRoo, T., 63, 67
Dietzsch, J., 283
Distichiasis, 94, 96
Ditchek, T., 68
Dorfman, R. F., 153
Douglas, B., 213, 218
Drinker, C. K., 1, 4–5, 59, 105
Dukes, C. E., 254
Dumont, A. E., 59
Dutcher body, 148
Dyes, 6, 61–62

E

Eaves, G., 58
EB virus, 143
Edema. *See* Lymphedema
Edwards, C. L., 305
Embolization of oil, 111, 275–280
Endoscopy, 303
Engeset, A., 64, 137, 198, 226, 282
Epstein, A. L., 153
Erhich, P., 316
Esterly, J. R., 94
Ethiodol, 64–67, 274–281
Eustace, P. W., 95
Eustachius, 1
Extravasation, 76, 108
Extremities
  lower, 18–21, 103
  upper, 52–55
  See also Lymphedema

F

Farrell, W. J., 160
Femoral nodes, 296–297
Fibrolipoma, 45, 131
Fibrosis
  in chyluria, 106
  in chronic lymphedema, 90–91, 97, 99, 100
  in nodes, 80, 170
  See also Idiopathic retroperitoneal fibrosis
Field, M. E., 105
Filariasis, 97, 103
Finland, M., 316
Fisch, U., 53
Fischer, H. W., 65
Fistula, 114–116
Foldi, M., 59, 113
Fornier, A. M., 124
Forsgren, L., 170
Fraimow, W., 275–276
Freedman, S. O., 317
Frommhold, H., 51
Fuchs, W. A., 108
Fuks, Z., 153
Funacka, S., 5
Fussek, H., 252

G

Gallium-67 citrate, 288, 297–298, 305–
    312
George, P., 91, 97
Gerhard, L., 281
Gerota, D., 4
Gerteis, W., 213
Gilchrist, M. R., 67
Gillies procedure, 101
Glatstein, E., 170
Glick, A. D., 153
Goiter, 68
Gold-198, 285, 288–289
Gold, P., 317
Gold, W. M., 275–276
Goldsmith, H. S., 101
Gonadal dysgenesis, 94
Good, R. A., 142
Gooneratne, B. W. M., 91
Gregl, A., 133, 173–174
Gross, R., 104
Grossman, I., 252
Gruart, F. J., 68

H

Hall, J. G., 137
Handley, W. S., 100
Hanks, G. E., 222
Hansen, J. A., 142
Harvey, W., 1
Hashimoto's disease, 155
Hayes, R. L., 305
Heart
    congestive failure, 59, 118
    lesions associated with lymphedema,
        94
    pericarditis, 59, 118
Heidenhain, R., 4
Heineke, H., 136
Hellman, S., 300
Herman, P. G., 23, 24
Herophilus, 3
Hirzfeld, L., 317
His, W., 3
Histoplasmosis, 134–136
Hodgkin's disease
    cell type, 149–150
    classification, 146–147
    clinical correlation, 156
    functional studies, 153
    hyperplasia in, 84
    laparotomy for, 170–171
    lymphography, 169
    radionuclide studies, 298, 300
    staging, 160
Hohenfellner, R., 281
Holsten, D. R., 137
Homans, J., 102
Horsefall, F. L., 316
Howland, W. J., 63
Hreschyshyn, M. M., 11
Hudack, S., 6, 61
Hueck, W., 58
Hughes, J. H., 91, 97, 102
Hunter, W., 3, 4
Huntington, G. S., 14, 58
Hygroma, 106–107
Hyperkeratosis in lymphedema, 94
Hyperplasia of lymph nodes

    follicular, 45, 122–124, 125, 170
    mediastinal nodes, 126
    reactive, 81–84, 124–126, 170
Hypersensitivity to lymphographic oils
    and dyes, 281–283
Hypogastric nodes, 26–28, 209–210, 224,
    243, 250, 254

I

Idiopathic retroperitoneal fibrosis, 109,
    118, 128
Illiac nodes
    acute inflammation, 122
    hyperplastic, 84
    in carcinoma, 217–218, 250–251
    in fibrolipomatosis, 131
    lymphographic appearance, 80
    normal
        common, 28–33, 243
        external, 23–26, 209–210, 212, 224,
            225–226, 243, 249
        internal, 26–28, 250
Indium-111, 285–289
Infection
    differentiation from carcinoma, 84
    role in lymphedema, 91
Inflammation
    acute, 122–124
    granulomatous epithelioid, 133–136
    in lymphedema, 91
    lymphographic appearance, 80–81
Inguinal nodes
    biopsy, 114
    hyperplastic, 84, 124
    in carcinoma, 251, 254
    in fibrolipomatosis, 131
    interpretation, 80
    normal, 22, 76, 212, 224
    obstructed, 108, 111
    on radiocolloid studies, 291, 296–297
Intestine, carcinoma of, 254–255
Intra-adventitial space, 112, 113–114
Iodopin, 64
Iriarte, P., 62
Ivanov, G. F., 113–114

J

Jackson, B. T., 47
Jackson, J., Jr., 298
Jaffe, E. S., 153
Jamieson, C. W., 103–104
Jay, J. C., 281
Jewett, H. J., 244
Jing, B. S., 62, 67, 109
Joduron, 6
Jossifow, G. M., 4
Juttner, H., 163

K

Kampmier, O. F., 14
Kaplan, H. S., 153
Kaposi's sarcoma, 106–107
Kaspar, Z., 91, 97
Kay, D. N., 305, 310, 312
Kett, K., 68
Kidney transplantation, 114
Kiel classification of lymphomas, 142
Kienle, J., 133
Kikuchi, T., 68

Kinmonth, J. B., 6, 11, 18, 47, 61, 89,
    91, 94, 95, 96–97, 100, 101, 103,
    104
Koehler, P. R., 65, 274, 280, 282
Kohler, I., 283
Kojima, M., 145, 153
Kondoleon, E., 100
Kountz, S. I., 90
Kreel, L., 73, 91, 97
Kropholler, R. W., 62, 281

L

Lacunar node, 23
LaMarque, J. L., 133, 134
Langhammer, H., 305
Laparotomy, 170–173
Laplante, M., 248
Larson, D. L., 112–113
Larson, N. E., 91, 102
Lawrentjew, A. P., 3
Leak, L. V., 4, 11
Lee, F. C., 106
Lee, K. F., 62
Leitsmann, H., 283
Lennert, K., 153
Lenzi, M., 138
Leukemia
    cell type, 147
    clinical and morphologic aspects,
        153–156
    functional studies, 151–153
    lymphographic appearance, 81–84
Levine, G. D., 153
Lewis, T. R., 104
Lichenification in lymphedema, 93–94
Lipiodol, 6, 64
Liver, 59, 171–172
Ludington, L. G., 281
Ludvik, W., 281
Ludwig, J., 4
Lukes, R. J., 141
Lukes-Butler classification, 147
Lumbar lymphatics, 38–39, 40–43, 76,
    225–226
Lupus erythematosus, 155
Lymph nodes, 1–4, 15, 16–18. See also
        specific disease or anatomic area
Lymphadenopathy, 133, 155
Lymphangiectasia, 117–118
Lymphangioma, 106–107
Lymphangitis
    complication of lymphography, 283
    in chyluria, 104
    in lymphedema, 91, 92, 97, 100
Lymphatic system
    anatomy, 15–18, 58–59
    embryogenesis, 14–15, 58
    function, 4, 15, 58–59
    See also specific disease or anatomic
        area
Lymphatic vessels
    anatomy, 15–16
    embryogenesis, 14
    history, 1–4
    tumors, 106–107
    See also specific disease or anatomic
        area
Lymphaticovenous   communications,
    109–111, 138, 167, 186, 199–208

Lymphedema
  lower extremity
    classifications, 89
    clinical considerations, 91–94
    diagnosis, 94–99, 112, 296–297
    etiology, 89–91
    treatment, 99–103
  upper extremity, 264–270
Lymphoblastoma, 125
Lymphocele, 114–116
Lymphocytes
  systems, 142–143
  transformation, 143–144
  types, 147–150
Lymphocytopenia in lymphangiecta-
    sia, 117
Lymphography, 61–74, 274–283, 285–
    312
  applications, 14
  cannulation, 62–64
  comparison with other techniques,
    73–74
  complications, 274–283
  contraindications, 61
  contrast media, 64–67
  filming, 67–68
  history, 5–11
  immunoglobulin studies, 316–321
  indications, 52
  interpretation, 76–87
  premedication, 61
  radionuclide studies, 285–312
  technique, 61–74
  vital dyes, 61–62
  See also specific diseases
Lymphology, 4–5
Lymphoma
  appearance of retroperitoneal nodes,
    44–45
  classification, 141–142, 146–150
  clinical and morphologic aspects,
    153–156
  diagnosis, 165–174
  differentiation from reactive hyper-
    plasia, 125–126
  functional studies, 151–153
  immunology and morphology, 142–
    146
  indications for lymphography, 160–
    165
  interpretation of lymphangiograms,
    81–84
  radionuclide studies, 292–293, 298–
    307, 310–312
Lymphosarcoma, 155, 160, 293

M

Magnification, 67–68, 77
Malabsorption disease, 155
Malek, P., 11
Mammary nodes, 260–261, 264, 291
Mandi, L., 133
Manson, P., 104
Marcille, M., 217, 218
Marshall, V. F., 244
Mascagni, P., 3
Mason, D. Y., 145, 152
Mathé, G., 155
Matoba, N., 68

Mayerson, P., 110
McClure, C. F. W., 14, 58
McClure, S., 133
McCready, V. R., 305, 310, 312
McMaster, P. D., 6, 61
Measles, 122
Mediastinal nodes, 264
Megalymphatics, 96, 103
Mesenteric nodes, 254
Metastases
  differentiation from inflammation,
    122
  nodal, 77–87
  in carcinoma of large intestine, 254
  in prostatic carcinoma, 252
  radionuclide studies, 292–293
  spread, 191–199
Millett, Y. L., 155
Milroy, W. F., 94
Milroy's disease, 94
Molen, H. R., 99
Morehead, R., 133
Morris, B., 137
Mortazavi, S. H., 62, 281
Mulholland, J. H., 59
Mycosis fungoides, 146, 147, 152, 154–
    155

N

Nathwani, B. N., 153
Negus, D., 90
Nelson, B., 281
Ngu, V. A., 21
Nielubowicz, J., 100
Nocardia apaca, 143
Nossal, G. J. V., 144
Nuck, A., 1, 3, 5–7

O

Obstruction of lymphatics, 108–111
Obturator node, 26
O'Connor, F. W., 105
Ohnuma, T., 155–156
Olin, T., 67
Olszewski, W., 89–90, 100
Order, S. E., 317
O'Reilly, K., 100
Orell, S., 70
Ormond, J. K., 128
Ottoviani, G., 112
Ovary, carcinoma of, 216–223

P

Pancreatitis, 118
Panniculitis, 130
Panning, W. P., 67
Papp, M., 59
Pappenheimer, J. R., 15–16
Pappenheimer pores, 16, 59
Para-aortic nodes
  acute inflammation, 122
  hyperplastic, 84
  in carcinoma, 213, 217–218, 250–251
  in lymphadenopathy, 133
  in lymphoma, 166–167
  interpretation, 80
  normal, 38–40, 43–46, 225–226
Paralumbar lymphatics, 38–39, 44–45,
    47, 265

Paralymphatic system, 112–113, 199
Parker, B. R., 84, 125–126
Parker, J., Jr., 298
Patel, A. R., 91, 97, 102
Patent blue violet dye, 6, 61, 281–282
Patent ductus arteriosus, 94
Peau d'orange, 93
Pecquet, J., 1, 3
Pelu, G., 68
Pelvic nodes
  in carcinoma, 213, 252
  normal, 23–38, 76, 292–293
  See also specific nodal group or dis-
    ease
Periaortic nodes, 38–39
Pericarditis, 59, 118
Perineural space, 111–114
Perivascular space, 111–114
Pes cavus, 94
Peyer's patches, 17, 142
Pfahler, G. G., 6
Phytohemagglutinin, 143
Pirogow, node of, 22
Platzbekder, H., 133
Pneumoconiosis, 310
Pneumonia, 280, 310
Pokeweed, 143
Poliomyelitis, 122
Pomerantz, M., 118
Post-thrombotic syndrome, 91
Preaortic nodes, 254
Pressman, J. J., 110
Projection difference index, 44
Promontory nodes, 33, 250
Prostate, carcinoma of, 249–254
Puckett, J., 100
Pulmonic stenosis, 94
Pyelography. See Urography
Pyelonephritis, 310

R

Radiocolloids, 285–297
Radiotherapy, 91, 136–138, 189
Randolph, J., 104
Rappaport, H., 141–142, 153, 156, 298
Rappaport classification, 141–142, 153,
    156, 298
Rasmussen, K. E., 281
Rauste, J., 133
Reed-Sternberg cell, 143–144, 149–150,
    298
Reichert, F. L., 108
Rejection of graft, 155
Retrocrural nodes, 23, 243
Retroperitoneal fibrosis. See Idiopathic
    retroperitoneal fibrosis
Richter syndrome, 154
Rigas, A., 90
Rim sign, 166
Rosenberger, A., 51
Rosenmüller, node of, 22, 24
Rouvièr, H., 4, 24, 33, 39–40, 53, 225
Rudbeck, O., 1, 3
Rummelhardt, S., 252
Rusznyak, I., 58–59
Ruttner, J. R., 122–125
Ruysch, F., 3, 8
Rye Conference classification, 147,
    149–150, 298, 303

S

Sabin, F., 14
Sachdeva, H. S., 68
Salvioli, G., 59
Sarcoidosis, 133, 310
Sarcoma
    immunoblastic, 147, 149, 153–156
    Kaposi's, 106–107
    reticulum cell, 160, 293
Sawney, C. P., 101
Scalene node, 114
Scanlon, G. T., 68
Schaffer, B., 280
Scharkoff, T., 133
Schlossman, S. F., 152
Schwann, T., 4
Schwarz, G., 160
Selenium-75 (selenomethionine), 287–288
Selle, J. G., 104
Seminoma, 125
Sentinel nodes, 261
Servelle, M., 6
Sézary's syndrome, 143, 146, 147, 152, 154–155
Shanbrom, E., 64, 110
Shimkin, P. M., 118
Sigurjonsson, K., 62
Silver, D., 100
Silvester, C. F., 110
Sistrunk, W. E., 100
Sjögren's syndrome, 155
Smalley, R. H., 133
Smith, E. B., 136
Sokolowski, J., 282
Spleen, 171–172
Spondylitis, 122–123
Sprue, 155
Starling, E. H., 4, 59
Stein, H., 152
Stevens, R. C., 63
Stoppani, F., 6
Storen, E. J., 114
Strickstrock, K. H., 133
Strong, G. H., 244
Subaortic nodes, 33
Supraclavicular nodes, 261, 263–264
Suramo, I., 134
Sutliff, W. D., 316
Syphilis, 134–136

T

T cells, 142–147, 151–152
Takahashi, M., 40, 44, 108, 166–167
Takashima, T., 118
Takekoshi, N., 118
Tapper, R. I., 104
Taylor, C. R., 145, 152
Taylor, G. W., 91
Technetium-99m, 285, 289, 293–295
Tegtmeyer, C. J., 63
Teneff, S., 6
Terrier, H., 100
Testes, carcinoma of, 225–242
Testicular lymphatics, 33–38, 81, 84
Thompson, N., 101, 102
Thompson procedure, 101, 102
Thoracic duct
    embryogenesis, 14–15, 51, 58
    history, 1–4
    injury, 114
    normal, 49–52, 58
Thorotrast, 5–6, 11
Threefoot, S. A., 65, 110, 274–275
Thyroid, 68
Tilghman, R. C., 316
Tjernberg, B., 122
Tomography
    computed, 73, 244
    conventional, 77
Tong, E. C. K., 62
Transplantation, renal, 114
Trowell, O. A., 136
Tsunoda, R., 145
Tuberculosis, 84, 133–134
Turner, A. F., 63
Turner, D. A., 305
Turner's syndrome, 94

U

U cells, 142–143
Ujiki, G. T., 138
Ultrasound, 73–74, 244
Urografin, 6, 11
Urography, 160, 186–187, 236, 303
Uterus, carcinoma of, 212–215

V

Van Den Brenk, H. A. S., 138
Van der T'oth, L. M., 99

Van Horne, J., 1
Vasko, J. S., 104
Veins, obstruction of, 91, 266–270
Venography, 187–191, 236, 244, 250, 264, 303
Viamonte, M., 63, 67, 122, 133, 136, 170
Vieussens, R., 4
Virchow, R., 4, 58, 137
Virchow-Robbins space, 112
Vitek, J., 91, 97
Volwiler, W., 59
Von Behring, E., 316
Von Recklinghausen, F. D., 4
Vulva, carcinoma of, 224

W

Waldenström's syndrome, 146, 148, 155
Waldeyer's ring, 55
Waldmann, T. A., 118
Wallace, S., 11, 67, 109, 110, 112–113
Wégria, R., 59
Weichert, R. F., 103–104
Weissleder, H., 133
White, R. J., 276
Wiertz, L. M., 283
Wiljasalo, M., 44, 122, 124
Winchester, R. J., 152
Wirth, W., 51
Witebsky, E., 317
Wolfel, D. A., 110, 133
Wrisberg, H., 3
Wücherer, O., 104
Wutzer, C. W., 109

X

Xeroradiography, 99
Xylocaine, role in dye complications, 281–282

Y

Yam, L. T., 152
Youker, J. E., 63

Z

Zalar, J., 133
Zeissler, R. M., 99
Zheutlin, N., 64, 110
Zuppinger, A., 108